Acknowledgments

The editors wish to thank a number of individuals who were instrumental in the development and production of this volume. Sincere thanks to Emily Smith, LERA's executive director, for her guidance and support throughout the process. Many thanks to Peggy Currid for her amazing editorial work on the volume and for her admirable efforts to keep the project on schedule. We are also very appreciative of WonJoon Chung's terrific research assistance as we prepared the volume's introduction. Finally, a very big thanks to the authors of the volume's chapters. We thank each of them for sharing their knowledge, insights, and expertise and for helping to advance the study of work and organization in the health care industry.

Contents

Complexity and Its Consequences: The Evolving Landscape of Health Care

ARIEL C. AVGAR
ILR School
Cornell University

TIMOTHY J. VOGUS
Owen Graduate School of Management
Vanderbilt University

THE ARRAY OF CHALLENGES FACING HEALTH CARE ORGANIZATIONS

This volume introduces the reader to a host of innovations being experimented with across the health care industries in the United States and in the United Kingdom. Each of the chapters included in this volume offers an in-depth analysis of the ways in which regulators, organizations, professions, unions, or employees are confronting the increasing and multifaceted pressures and challenges bearing down on the health care industry as a whole and on its key stakeholders. These pressures and challenges include growing complexity, optimizing multiple performance outcomes simultaneously, and (radically) changing regulatory regimes.

Addressing these pressures has required innovative responses by each group of stakeholders. Before specifying responses, we provide an overview of the dominant and often conflicting pressures and challenges that have driven health care industry actors to seek out new practices and arrangements across a host of clinical, technological, employment, and financial domains.

Although these pressures are varied, there are three categories of challenges that have played an especially central role in affecting health care industry actors as they attempt to change and innovate. Specifically, health care organizations face an industry characterized by (1) increased complexity, (2) the need to satisfy and deliver on multiple performance outcome metrics simultaneously, and (3) changing environmental and regulatory conditions. In what follows, we briefly summarize each of these pressures and the effect that they are likely having on the responses of health care industry stakeholders.

The Growing Complexity of Health Care

Health care has always been an incredibly complex industry. It engages multiple stakeholders and attempts to address and reconcile myriad divergent interests and needs; therefore, it requires an extremely high level of coordination across systems, organizations, occupational groups, units, areas of specialization, and providers (Gittell, Seidner, and Wimbush 2010). In addition, the work of health care delivery is inherently complex because of the range of conditions being treated coupled with the persistent uncertainty regarding any particular patient's diagnosis and the appropriateness of potential interventions (Argote 1982).

Nevertheless, the level of complexity in health care has only increased over the past decades as a result of a number of factors, including, but not limited to, demographic and population changes and associated chronic disease conditions, technological advances, and organizational and system-level restructuring. As a result of some of these changes, health care organizations are facing the prospect of caring for patients with increasingly complex needs and conditions (Ory et al. 2013), the clinical and administrative tools being used to treat these patients are progressively more sophisticated, and the organizational configurations in which care is provided are varied and constantly evolving (Avgar, Givan, and Liu 2011).

Health care organizations and providers, therefore, confront a reality in which the primary objective of delivering high-quality and affordable care is becoming increasingly difficult to attain on a consistent and reliable basis. In fact, recent evidence on the quality of care provided in health care systems in developing countries raises significant concerns about the outcomes delivered (for recent evidence on the shortcomings of the U.S. health care system, see James 2013). Barriers to delivering high-quality patient care can be attributed, among other factors, to the high level of complexity common in this industry and the product of a host of interconnected patterns of change.

The aging of populations in most developed countries is likely to place further strain on health care systems, which may not be prepared for the clinical, organizational, and workforce-related implications associated with the demands that this demographic shift will entail (see, for example, Angus et al. 2000 and Schneider and Guralnik 1990). In a recent study by Dall and colleagues (2013), the authors project dramatic changes in the composition of the health care workforce in the United States by the year 2025 as a result of population aging and changing levels of insurance coverage. Specifically, the authors expect a greater need for specialists because of the chronic conditions that are more common among aging patients, such as hypertension, heart disease, and diabetes (Dall et al. 2013).

Alongside demographic changes, health care organizations are confronted with the availability of increasingly sophisticated clinical and information technologies (Avgar, Eaton, Givan, and Litwin 2016). On the one hand, these new technologies offer the promise of greater clinical capabilities and timely access to complex and diffused information. The proliferation of new health information technology (HIT), for example, has been lauded for its potential to increase coordination of care, reduce medical and medication errors, and decrease patient care costs (Avgar, Eaton, Givan, and Litwin 2016).

On the other hand, the introduction of new technologies has not been without its challenges. New technologies require greater organizational learning capabilities (Avgar, Tambe, and Hitt 2016), call for an upskilling of segments of the workforce, necessitate new organizational routines and work arrangements, and alter the mode of interaction patients have with their providers (see, for example, Litwin 2011). This is not to say that new clinical and information technologies are not worthwhile investments. Rather, the introduction of powerful new tools throughout the health care delivery system is yet another source of complexity facing the industry and its stakeholders.

Finally, in addition to growing clinical and technological complexities, health care organizations are, by their very nature, an arena characterized by extremely complex interactions and interdependencies within and between units, occupational groups, and organizations and across stakeholders including patients (Begun, Zimmerman, and Dooley 2003). Exacerbating this complexity is the large array of emerging employment models that bind different stakeholders, such as physicians and nurses, to the organization. Thus, for example, hospitals have seen a growing use of alternative employment arrangements, such as contracting and outsourcing (Litwin, Avgar, and Becker 2016). As such, health care organizations attempt to coordinate complex interactions between stakeholders who have fundamentally different ties and modes of interaction with the organization. The varied nature of employment relationship in the health care industry makes the task of managing the workforce especially complicated.

Satisfying and Improving Multiple Performance Outcomes

In other industries, the complexity previously described can be managed in part by focusing on a specific outcome (e.g., efficiency; Cyert and March 1963). However, health care organizations are facing growing pressures to advance multiple and competing outcomes simultaneously. In the United States, this has been articulated as the so-called triple aim of higher-quality patient-centered care, better population health, and lower per capita costs (Berwick, Nolan, and Whittington 2008). The simultaneous pursuit of improvement on multiple dimensions is, in large part, the result of the fact that health care organizations and the industry overall have historically struggled to achieve high-quality and error-free care, improve population health outcomes, and contain the escalating costs of delivering care (Berwick, Nolan, and Whittington 2008; Institute of Medicine 1999, 2001, 2004).

For example, in the United States, concerns about the adequacy of the quality and safety of patient care continue to persist many years after publication of the Institute on Medicine's seminal report estimating that at least 98,000 preventable patient deaths occur each year (Institute of Medicine 2001). In the United Kingdom, recent estimates put the number of preventable patient deaths at nearly 12,000 per year (Hogan et al. 2012). Recent research suggests that the severity of this problem has, if anything, been underestimated and responses have been slow and insufficient (for recent estimates, see James 2013).

Health care systems around the world have also been struggling to contain the escalating costs of delivering care (Keehan et al. 2012; World Health Organization 2014). It is estimated, for example, that health care costs account for 18% of GDP in the United States (Institute of Medicine 2012), whereas in the United Kingdom the number is closer to 9% of GDP (Organisation for Economic Co-operation and Development, no date). As such, hospitals and other health care organizations face considerable regulatory and competitive pressures to contain costs and improve efficiency (Avgar, Eaton, Givan, and Litwin 2016; Weinberg 2003). Not surprisingly, this cost-containment pressure can often serve to exacerbate health care organizations' difficulties in attaining the required quality and safety improvements discussed above (Weinberg 2003).

Further complicating this delicate balancing act between cost and quality, health care organizations are attempting to attain these aims while, at the same time, enhancing their ability to attract and retain skilled clinical professionals amidst looming workforce shortages (Avgar, Eaton, Givan, and Litwin 2016; Dall et al. 2013). The prospect of a workforce shortage has been debated in the literature (Lafer 2005), but it appears as though health care organizations are reacting to this threat regardless of whether it is real or perceived (for a similar discussion, see Avgar, Eaton, Givan, and Litwin 2016). Addressing potential workforce shortages is made more difficult by the nature of health care work, which is demanding, stressful, and characterized by high levels of turnover and burnout (Aiken et al. 2002; Avgar, Eaton, Givan, and Litwin 2016; Gillespie and Melby 2003). Taken together, health care organizations are attempting to improve care, while reducing costs and while also confronting workforce challenges that, if not dealt with, could jeopardize both efforts.

Changing Regulatory Regimes

Alongside the complexity inherent to the health care setting and the challenge of balancing multiple and competing outcomes, health care organizations also operate in an evolving regulatory landscape. Changing regulatory regimes have been motivated, largely, by public policy makers' efforts to incentivize new models for delivering patient care and for financing it.

Most notably in the United States, the passage of the Affordable Care Act (ACA) in 2010 has, in some key respects, transformed the regulatory framework governing access, delivery, and financing of patient care. As such, it has fundamentally altered the environment in which health care organizations operate. The ACA has affected health care organization in a host of complex ways, with additional consequences that have yet to fully materialize. There are three key ways in which the ACA has clearly and dramatically changed the environment in which health care organizations deliver care.

First, one of the primary objectives of the law was to provide health care insurance coverage to millions of uninsured or underinsured Americans (Sommers et al. 2013). The ACA increases coverage in a number of different ways including the expansion of Medicaid, the establishment of subsidies for low-income individuals, extending young adult coverage on their parents' plans, and mandating individual coverage (Clemans-Cope et al. 2013; Hofer, Abraham, and Moscovice 2011; Schoen, Doty, Robertson, and Collins 2011; Sommers et al. 2013). Achieving the important goal of providing expanded access to the U.S. health care system will, in all likelihood, create an increase in demand for services across the spectrum of patient care institutions, including primary, acute, and long-term settings (Dall et al. 2013; Hofer, Abraham, and Moscovice 2011). Some estimates project that by 2019 the ACA will extend coverage to an additional 25 million Americans (Shaw, Asomugha, Conway, and Rein 2014). Hofer and colleagues (2011) estimate that by 2019 expanded coverage will lead to between 15 and 24 million additional primary care visits annually. The likely increase in demand for services has clear implications for health care organizations' workforce, logistical, and clinical preparedness, which has motivated health care organizations to experiment with a host of workplace innovations.

Second, the ACA also seeks to improve patient care quality and to reduce costs by promoting new organizational models that alter the level of coordination and collaboration across health care institutions and providers (DeVore and Champion 2011; Fisher and Shortell 2010). In particular, the ACA establishes a new institutional arrangement referred to as an accountable care organization (ACO), which is a voluntary partnership among a number of hospitals, physicians, and health care providers designed to deliver high-quality and affordable care by linking reimbursements to quality and cost-related metrics.

The goal of the ACO is to incentivize health care organizations and providers to work together in caring for patients across traditional institutional and disciplinary boundaries that have often prevented integration and coordination (Berwick 2011; Fisher and Shortell 2010). According to some estimates, more than 700 organizations have been recognized as ACOs since 2011 and serve over 23 million Americans (Kaiser Health News 2015). ACOs, therefore, represent an effort on the part of policy makers to promote both quality of care improvements and cost containment by establishing new incentives and institutional structures. As such, ACOs constrain the ability of participating organizations from privileging one outcome—quality or cost—over the other. ACOs, like other elements of the ACA, were introduced as an attempt to align both of those objectives, which are often deemed to be in tension and incompatible.

Health care organizations participating in an ACO are, therefore, likely to seek out new ways of advancing both quality and cost reductions as clearly depicted by how they build the infrastructure to operate differently in the chapter in this volume by Hilligoss, McAlearney, and Song. Systems such as the National Health Service (NHS) in the United Kingdom that are single payer (i.e., central government run) and provide universal coverage have pushed in a different direction. Specifically, the NHS, which employs 1.7 million people and treats 1,000,000 patients daily, has recently as a result of the 2012 Health and Social Care Act begun to pursue cost reduction by putting the local general practitioner (i.e., primary care physician) more at the center and otherwise devolving decision making to the more local level by moving decisions "closer to the patient." At the same time, market forces are being introduced to allow for private sector entrants into the market to foster choice, competition, efficiency, and some movement away from central government health care provision. This has not been smooth or uncontroversial, but it is an example of how a system comes to wrestle with mounting cost pressures while attempting to preserve access and quality.

Finally, and building on this idea of aligning quality and cost-containment objectives, the ACA also introduced the value-based purchasing (VBP) program, which is designed to replace the fee-for-service model in the acute hospital setting (U.S. Department of Health and Human Services 2015). In doing so, hospitals do not receive Medicare payments solely based on the number of services they provide. Rather, hospitals are required to meet benchmarks, introduced over time, related to quality of care, safety, patient and caregiver perceptions of care, population health, efficiency, and cost reductions (U.S. Department of Health and Human Services 2015; VanLare and Conway 2012). Hospitals are scored across a host of measures that capture different dimensions associated with each of those domains and are assessed both in terms of their current performance and their level of improvement. Performance and improvement scores are used to allocate incentive payments to hospitals treating Medicare patients. As with the introduction of ACOs, the VBP provisions of the

ACA reshape the reimbursement model of participating organizations—thereby pushing for greater alignment between efforts to improve patient quality and the cost of delivering this care. VBPs are intended to establish greater accountability on the part of hospitals treating Medicare patients. Taken together, these sets of pressures have limited health care organizations' ability to engage in traditional trade-offs across different outcomes, especially between quality and cost. If they can't segment their responses and have to navigate increasing complexity in a manner that optimizes performance on multiple dimensions (cost, quality, and health) or face regulatory or competitive penalties, the key question then becomes "How can health care organizations respond to these significant mounting challenges simultaneously?"

It is precisely this question that animates this volume. To address it, we draw on explorations of a range of innovative models of collaborative (e.g., labor–management partnership), structural (e.g., organization design and practices), and process (e.g., attending to the mindset reflected in organizational climate) approaches to building workforce capacity and skill, engaging in efforts to improve quality of patient care, and seeking out ways to contain the escalation of costs.

CULTIVATING REQUISITE VARIETY: ORGANIZATIONAL EFFORTS TO RESPOND TO MOUNTING CHALLENGES

At a conceptual level, responding to the challenges of the evolving health care landscape through a range of innovative approaches reflects the pursuit of "requisite variety" (Ashby 1956) to address the complexity of health care delivery. The law of requisite variety comes from work on cybernetic systems and early systems theory and posits that the variety of a system (such as an organization, team, or individual) must be as great as the variety of the environment that it is trying to regulate (Ashby 1956). Importantly for health care, "the environment" theorized in requisite variety can actually be a vector of environments with a number of different components requiring different forms of variety to regulate it (Ashby 1956: 217)—that is, the complex health care landscape (i.e., the challenges of performing well on multiple dimensions simultaneously, changing and demanding regulatory regimes, growing complexity, and a workforce pushed to the limit) necessitates organizations that can absorb and process the complexity.

In other words, if such complex and equivocal inputs such as the changing regulatory regimes and the simultaneous pursuit of difficult goals are to be effectively managed, they must be fully registered and understood (Weick 1979). "Fully registered" means depicted accurately, and doing so requires practices and processes that can register the complexity, which means that simple solutions that are narrowly tailored (i.e., medicalized;

Wears, Perry, and Sutcliffe 2005) are insufficient and that one needs to pursue more comprehensive and multi-faceted approaches (Singer and Vogus 2013). To argue for requisite variety is not to argue for unlimited variety—just enough to match the environment(s)—because there are diminishing returns to variety even in turbulent environments like health care (Weick 1979). Similarly, requisite variety is also not random variety; adding random variety is a dangerous strategy that helps only in extremely rare "garbage can" settings where an organization does not know what it's doing (Cohen 1986).

More accurate representation of the complex, evolving health care landscape also requires pursuing requisite variety by increasing the variety of the range of individuals studying and attempting to address the problems. Consequently, we assembled a set of authors who span health services research/health policy, human resource management, industrial relations, management, sociology, and engaged health care practitioners. It is through these varied perspectives that the persistent problems of contemporary health care delivery are represented in a more complex and nuanced manner and the corresponding interventions brought to bear on the problem are more comprehensive and integrative. Thus, to best meet the challenges facing health care calls for requisite variety from health care organizations and the researchers who study them (and often intervene in them).

The chapters that follow in this volume are intended to depict the requisite variety to meet the multifaceted and intertwined challenges facing health care organizations. We begin with a set of chapters that richly depict the complexity of the health care context in the United Kingdom and the United States and illustrate the range of ways organizations are responding to it.

The next set of chapters explores labor–management partnerships as a means of matching the environmental challenges by developing and making fuller use of the expertise of those on the front line such that all organizational resources are marshaled to produce more cost-effective, higher-quality, and health-promoting care.

We then move to a set of chapters that illustrate specific structural innovations to facilitate greater competition and flexibility, place the patient at the center of care delivery (as opposed to the provider), fundamentally rethink relational practices and processes to foster greater coordination, and illustrate the role of information technology in meeting the challenges.

Last, we close with two chapters that illustrate how rethinking and reshaping the mindsets applied to care delivery in the form of organizational climate can enhance efficiency, quality, and safety. We describe each of these chapters in more detail next.

In their chapter, *Beyond Pay for Performance: An Ownership Perspective for Providing Quality Primary Health Care at a Sustainable Cost*, Benjamin R. Pratt, Benjamin B. Dunford, and Matthew B. Perrigino apply a human resource management perspective in analyzing key features of the U.S. health care system and the reform enacted in the 2010 Affordable Care Act (ACA). The chapter analyzes the prospects of the ACA to improve patient-care quality while containing cost by examining the incentive structures the act sets up and the consequences that these have for provider behaviors. Pratt and colleagues maintain that the challenge of delivering high-quality care at a sustainable cost is, among other factors, driven by the difficulty in aligning the interests of principals and agents—in this case, providers. Aligning interests in a way that delivers better care at affordable costs is, according to the authors, a function of properly structured incentives. The chapter assesses both the traditional managed care model and the extent to which the ACA's attempt to move away from a fee-for-service model has, in fact, created a better alignment between physician and patient interest. To do so, the authors leverage psychological ownership theory as a lens through which to assess shortcomings associated with the existing managed care model and prospect for improvement under the ACA. Pratt and colleagues analyze the degree to which different models of care engender psychological ownership. The chapter offers a unique view of health care reform in the United States and the features that will most likely lead to providers' psychological ownership, thereby aligning their interests with those of patients.

Stephen Bach's chapter, *New Models of Care and Workforce Change in the NHS in England*, provides the reader with a comprehensive review and analysis of the current state and patterns of change within England's National Health System (NHS). The chapter offers an overview of the NHS's inner workings, the challenges and pressures it faces, the innovations designed to address these, and the implications that they have for key stakeholders. As such, the chapter focuses on the central factors that have influenced efforts to restructure and reform the NHS. Bach identifies four overarching challenges that have shaped the ways in which public policy makers have approached the system's restructuring: increased fragmentation of a traditionally integrated system, patient safety shortcomings, efforts to curtail health care funding, and workforce capacity. One of the themes that stems from this description is the growing fragmentation of a system that used to be characterized by a high level of integration and the implications this has had on coordination in an already complex environment. Alongside this fragmentation, Bach highlights the increasingly visible role that private sector institutions are playing within the NHS. The portrait that emerges is of a system in which core and long-standing features and building blocks are being reconsidered and restructured, thereby adding to the already

existing challenges facing the health care industry. The chapter adds greatly to this volume by allowing for a well-developed comparative perspective,
which complements the detailed evidence on the patterns and trends in the
health care industry in the United States.

In their chapter, *Building the Infrastructures of Accountable Care: Early
Lessons from Four Commercial ACOs*, Brian Hilligoss, Ann Scheck
McAlearney, and Paula H. Song use qualitative case studies of four ACOs
to illustrate what is required to implement a new organizational form to
respond to a shifting regulatory regime in the United States and to the
pursuit of the so-called triple aim. They richly describe the significant investment in four distinct, yet related, infrastructures required to opera-
tionalize the ACO and put this new model into practice. Specifically, they
identify economic (i.e., financial incentives for the organization and its
employees) and sociocultural (i.e., shared values and trust-based relationships) factors needed to foster change, engagement, and continuous
performance improvement. They also describe the importance of an
information infrastructure that combines networked information technologies and robust data analysis capabilities needed to manage risk, monitor performance, and allocate rewards to motivate performance. Last, at
the core of the ACO model, is coordination across the care continuum for
a defined population of patients. Building this infrastructure allows for
appropriate utilization of services that are both more efficient and effective.
Taken together, these four infrastructures work to slow spending growth
while improving quality and population health.

Rebecca Kolins Givan's chapter, *Who Regulates? Physicians and the
Regulation of Health Care*, introduces the reader to the intricacies and nuances inherent to the regulation of health care delivery. In doing so, she
points to the consequential implications associated with fundamentally
different regulatory regimes. The state of health care in the United States
and in the United Kingdom is not simply a function of unexpected or
unpredictable forces and pressures. Rather, the very ability of these health
care systems to confront the many pressures they face is, among other
factors, the product of the regulatory systems put in place and the balance
of power that they create. Givan offers the reader a detailed roadmap necessary for a comprehensive understanding of the regulatory systems in
health care, the central actors, and the voice and power and influence that
they have. The chapter's focus on both the United States and United
Kingdom regulatory patterns allows Givan to provide a comparative perspective on an issue that is central to understanding industry and organizational responses to mounting challenges. She points to the margin-
alization of the role that physicians play in the regulation of health care
in the United States. Furthermore, the chapter draws the reader's attention
to the ways in which the regulatory framework in the United States con-

strains and restricts front-line physician autonomy in the delivery of patient care. Finally, Givan identifies the primary public and private mechanisms through which these regulatory systems govern and incentivize stakeholder strategies and actions. Paul F. Clark's chapter, *Nurse Union Strategies for Improving the Quality of Patient Care*, presents a carefully crafted description of the different tools leveraged by unions in an effort to expand front-line employee voice and to improve patient care. At the heart of the chapter is a forceful argument about the central role that the nurses' voice plays in advancing key health care outcomes. Nurses, according to Clark, do not simply use their voice to improve wages, benefits, and working conditions. Rather, union-enabled voice is viewed by nurses and their unions as a way to highlight organizational shortcomings that challenge their ability to deliver high-quality patient care. Clark contributes to the study of health care unions and patient care outcomes by distinguishing among the various strategies employed by labor in its efforts to advance members' interests while also improving the organizational conditions in which they deliver care to their patients. The chapter distinguishes among collective bargaining, joint consultation, and lobbying and legislative action. Clark analyzes the adequacy of each of these strategies as a means of safeguarding appropriate staffing levels, limiting use of mandatory overtime, and restricting floating of nurses across units. The author also presents a review of four innovative labor–management initiatives designed to enhance front-line voice and to improve patient care. In sum, the chapter provides the reader with a clear understanding of the different ways unions can play an instrumental role as champions for both workers and patients.

In their chapter, *Labor–Management Partnerships in Health Care: Responding to the Evolving Landscape*, Adrienne E. Eaton, Rebecca Kolins Givan, and Peter Lazes provide an in-depth analysis of six partnership cases that highlight both the challenges and promises associated with this labor relations institution. The chapter offers the reader a window into the complexities inherent to labor and management efforts to engage in a collaborative, problem-solving relationship. The authors detail the variation in the antecedents to partnership, in the patterns of interactions among key stakeholders, and in the outcomes associated with this effort. In doing so, their chapter contributes to existing evidence on partnership in the health care setting by introducing the reader to multiple rich portraits of this potentially powerful approach to addressing many of the clinical and workforce challenges discussed above. Eaton and colleagues leverage their description of these six cases to tease out common themes that emerge and to highlight overarching lessons for scholars and practitioners. They do so while comparing and contrasting their evidence on partnership in the health care context to the literature on partnership in other settings. Taken together, the chapter showcases the ability of labor–management partnership to serve as a vehicle through which health care organizations can confront the strong headwinds they face while also acknowledging the inherent difficulties and challenges associated with its adoption and implementation.

In the chapter, *Leading Change Together: Kaiser Permanente's Partnership Strategy for Innovation*, Jim Pruitt and Paul M. Cohen offer an insider's view into what has been viewed by many as the most comprehensive and successful labor–management partnership in the health care arena. The authors provide the reader with an overview of the partnership's historical background and context, detailing the parties involved and the steps taken to implement and institutionalize this labor–management relationship across a large and diverse health care system. Pruitt and Cohen's analysis of the Kaiser Permanente labor–management partnership adds to the evidence regarding the links between partnership and outcomes for employees, the organization, and patients. The authors also highlight the importance of attention to partnership at the workplace level as a way to increase organizational innovation and improve patient care. Part and parcel of this front-line orientation, according to Pruitt and Cohen, is the use of self-directed teams. Finally, the authors make an argument about the link between Kaiser Permanente's investments in partnership and the organizational performance.

Cheryl Rathert, Jessica N. Mittler, and Laura E. McClelland's chapter, *Caring Health Care Work Environments and Patient-Centered Care*, convincingly details the ways in which health care organizations have responded to changing regulatory regimes initiated by the ACA and value-based purchasing through designs that refocus attention on the quality of the work environment for care providers, or the extent to which care providers are facilitated in developing therapeutic relationships with patients. In other words, they unpack what it really means to be "patient centered" and argue that it requires establishing a therapeutic alliance with patients that is compassionate and caring and reduces patient vulnerabilities. In other words, patient-centered care providers are able to get to know "the patient as a person" and engage the patient as an active participant in his or her own care. The authors detail a range of organizational practices that create work environments that support caregivers in the pursuit of truly patient-centered care (e.g., compassion practices and Magnet® status) and allow for careful tailoring of care to a particular patient, including a strong service climate that prioritizes the patient, high-performance work environments that allow for customization, and voice climate that fosters speaking up in the name of enhancing patient experience.

In their chapter, *Changing Forms of Organization and Implications for Managing Across Boundaries*, Simon Bishop and Justin Waring discuss how recent attempts to control costs in the U.K.'s National Health Service through a set of regulatory changes intended to stimulate competition and innovation among health service providers has had cascading organizational implications. First, the change gave rise to new clinical commissioning groups that allow primary care physicians to purchase care services on behalf of their patient groups—the idea being to devolve decision making to the more local level to make room for competition. Consequently, a number of new organizational forms and provider models have been established, including increasing participation by for-profit entities, public–private partnerships, regional specialist centers, and nongovernmental social enterprises. They distill the implications of the proliferation of new organizational forms for regional and national governance as well as the important implications for health care workforces as new arrangements upend relations among professions (as new winners and losers emerge) and create unrest by professional organizations.

Joan Resnick, Sarah Lax, Eliana Temkin, and Jody Hoffer Gittell's chapter, *Building Relational Coordination Across Front-Line Work Groups: A Case from Kaiser Permanente Northwest*, describes a mixed-method study of how Kaiser Permanente implemented a set of interventions to enhance relational coordination among front-line employees in six work groups in four medical office buildings. Kaiser specifically focused on targeting relational coordination—or frequent, timely, accurate, problem-solving communication across work groups, supported by relationships of shared goals, shared knowledge, and mutual respect—to better coordinate their highly interdependent, uncertain, and time-constrained work. The author present case studies demonstrating that at the core of relational coordination is a shared sense of "teamness" cultivated through a series of interventions such as seminars, trainings, and facilitated discussions of relational coordination survey data. These initial conversations fostered additional interventions such as the "living room huddle," which brought all staff together outside their departments to learn about each other's roles, and "starter conversations, which did the same for leaders. These interventions grew into broader relational coordination summits. After the multifaceted interventions were implemented, the teams saw benefits in terms of employee engagement, patient satisfaction, and relational coordination. In doing so, the authors showcase the promise and the discipline required to realize the promise of relational interventions.

Edmund R. Becker and Jaeyong Bae's chapter, *Impact of Electronic Health Records on Hospital Patient Satisfaction: What Is the Influence of*

Organizational Characteristics?, integrates health information technology (HIT) into the discussion of health care reform. This is important given the expectations placed on HIT as a vehicle to improve a host of outcomes in health care and the absence of conclusive evidence as to whether these expectations are being met. The authors make two important contributions. First, they examine the effect that different levels of electronic health record (EHR) implementation has on patient satisfaction in acute care hospitals. Second, and central to the theme of this volume, Becker and Bae examine the role that organizational factors play in explaining EHR implementation and in affecting the relationship between this new technology and patient satisfaction. They test the interactions among four organizational factors and their impacts on EHR implementation using a unique database with merged data from a number of sources representing approximately 25% of all acute care hospitals in the United States. As a whole, the chapter highlights the role that HIT can play in advancing an important health care outcome—patient satisfaction. The chapter provides additional support for the argument that the study of health care innovations, like new technology, needs to account for the organizational context in which those innovations are embedded.

In their chapter, *A New Perspective on Organizational Climate as a Boundary Spanner: Integrating a Fragmented Health Care System*, Tal Katz-Navon and Eitan Naveh develop a provocative conceptual argument regarding how the benefits of integrated health care systems can be realized—organizational climate or the shared meanings people attach to interrelated experiences they have at work. They posit that climate serves as an "organizational canopy" that integrates dispersed people and organizations by instilling a view of organizations as permeable and otherwise changing perceptions of boundaries, serving a transformational function whereby employees internalize organizational values that are more likely to span boundaries, a control function (e.g., instilling a service orientation even when unsupervised), spillover (personal behavior transfers across contexts), and crossover (interpersonal contagion).

Deirdre McCaughey and Gwen McGhan's chapter, *Health Care Providers and Patients in Sync: Antecedents for Optimizing Provider and Patient Safety Outcomes*, illustrates how scholarly fragmentation among researchers of employee and patient safety has been suboptimal for each in practice. Notably, it has resulted in comparatively less attention to employee safety. This is especially problematic because, the authors argue, patient safety and employee safety are inextricably linked because delivering the highest-quality, safest care relies on a healthy and safe workforce. They show how the concept of safety climate—a snapshot of employee beliefs about safety linked to identifiable policies and practices—can work to bring together research and practice regarding patient and employee safety. Specifically, they adapt two models of safety to simultaneously enhance patient and employee safety by cultivating a strong safety climate at the organization and department levels through redesigning organizational practices and work processes to reduce exposure to psychological and physical hazards, enhance safety motivation, and reduce unsafe behaviors.

REFERENCES

Aiken, L. H., S. P. Clarke, D. M. Sloane, J. Sochalski, and J. H. Silber. 2002. "Hospital Nurse Staffing and Patient Mortality, Nurse Burnout, and Job Dissatisfaction." *Journal of the American Medical Association* 288, no. 16: 1987–93. doi:10.1001/jama.288.16.1987.

Angus, D. C., M. A. Kelley, R. J. Schmitz, A. White, and J. Popovich. 2000. "Current and Projected Workforce Requirements for Care of the Critically Ill and Patients with Pulmonary Disease—Can We Meet the Requirements of an Aging Population?" *Journal of the American Medical Association* 284, no. 21: 2762–70. doi:10.1001/jama.284.21.2762.

Argote, L. 1982. "Input Uncertainty and Organizational Coordination in Hospital Emergency Units." *Administrative Science Quarterly* 27, no. 3: 420–34. doi:10.2307/2392320.

Ashby, W. R. 1956. *An Introduction to Cybernetics.* Eastford, CT: Martino Fine Books.

Avgar, A. C., A. E. Eaton, R. K. Givan, and A. S. Litwin. 2016. "Editorial Essay: Introduction to a Special Issue on Work and Employment Relations in Health Care." *Industrial and Labor Relations Review* 69, no. 4: 787–802. doi:10.1177/0019793916649171.

Avgar, A. C., P. Tambe, and L. Hitt. 2016. "IT Implementation, Workplace Organization, and Employee Skill Acquisition: Evidence from Electronic Medical Records." Working paper.

Avgar, A. C., R. K. Givan, and M. Liu. 2011. "Patient-Centered but Employee Delivered: Patient Care Innovation, Turnover Intentions, and Organizational Outcomes in Hospitals." *Industrial and Labor Relations Review* 64, no. 3: 423–40. doi:10.1177/001979391106400301.

Begun, J. W., B. Zimmerman, and K. Dooley. 2003. "Health Care Organizations as Complex Adaptive Systems." In *Advances in Health Care Organization Theory.* Edited by Stephen S. Mick and Mindy E. Wyttenbach. San Francisco, CA: Jossey-Bass.

Berwick, D. M. 2011. "Launching Accountable Care Organizations—The Proposed Rule for the Medicare Shared Savings Program." *New England Journal of Medicine* 364, no. e32: 1–4. doi:10.1056/nejmp1103602.

Berwick, D. M., T. W. Nolan, and J. Whittington. 2008. "The Triple Aim: Care, Health, and Cost." *Health Affairs* 27, no. 3: 759–69. doi:10.1377/hlthaff.27.3.759.

Clemans-Cope, L., S. K. Long, T. A. Coughlin, A. Yemane, and D. Resnick. 2013. "The Expansion of Medicaid Coverage Under the ACA: Implications for Health Care Access, Use, and Spending for Vulnerable Low-Income Adults." *INQUIRY: The Journal of Health Care Organization, Provision, and Financing* 5, no. 2: 135–49. doi:10.1177/0046958013513675.

Cohen, M. D. 1986. "Artificial Intelligence and the Dynamic Performance of Organizational Designs." In *Ambiguity and Command: Organizational Perspectives on Military Decision Making.* Edited by J. G. March and R. Weissinger-Baylon. Boston, MA: Pitman.

Cyert, R. M., and J. G. March. 1963. *A Behavioral Theory of the Firm*. Englewood Cliffs, NJ: Prentice-Hall.

Dall, T. M., P. D. Gallo, R. Chakrabarti, T. West, A. P. Semilla, and M. V. Storm. 2013. "An Aging Population and Growing Disease Burden Will Require a Large and Specialized Health Care Workforce by 2025." *Health Affairs* 32, no. 11: 2013–20. doi:10.1377/hlthaff.2013.0714.

DeVore, S., and R. W. Champion. 2011. "Driving Population Health Through Accountable Care Organizations." *Health Affairs* 30, no. 1: 41–50. doi:10.1377/hlthaff.2010.0935.

Fisher, E. S., and S. M. Shortell. 2010. "Accountable Care Organizations: Accountable for What, to Whom and How." *Journal of the American Medical Association* 304, no. 15: 1715–16. doi:10.1001/jama.2010.1513.

Gillespie, M., and V. Melby. 2003. "Burnout Among Nursing Staff in Accident and Emergency and Acute Medicine: A Comparative Study." *Journal of Clinical Nursing* 12, no. 6: 842–51. doi:10.1046/j.1365-2702.2003.00802.x.

Gittell, J. H., R. Seidner, and J. Wimbush. 2010. "A Relational Model of How High-Performance Work Systems Work." *Organization Science* 21, no. 2: 490–506. doi:10.1287/orsc.1090.0446.

Hofer, A. N., J. M. Abraham, and I. Moscovice. 2011. "Expansion of Coverage Under the Patient Protection and Affordable Care Act and Primary Care Utilization." *Milbank Quarterly* 89, no. 1: 69–89. doi:10.1111/j.1468-0009.2011.00620.x.

Hogan, H., F. Healey, G. Neale, R. Thomson, C. Vincent, and N. Black. 2012. "Preventable Deaths Due to Problems in Care in English Acute Hospitals: A Retrospective Case Record Review Study." *BMJ Quality and Safety* 21, no. 9: 737–45. doi:10.1136/bmjqs-2011-001159.

Institute of Medicine. 1999. *To Err Is Human: Building a Safer Health System*. Washington, DC: The National Academies Press.

Institute of Medicine. 2001. *Crossing the Quality Chasm: A New Health System for the 21st Century*. Washington, DC: The National Academies Press.

Institute of Medicine. 2004. *Health Literacy: a Prescription to End Confusion*. Washington, DC: The National Academies Press.

Institute of Medicine. 2013. *Best Care at Lower Cost: The Path to Continuously Learning Health Care in America*. Washington, DC: The National Academies Press.

James, J. T. 2013. "A New, Evidence-Based Estimate of Patient Harms Associated with Hospital Care." *Journal of Patient Safety* 9, no. 3: 122–28. doi:10.1097/pts.0b013e3182948a69.

Kaiser Health News. 2015. "Accountable Care Organizations, Explained." http://bit.ly/2ectgoz.

Keehan, S. P., A. M. Sisko, C. J. Truffer, J. A. Poisal, G. A. Cuckler, A. J. Madison, J. M. Lizonitz, and S. D. Smith. 2011. "National Health Spending Projections Through 2020: Economic Recovery and Reform Drive Faster Spending Growth." *Health Affairs* 30, no. 8: 1594–1605. doi:10.1377/hlthaff.2011.0662.

Lafer, G. 2005. "Hospital Speedups and the Fiction of a Nursing Shortage." *Labor Studies Journal* 30, no. 1: 27–46. doi:10.1353/lab.2005.0029.

Litwin, A. S. 2011. "Technological Change at Work: The Impact of Employee Involvement on the Effectiveness of Health Information Technology." *Industrial and Labor Relations Review* 64, no. 5: 863–88. doi:10.1177/001979391106400502.

Litwin, A. S., A. C. Avgar, and E. R. Becker. 2016 (Jun. 22). "Superbugs Versus Outsourced Cleaners: Employment Arrangements and the Spread of Health Care–Associated Infections." *Industrial and Labor Relations Review* (published online in advance). doi:10.1177/0019793916654482.

Organisation for Economic Co-operation and Development. No date. "OECD Health Statistics." http://bit.ly/2etZCHb.

Ory, M. G., S. Ahn, l. Jiang, M. L. Smith, P. L. Ritter, N. Whitelaw, and K. Lorig. 2013. "Successes of a National Study of the Chronic Disease Self-Management Program." *Medical Care* 51, no. 11: 992–98. doi:10.1097/mlr.0b013e3182a95dd1.

Schneider, E. L., and J. M. Guralnik. 1990. "The Aging of America. Impact on Health Care Costs." *Journal of the American Medical Association* 263, no. 17: 2335–40. doi:10.1001/jama.263.17.2335.

Schoen, C., M. M. Doty, R. H. Robertson, and S. R. Collins. 2011. "Affordable Care Act Reforms Could Reduce the Number of Underinsured US Adults by 70 Percent." *Health Affairs* 30, no. 9: 1762–71. doi:10.1377/hlthaff.2011.0335.

Shaw, F. E., C. N. Asomugha, P. H. Conway, and A. S. Rein. 2014. "The Patient Protection and Affordable Care Act: Opportunities for Prevention and Public Health." *The Lancet* 384, no. 9937: 75–82. doi:10.1016/s0140-6736(14)60259-2.

Singer, S, J., and T. J. Vogus. 2013. "Reducing Hospital Errors: Interventions That Build Safety Culture." *Annual Review of Public Health* 34: 373–96. doi:10.1146/annurev-publhealth-031912-114439.

Sommers, B. D., T. Buchmueller, S. L. Decker, C. Carey, and R. Kronick. 2012. "The Affordable Care Act Has Led to Significant Gains in Health Insurance and Access to Care for Young Adults." *Health Affairs* 32, no. 1: 165–74. doi:10.1377/hlthaff.2012.0552.

U.S. Department of Health and Human Services. 2015 (Sep.) "Hospital Value-Based Purchasing." http://go.cms.gov/2ecsiIY.

VanLare, J. M., and P. H. Conway. 2012. "Value-Based Purchasing—National Programs to Move from Volume to Value." *New England Journal of Medicine* 367, no. 4: 292–95. doi:10.1056/nejmp1204939.

Wears, R. L., S. J. Perry, and K. M. Sutcliffe. 2005. "The Medicalization of Patient Safety." *Journal of Patient Safety* 1, no. 1: 4–6. doi:10.1097/01209203-200503000-00003.

Weick, K. E. 1979. *The Social Psychology of Organizing* (2nd edition). Reading, MA: Addison-Wesley.

Weinberg, D. B. 2003. *Code Green: Money-Driven Hospitals and the Dismantling of Nursing*. Ithaca, NY: Cornell University Press.

World Health Organization. 2014. "Global Status Report on Alcohol and Health." http://bit.ly/29ivhM2.

CHAPTER 1

Beyond Pay for Performance: An Ownership Perspective for Providing Quality Primary Health Care at a Sustainable Cost

BENJAMIN R. PRATT
BENJAMIN B. DUNFORD
MATTHEW B. PERRIGINO

Krannert Graduate School of Management
Regenstrief Center for Healthcare Engineering
Purdue University

INTRODUCTION

Since the origins of medicine, physicians have shouldered the responsibility of serving the interests of multiple stakeholders. For example, the Hippocratic Oath charges physicians to uphold the well-being of their patients in addition to upholding the interests of their practice and profession (Arnold and Stern 2006; Dharamsi, Ho, Spadafora, and Woollard 2011; Katz 2002). This mandate to balance the needs of multiple stakeholders sometimes creates challenging trade-offs that can present conflicts of interest or even ethical dilemmas. Sometimes decisions that favor the practice lead to low-quality patient care, yet other times decisions that serve the interests of patients at the expense of the practice place the practice or physician livelihood at risk (Brennan et al. 2006; Khushf and Gifford 1998).

Historically, the interests of patients and the interests of the practice were integrated by a variety of "pay for performance" systems in primary care. Initially, physicians were paid by patients (or patients' kin) themselves, according to their efforts in diagnostics and treatment (Petersen et al. 2006; Rosenthal 2008; Rosenthal, Frank, Li, and Epstein 2005). This pay-for-performance framework allowed physicians the autonomy to balance the interests of patients with the business of medicine, while also effectively aligning the clinical interests of patients with economic gain because low-quality patient care would lead to disputes over payment and negative publicity for the physician or practice.

During the 1970s, the vast majority of businesses and consumers shifted to a managed care model, which introduced a fee-for-service framework. In this model, insurance companies assumed payment responsibilities for consumers, created guidelines of sound practice that revoked provider autonomy over patient care, and negotiated standardized payment rates from providers (Baker 1997; Ransom et al. 1996; Safran, Tarlov, and Rogers 1994). While the three-party, fee-for-service framework (which we will refer to as the managed care model) imbued primary care physicians (also known as primary care providers and PCPs) with authority as the gate-keepers of medical care in the United States, it also de-prioritized the interests of patients by decoupling rewards from care quality (Golden, Ortiz, and Wan 2013; Marcotte, Moriates, and Milstein 2014). The managed care model also exacerbated the tension between the interests of patients and the financial interests of physicians (Ancane, Palmowski, and Ancans 2015; Brennan et al. 2006; Thompson 1993) by rewarding physicians according to quantity of patients seen rather than the quality of diagnosis, medical intervention, or medical counsel given to patients (see Grumbach, Keane, and Bindman 1993 for reviews).

In an effort to reverse the diminished quality of primary care attributable to the managed care model, the Patient Protection and Affordable Care Act of 2010 (hereafter Affordable Care Act or ACA) was designed to help physicians provide high-quality patient care at a sustainable cost by giving physicians financial incentives for meeting patient care outcomes, for participating in new health care delivery models [such as the patient-centered medical home (PCMH) model and the accountable care organization (ACO) model], and implementing preventive services (Blumenthal, Abrams, and Nuzum 2015; Kocher, Emmanuel, and DeParle 2010). While it still may be too early to evaluate the extent to which the ACA has met its objectives, the ACA's overall impact on primary care quality has been mixed thus far (Bendix 2013; Blumenthal, Abrams, and Nuzum 2015; Hall and Lord 2014).

We argue that, despite a strong framework and the shift to outcome-based economic incentives, the ACA's potential impact is limited because of remaining barriers to high-quality patient care. For example, research shows that PCPs spend an inadequate amount of time with patients largely because of a heavy workload and time demands (Koh and Sebelius 2010; Luquis and Paz 2015). Despite recent efforts to improve health care delivery with pay-for-performance models that focus on outcomes rather than services—thus better aligning patient, physician, and public interests—many quality and cost challenges remain, prompting government and private sector leaders to seek solutions from various disciplines (Blumenthal, Abrams, and Nuzum 2015).

To that end, we apply insights from the human resource management literature. We note that corporations have long wrestled with the often conflicting interests of managers and shareholders, and the human resources (HR) field has produced a vast body of knowledge regarding incentive alignment and pay for performance that has direct and potentially fruitful applications to health care. Specifically, we assert that ownership theory from the HR discipline offers substantive insight on how to align the interests of various stakeholders. Ownership theory (Avey, Avolio, Crossley, and Luthans; Klein 1987; Pierce, Kostova, and Dirks 2001; Rosen and Quarrey 1987; Van Dyne and Pierce 2004) asserts that goal alignment is best achieved by more than just financial incentives, requiring also the provision of control and information (Dunford, Schleicher, and Zhu 2009). In this chapter, we draw on ownership theory to offer an analysis of current health care policy, where it performs well, and where it can be improved to help physicians achieve their dual purpose of maximizing patient well-being at sustainable costs. As stated in the Hippocratic Oath, the doctor–patient relationship is invaluable to high-quality medical care, and it is the key outcome for which effective PCPs strive (Dharamsi, Ho, Spadafora, and Woollard 2011; Katz 2002).

Our central thesis is that while the ACA offers measures that improve the primary care environment by rewarding physicians for improving patient outcomes, it has not completely solved the primary care quality problem and has, in some cases, inadvertently created barriers to quality. Thus, the purpose of this chapter is to draw on ownership theory to make policy recommendation about how the U.S. health care system could be altered to help physicians accomplish their mandate to provide outstanding patient care at a sustainable cost.

We begin with a review of ownership theory and the insights it offers on goal alignment (above and beyond goal alignment paradigms that underlie the ACA). We then apply ownership theory to the ACA to demonstrate not only how the act reinforces obstacles to high-quality health care but also how some of the provisions that it contains—if further developed and augmented—have the potential to revolutionize health care in a way that makes it both high-quality and economically sustainable. We conclude with theory-based policy recommendations and suggested areas for future research.

THEORETICAL PERSPECTIVES ON INTEREST ALIGNMENT FROM THE HUMAN RESOURCE DISCIPLINE

For decades, health care thought leaders, lawmakers, and practitioners have wrestled with what is known as the principal–agent problem described by agency theory (Jensen and Meckling 1976). This problem results when one person or entity (principal) gives authority to another person or entity (agent) to make decisions on the principal's behalf. For example, in the negotiation of a collective bargaining agreement, rank-and-file workers (principals) are represented at the bargaining table by labor union leaders (agents) to negotiate the best possible wages, benefits, and working conditions on their behalf. In corporations, shareholders (principals) delegate the day-to-day management and control of the firm to a CEO (agent). Finally, patients (principals) seek the services of physicians (agents) and authorize them to make recommendations about how to optimize their health and well-being. Principal–agent problems occur when principals don't act in the best interest of agents because of divergent self-interests (Jensen and Meckling 1976). The principal–agent problem is regarded to be more common when monitoring of the agent is difficult or when principals lack the capability or expertise to understand whether agents are truly acting in their best interests (Eisenhardt 1989). A fundamental tenet of agency theory is that the optimal way to align the interests of principals and agents is through outcome-based contracts, such as pay-for-performance plans (Jensen and Meckling 1976). The principal–agent problem has been identified in numerous management disciplines (finance, marketing, accounting, economics, political science, and organizational behavior) and is also prominent in health care (Smith, Stepan, Valdmanis, and Verheyen 1997).

Over time, various approaches have been developed for solving the principal–agent problem. In this section of the chapter, we identify two approaches—financial and psychological.

Financial Approaches to Interest Alignment
The most common approach to aligning the interests of principals and agents is to use financial incentives that link the agent's pay to performance outcomes that principals value highly (Eisenhardt 1989; Jensen and Meckling 1976). For example, in corporations, stock-based rewards are commonly granted to align the interests of executives and shareholders (e.g., Bartol, Locke, Rynes, and Gerhart 2000; Hall and Liebman 1998; Hall and Murphy 2002). They align CEO and shareholder interests because they reward executives when they boost shareholder value and punish them when they diminish shareholder value. Hall and Murphy observed that stock-based rewards "motivate executives by providing a direct link between company performance and executive wealth, thereby providing incentives for executives to take actions that increase share prices" (2002: 4). In health care, outcome-based contracts are also common (Pontes 1995). For example, as noted earlier, one of the most significant advancements associated with the ACA is the creation of outcome-based incentives that more closely align the interests of physicians and patients.

The managed care model incentive structure that has dominated the health care landscape for the past few decades has exacerbated the principal–agent problem tremendously because it has rewarded doctors for the *volume* of services that they provide rather than patient health outcomes they achieve. The ACA seeks to overcome this problem by changing some of the metrics by which physicians are rewarded so that they are more closely aligned with the well-being and true interests of patients, such as health outcome bonuses and quality measures that ensure patients don't needlessly end up in the hospital (Anderson, Davis, and Guterman 2015; Blumenthal, Abrams, and Nuzum 2015; Kocher, Emanuel, and DeParle 2010). Additionally, the ACA provides quality standards regarding care coordination, the utilization of preventive services, the avoidance of unnecessary procedures and hospitalizations, and the avoidance of hospital-related medical complications (Davis, Abrams, and Stremikis 2011; Kocher, Emanuel, and DeParle 2010; Koh and Sebelius 2010).

Psychological Approaches to Interest Alignment: An Ownership Theory Perspective

Psychological ownership theory offers a second approach to aligning the interests of patients and physicians (Klein 1987; Pierce, Kostova, and Dirks 2003). Like agency theory, psychological ownership theory argues that pay for performance is a key element of incentive alignment. However, ownership theory goes beyond agency theory to offer additional insight in suggesting that financial incentives alone are not sufficient to align interests between parties.

Psychological ownership is conceptually defined as "the state in which individuals feel as though the target of ownership or a piece of that target is 'theirs' (i.e., 'It is mine')" (Pierce, Kostova, and Dirks, 2003: 86). The nuances of the psychological ownership construct stem from a synthesis of literatures in sociology, philosophy, psychology, and human development (Dawkins, Tian, Newman, and Martin 2015; Pierce, Kostova, and Dirks 2001). By its nature, psychological ownership is both cognitive and affective, aligning with the logic through which one perceives the world and creating an emotional attachment between the individual and the target (Dawkins, Tian, Newman, and Martin 2015). Within the management and labor relations literatures, the target is typically some aspect of the employing organization and can be as specific as a job, a set of tasks, or the organization itself (Chi and Han 2008; Rousseau and Shperling 2003).

According to psychological ownership theory, there are three key perceptions that fuel a person's development of psychological ownership, which are illustrated in Figure 1 on the following page. First, to develop psychological ownership, a person must believe that he or she has control over the target that he or she seeks to own (Pierce, Kostova, and Dirks 2001). In an organizational setting, those things that an employee can control, such as processes, tasks, resources, and subordinates, are things for which that employee can develop psychological ownership. With control often comes a sense of responsibility for or to the target being controlled, and that responsibility can easily morph into perceptions of ownership.

FIGURE 1
The Roots and Routes of Psychological Ownership

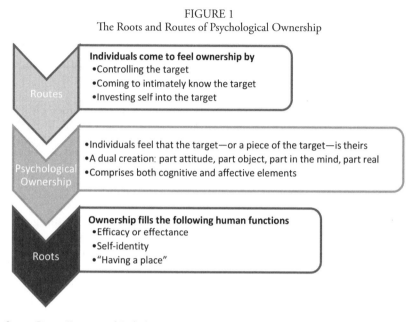

Individuals come to feel ownership by
- Controlling the target
- Coming to intimately know the target
- Investing self into the target

Routes

- Individuals feel that the target—or a piece of the target—is theirs
- A dual creation: part attitude, part object, part in the mind, part real
- Comprises both cognitive and affective elements

Psychological Ownership

Ownership fills the following human functions
- Efficacy or effectance
- Self-identity
- "Having a place"

Roots

Source: Pierce, Kostova, and Dirks (2001, 2003).

Second, the individual must believe that he or she has adequate information about the target, or that he or she knows the target intimately in order to develop perceptions of ownership over that target. As stated by Pierce and his colleagues, "People come to find themselves psychologically tied to things as a result of their active participation or association with those things" (2003: 92). Through such familiarity with the target, an individual perceives that he or she is one of the few people (perhaps even the only person) who knows what is needed to make the target function efficiently, keep the target safe, etc. Finally, psychological ownership requires an individual's perception of having "skin in the game," or an investment of oneself into the target (Pierce, Kostova, and Dirks 2001), either through financial resources or some investment of one's physical or emotional resources. Consistent effort over a range of time leads to a perceived (and sometimes even real) transfer of oneself into the target.

Pierce and his associates (2001, 2003) also describe the "roots" of psychological ownership, or the reason it exists and the functions it performs for individuals. First, they argue that psychological ownership brings about a feeling of self-efficacy for the individual. By successfully "owning" some aspect of work life, the individual experiences "causal efficacy in altering the environment" in which he or she exists (2001: 300). Second, people accentuate their sense of self-identity through psychological ownership. In essence, Pierce and his colleagues posit, "People use ownership for the purpose of defining themselves, expressing their self-identity to others, and ensuring the continuity of the self across time (2001: 300). Finally, the authors contend that it is necessary for every human to have a place, which is brought about by psychological ownership. Through possession of certain work practices, positions, and processes, individuals are able to create either a real or imagined space that can become a home—a familiar space in which the person feels comfort and belonging (Pierce, Kostova, and Dirks 2001).

As demonstrated in Figure 2, the relationship between psychological ownership, its routes, and its roots is cyclical. Control of the target, intimate knowledge of the target, and the investment of self into the target facilitate an individual's cognitive and affective perceptions of ownership over that target. This perceived ownership strengthens the individual's self-efficacy related to that target and facilitates his or her identity in relation to that target while providing a sense of belongingness to the immediate environment in which the target is located. These perceptions of self, bolstered by the self-efficacy, identity, and belongingness produced by psychological ownership, further enhance the individual's desires for control of the target, an even more intimate knowledge of the target, and a deeper personal investment into the target, thus perpetuating the cycle of psychological ownership (Pierce, Kostova, and Dirks 2001, 2003).

The Relative Importance of Information and Control

A defining characteristic of ownership theory is that all routes are not equal in the strength of their relationship with interest alignment. Multiple

FIGURE 2
The Cyclical Nature of Psychological Ownership

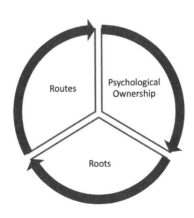

empirical studies show that relative to an agent's level of pay linked to a principal's performance outcomes, perceptions of control and access to information are much stronger predictors of agents' attitudes and behavior (Dunford, Schleicher, and Zhu 2009). In short, the most effective routes for motivating agents to act in the best interests of principals is to give them information about and control over the work delegated to them by a principal (e.g., Bakan, Suseno, Pinnington, and Money 2004; Klein 1987; Rosen, Case, and Staubus 2005; Rosen and Quarrey 1987; Rousseau and Shperling 2003).

One reason that employee perceptions of information and control may be more salient than pay-for-performance investment involves what has been referred to as the "1/n problem" (Benartzti, Thaler, Utkus, and Sunstein 2007). Critics question the motivational aspects of pay for performance, arguing that for most workers there is a poor line of sight between their day-to-day activities and an organization's performance (Benartzti, Thaler, Utkus, and Sunstein 2007). As companies get larger, the relative impact of one individual on the firm's overall performance becomes smaller, and the more trivial the individual's portion of the firms' overall profit (hence, the "1/n" terminology). Together these forces are likely to weaken the link between pay-for-performance systems and attitudes and behaviors.

In summary, psychological ownership theory suggests that while pay for performance is a useful method for aligning the interests of agents with the interests of principals, pay for performance may be less efficacious if used in isolation. To complement pay for performance, psychological ownership theory suggests that agents should perceive a high level of knowledge about and a high level of control over the work they do on behalf of principals (Bakan, Suseno, Pinnington, and Money 2004; Dunford, Schleicher, and Zhu 2009; Klein 1987; Rosen, Case, and Staubus 2005; Rosen and Quarrey 1987). When perceived information and control are high, agents are more likely to make decisions and act in ways most beneficial to principals. We assert that these insights provide a key to helping primary care physicians meet the needs of patients and society in providing high-quality health care at a sustainable cost. In the section that follows, we will leverage ownership theory to analyze the current U.S. health care system in terms of the barriers it places on primary care physicians' perceptions of information and control.

THE IMPACT OF MANAGED CARE ON PCP OWNERSHIP OF PATIENT CARE

While a strong body of evidence indicates that the managed care model has slowed the rate of rising private health care expenses in the United States (Dranove 2000), managed care has also had less perceptible, but equally important, impacts on the way in which doctors and patients work together (Silver 1997). This section starts with a brief history of managed care within the U.S. health care system. We will then describe how managed care has, perhaps unwittingly, blocked primary care physician routes to ownership of patient care by limiting physician control over and information regarding patient care, and impeding physician investment in patient care. We will explain how these route blockages sever physicians' roots of ownership regarding patient care, causing lower physician satisfaction and resulting in a smaller primary care physician workforce. Finally, we will articulate the impacts of the Affordable Care Act on physician routes and roots of patient care ownership. Although the ACA has reinforced many managed care elements that alienated PCPs from the ownership of patient care in the first place, it has also introduced innovative mechanisms through which the quality of primary care can improve dramatically while costs can be kept at sustainable levels.

The Rapid Ascent of Managed Care

While managed care has existed in some form or another for nearly 100 years in the U.S. health care system (Dranove 2009), the passage of the Health Maintenance Organization Act of 1973 signaled a dramatic shift from indemnity health insurance to the proliferation of managed care insurance plans in the United States (Iglehart 1994). Health maintenance organizations (typically referred to as HMOs), which represented the first widely available form of managed care, grew dramatically during the 1970s and 1980s. HMOs reached their peak in 1996, when a study conducted by the Kaiser Institute and the Health Research and Educational Trust (HRET) showed that 31% of all employer health plans were HMOs, making HMOs the most readily available type of health care plan in the United States during that year (Claxton et al. 2015). As opposed to the traditional indemnity insurance model, in which policy holders recoup the direct expenses related to medical care that they receive from a licensed physician, HMOs manage costs by requiring policy holders to see physicians that work for the HMO. In this arrangement, doctors are accountable to the HMO to ensure that they are using the most cost-effective methods of treatment possible.

As the success of traditional HMOs waned in the 1990s, another form of managed care, known as preferred provider organizations (commonly called PPOs), became the most prominent form of health insurance in the U.S. health care system. Instead of hiring physicians to work for the insurance organization, PPOs contract with private health care providers to offer services at discounted rates for patients covered by specific PPO insurance plans (Gray, Lowery, and Benz 2013). The meteoric success of PPOs is unprecedented in the U.S. health care system. In 1988, only 11%

of all health care plans offered by employers were PPOs; by 2005, PPOs comprised 61% of all health care plans available through employers (Claxton et al. 2015). Since 2005, there have been more PPO plans available through employers than all other types of insurance combined, with PPO plans comprising 52% of all health care insurance plans offered by employers in 2015 (Claxton et al. 2015). While initially popular because of their lower cost to businesses and individual consumers (Iglehart 1994), the cost of PPO plans has increased significantly over the past 15 years (Claxton et al. 2015). In 2015, PPO family health insurance offered through an employer cost an average of $18,469, with employers shouldering an average of $13,253 of that total cost, while employees bore $5,430 of that annual cost (Claxton et al. 2015).

A more recent managed care plan type is the high-deductible health plan with savings option (often referred to as an HDHP/SO). In this type of plan, a portion of the premium is applied to an account to help offset the costs of deductibles and co-pays for medical visits, which have increased significantly across all types of medical insurance plans over the past 20 years as well (Claxton et al. 2015).

Predictably, the dramatic surge of managed care has co-occurred with the sudden disappearance of indemnity health insurance policies. While managed care plans now dominate the insurance marketplace, representing 99% of plans available through U.S. employers, indemnity health insurance plans make up less than 1% of the employer-based market (Claxton et al. 2015). As indemnity insurance has faded away, managed care organizations (MCOs) have changed form as well. Originally patterned as nonprofit entities serving a social need (e.g., Kaiser Permanente), MCOs have become more profit oriented since the early 1990s (Iglehart 1994). For example, in 1993, the national board of Blue Cross and Blue Shield approved the creation of for-profit HMOs within their system, allowing a number of state-run Blue Cross and Blue Shield plans to build for-profit HMOs in their system (Iglehart 1994). Corporatization of MCOs means the prioritization of stockholders and the responsibility to widen profit margins (Iglehart 1994), which further de-emphasizes the importance of serving consumers or doctors.

Despite their strong resistance to the unparalleled growth of MCOs in the U.S. health care market (Dworkin 2000; McMurray 1998; Silver 1997), the vast majority of primary care doctors—foreseeing the imminent financial risks of remaining outside of the managed care system—opted to join managed care networks as they grew in power and influence (Dranove 2000). Speaking of this decision made by so many doctors, economist Uwe E. Reinhart opined:

> I do not think that most physicians recognize that carving up
> the system into competing health plans is a road to serfdom

[for them]. … The private HMO managers have become literal bounty hunters who are unleashed on the system and are allowed to carve out for themselves, mainly from the hides of doctors, enormous profit margins. And government and payers take no notice. That is why outfits like U.S. Health Care are able to keep 30 cents of every premium dollar for administration, marketing and profit. Imagine if government burned 30 percent of the premium dollar. (In Iglehart 1994: 67)

Despite much of the cost savings boasted by managed care (Dranove 2000), it has fundamentally altered both the way in which primary care is offered in the United States and what it means to be a doctor. Perhaps most unfortunately, however, is that the "incentives of managed care have now put physicians' and patients' interests in more obvious conflict" (Mechanic 2000: 103).

Blocked Routes of Psychological Ownership

As mentioned earlier in this chapter, Pierce, Kostova, and Dirks (2001, 2003) identified three "routes" to the psychological ownership of a target, which are control, access to information, and investment in the ownership target. Owing to the standardization of health care required by the managed care model, physicians' routes to ownership have been constrained dramatically, which in turn have weakened the primary care system and limited primary care quality in the process.

As managed care progressed throughout the 1980s and 1990s, hospital administrators and insurance CEOs began to play a larger role in clinical decisions, specifically ensuring that doctors maximized cost effectiveness in treatment (Dranove 2000). Physician autonomy eroded rapidly, and doctors experienced a "proletarianizing" effect within their profession (McKinlay and Stoeckle 1988; Silver 1997). Both new and experienced physicians have been critical of managed care specifically because it limits the clinical judgment of doctors by requiring certain procedures in order to receive full reimbursement, by requiring MCO approval before referring to specialists, and even requiring doctors to get pre-approval from managed care organizations before performing certain interventions (Deom, Agoritsas, Bovier, and Perneger 2010; Dranove 2000; Simon et al. 1999). In an editorial piece framed as a call for doctors to adjust their expectations and become more supportive of managed care, Mechanic (2000) acknowledges the rancor felt not only among practicing physicians but among medical school faculty and administrators as well. The number one complaint among doctors cited by Mechanic (2000) was the amount of autonomy doctors lost in working with MCOs. A survey of 703 physicians in 1991 and 1996 corroborated the opinions of doctors cited by Mechanic: the surveys in 1996—which represented a health care system with significantly more managed care than could be found in the market in 1991—showed that doctors felt they didn't have enough time to meet basic patient care needs and that their autonomy to make even the most important of medical decisions had been curtailed (Burdi and Baker 1999). Particularly sobering to note was that 35.8% of providers surveyed in 1996 stated that, if they had the opportunity to do it again, they would elect not to go into medicine as a profession (Burdi and Baker 1999).

In a more nationally representative survey of more than 12,000 physicians, Stoddard and his colleagues (2001) found that physicians who worked frequently with patients who had managed care plans had less job satisfaction than physicians who worked less with managed care. Of particular note in that study was the fact that limits to physician autonomy mediated the relationship between work with managed care and job satisfaction, while lower salaries did not mediate this relationship. Essentially, these findings support ownership theory's proposition that the loss of clinical autonomy weighed heavier on physicians surveyed than did income reduction (Stoddard, Hargraves, Reed, and Vratil 2001). For many doctors, clinical autonomy is at the core of what it means to be a doctor (Dworkin 2000).

Information is the second required route to psychological ownership (Pierce, Kostova, and Dirks 2001, 2003). Without the ability to gain sufficient information about the target, individuals are not able to develop psychological ownership over (i.e., responsibility for) that target. In addition to complaints regarding diminished autonomy, physicians decry managed care's emphasis on the quantity of clinical work provided. Primary care physicians in HMOs and PPOs are given pay incentives to increase their panel size, with many providers increasing from panel sizes of 2,000 up to panel sizes of 4,000 patients or more (McMurray 1998). Not only do such enormous panel sizes increase patient wait time for getting appointments, as well as patient wait times while in the office, but they also require providers to meet with patients for shorter amounts of time, often with no prep time before the appointment. In the 1996 survey of physicians, of which nearly 83% were doctors with managed care contracts, only 70% felt like they got to spend enough time with most clients (Burdi and Baker 1999), which represented a 13.5% drop from the 83.5% who felt they got to spend enough time with most clients in 1991. The same survey showed that the number of physicians who carefully reviewed patient medical records and test results dropped from 92.6% in 1991 to about 72% in 1996—a staggering drop of 20% (Burdi and Baker 1999). Because there is rarely time between sessions for writing notes, PCPs often spend the bulk of what little time they have with patients writing notes on the exam room computer, rather than talking with and examining the patient (Bendix 2013). Many providers feel that they don't get enough time with patients to gather the information that they need to make accurate diagnoses, much less to get to know the patient and develop both rapport and a holistic approach to treating that patient (Burdi and Baker 1999; Dranove 2000; McMurray 1998).

Decreased autonomy and information about patient care, coupled with financial incentives aimed at increasing the quantity of medical visits and cost-cutting measures, strongly de-incentivize PCP investment in patient health and well-being. McMurray (1998: 315–16) explained the conflicting nature of the demands made on her in patient care within a managed care setting as follows:

> As the months go by, my established patients become more unhappy as it becomes more difficult for them to see me. My new patients are enraged at the more than 3 months' wait for a physical. … In the office, they sit with lists written on the backs of envelopes to remind them to discuss their headaches, constipation, elevated cholesterol, and hormone levels. There just doesn't seem to be enough time for them to begin to trust me, nor for me to understand the person behind the list. I dread looking at my daily schedule and long for the short, uncomplicated medical encounter.
>
> A new patient calls me on the phone. … The wait for an appointment is unacceptably long to her. Although I have never seen her, on paper I am already her physician, and she is angry and irritated. I call her back, having already added extra patients to my session that day. Sitting in my office with my elbows on a stack of charts that all bear notes asking me to call patients, I am overwhelmed and vaguely realize that our conversation hasn't gone well. Many weeks later, when we finally meet, my new patient forcefully condemns my lack of compassion on the phone and is uninterested in both my abject apologies and my explanations about "HMO panel sizes" and "time pressures." I know that she has labeled me arrogant and insensitive, and the sense of failure on my part is enormous. Although I spend time rationalizing and working through the experience, her diatribe against me remains one of the most painful moments in my 15 years of doctoring.

McMurray's account paints an unsustainable picture of primary care in a managed care setting. Though by her account she clearly wants to more deeply invest herself in meaningful patient care, McMurray feels an even stronger responsibility to the HMO and spreads herself so thin within her job that her burnout levels are palpable as she tells her story (McMurray 1998).

Though perhaps an extreme example, McMurray's story is not too different from that of many other providers, who have indicated in survey and research interviews that they just don't get to invest in the doctor–patient relationship like they used to (Bendix 2013; Burdi and Baker 1999; Deom, Agoritsas, Bovier, and Perneger 2010; Dranove 2000). Lack of investment in patient care, for whatever reason and despite doctors' best intentions, limits the ability of PCPs to take ownership of patient care. As implied by the Hippocratic Oath (Lasagna 1995) and demonstrated in research (Deom, Agoritsas, Bovier, and Perneger 2010, Stavropoulou 2011; Tarrant, Dixon-Woods, Colman, and Stokes 2010), lower-quality doctor–patient relationships are linked to lower-quality health care and poorer health outcomes for patients.

Severed Roots of Psychological Ownership

The routes of psychological ownership—control, information, and personal investment—lead to the formation of the roots of psychological ownership, which are self-efficacy, identity, and having a place (Pierce, Kostova, and Dirks 2001). While the routes of psychological ownership are vital for the creation of psychological ownership, the roots are what maintain and motivate this ownership (Dawkins, Tian, Newman, and Martin 2015; Pierce, Kostova, and Dirks 2003). Although economic incentives always play an important role in managing behavior, the plight of PCPs over the past 30 years shows that economic incentives alone are not sufficient to fix a health care model that so clearly prioritizes cost over quality.

Primary care doctors who experienced the sudden shift from indemnity insurance to managed care during the 1980s and 1990s resisted its growth because of its impact on the profession itself, as evidenced by this lament:

> What made medicine a profession in the modern sense of the term was the autonomy physicians enjoyed in their everyday work. Physicians were not "organization men." They did not have to be backslappers or joke-tellers or handshakers; they did not have to get along with the boss or be shrewdly political. Their healing skill was enough to attract patients and earn a comfortable living. Their job in life was largely to supervise themselves. *They answered to no one but their patients* [emphasis added]. …
>
> Years ago, physicians might have been satisfied with less income, since what they lacked in money was made up for in status. There was almost an ascetic nobility that went with being a doctor. But now that doctors get little more out of their work than a paycheck, the money is much more important to them and they increasingly try to make more of it. (Dworkin 2000: 37, 39)

Though many PCPs experienced only minimal salary reductions, the reduction in status—as evidenced by loss of autonomy, information, and opportunities for self-investment in patient care—experienced by doctors since the meteoric growth of managed care has had a negative outcome on PCPs. Primary care providers previously enjoyed a considerable amount of autonomy in providing high-quality care to patients with whom they had a great deal of rapport and mutual respect (Dranove 2000). However, macro-level political and economic changes reduced these same providers to being company men and women—required to give an accounting of all their efforts to corporate interests, and continuously stretched by ever-increasing patient panels. With expanding panel sizes and shrinking appointment times, it is difficult for primary care doctors to feel like they are making any difference at all. With the decreasing clinical and business autonomy, what it means to be a doctor has devolved significantly, leaving many doctors to question their professional identities. Finally, without the status previously afforded to doctors societally, many PCPs are left without the deference and respect that had been their psychological home in generations past.

Without firm roots, psychological ownership can't continue, and doctors may question why they are involved in this line of work. Indeed, in the wake of managed care's takeover of the U.S. health care system, many PCPs have retired early or transferred to other subspecialties of medicine (McKinlay and Marceau 2008; Schwartz 2012). Additionally, fewer medical students have chosen primary care as their specialty over the past two decades (Schwartz 2012), which means that the profession has been losing PCPs for a number of years now. This net loss has created a primary care shortage in the United States, which has made it difficult for many patients to be seen in primary care and, experts posit, may lead to a full-blown health care crisis by 2020 (U.S Department of Health and Human Services, Health Resources and Services Administration 2013). This PCP shortage and many other disturbing trends in the U.S. health care system over the past two decades were important considerations in creating the Affordable Care Act of 2011.

The ACA and Psychological Ownership

One of the three primary tasks of the ACA was to improve the quality of medical care in the U.S. health care system (Kocher, Emanuel, and DeParle 2010). While evidence already demonstrates the ACA's effectiveness in improving access to medical care for previously uninsured Americans, and while the ACA has succeeded in slowing the rate at which health care costs have been expanding in the United States, it is not yet clear whether it will achieve the quality of care improvement anticipated by its proponents (Blumenthal, Abrams, and Nuzum 2015). The ACA shows great promise in its ability to align the interests of multiple stakeholders for excellence in health care at a sustainable cost, particularly through its emphasis on pay for performance.

However, through our application of the prescriptions of ownership theory, we assert that the ACA also contains measures that limit its effectiveness in ensuring improved quality in primary care. Specifically, we argue that the ACA has unintentionally reinforced limitations to physician autonomy (control) and access to information, two key elements to solving the principal–agent problem. Consequently, under the ACA in its current form, PCPs are unlikely to develop a strong sense of psychological ownership regarding patient care. In the next section of the chapter, we outline some of the strengths and weaknesses of key provisions in the ACA, with an emphasis on how the act might be adjusted to reach its full potential.

Strengths and Limitations of the ACA

The ACA is an expansive act, with numerous provisions that have been carefully and systematically enacted over the five years since it became law (see Table 1, following the next page). While we support many of our assertions with research conducted in the time since the ACA was enacted, we readily acknowledge that it is still too early to formally evaluate the act. The statements made in this section, therefore, should be considered propositions based on theory and preliminary research findings.

A problematic and potentially detrimental provision within the ACA is its formal entrenchment of MCOs within the U.S. health care system. While third-party payer insurance systems have a long history in American health care, and while managed care has dominated the health insurance market over the past 20 years (Dranove 2000; Miller and Hudson-Thrall 2010), the ACA's insurance mandate further strengthens MCOs and allows them to exert more legitimate control over the U.S. primary care system (Hall and Lord 2014; Lathrop and Hodnicki 2014). Hall and Lord's recent evaluation of the ACA (2014) showed that since the insurance mandate was implemented, many MCOs have systematically lowered reimbursement rates for providers, often requesting that PCPs accept reimbursements as low as the Medicare reimbursement rate. In some cases, providers who have been unwilling to accept lower reimbursement rates have been dropped from provider networks (Hall and Lord 2014), which can debilitate provider panels and leave consumers in the undesirable quandary of choosing either a new PCP or a new health insurance plan. Additionally, the popular media has already begun to regularly recount tales of patients switching health care plans only to find out that their provider is not in their new network (Tozzi 2014).

Increased power for MCOs limits doctors' clinical autonomy and, consequently, the ownership they can possess over patient care. Though the national mandate for health insurance coverage will increase the overall number of patients available to PCPs, we assert that it also reallocates a significant portion of a provider's control—which is a key route to psychological ownership—to MCOs, whose goals are typically not aligned with either patients or providers. A recent survey of PCPs showed that one of eight providers was dropped from at least one insurance plan over the previous year, while an additional one of eight providers had an insurance company threaten to drop them from the network (Bendix 2013). Physicians who are unwilling to comply with the ever-tightening rules of insurance companies run the risk of significant economic detriment to their practices (Bendix 2013).

The accentuated reliance on health insurance created by the ACA has facilitated the creation of an incredible diversity of health insurance plans by MCOs, which are designed to maximize the variety of products offered to consumers in the increasingly competitive health marketplace (Bendix 2013). This expansive selection of plans gives consumers greater autonomy over the type of health insurance coverage they want, further demonstrating the positive impacts of the ACA on American health care consumers. However, the vast permutations of the health care insurance plans require PCPs and their staffs to allocate additional administrative time in determining which tests and procedures are covered on each patient's health insurance plan. A recent poll showed that more than 40% of PCPs surveyed feel that the ACA administrative mandates, such as pre-authorization requirements, threaten their relationships with patients by limiting the provider's autonomy in prescribing treatment and by focusing the provider on reimbursements rather than individualized care for patients (Bendix 2013).

The ACA takes a much more proactive stance on improving the information available to doctors by mandating that all PCPs implement electronic medical records. Electronic medical records make it much easier for PCPs to cooperate and coordinate with other providers in providing comprehensive care while avoiding service duplications, as well as dangerous medication combinations and contraindications (Kocher, Emanuel, and DeParle 2010). Furthermore, coordination facilitated by electronic medical records gives PCPs greater autonomy and information, which are key to owning patient care. Yet while electronic records undoubtedly facilitate provider communication and the gathering of information, the electronic record mandate outlined in the ACA has the potential to negatively impact many physicians' ownership of individual patient care.

TABLE 1
Positive and Negative Impacts of the ACA on Providers' Psychological Ownership Over Patient Care Quality

ACA provision	Positive impact on providers' psychological ownership	Negative impact on providers' psychological ownership
Mandates insurance coverage for all American citizens	Insurance coverage requires patients to choose a primary care provider (PCP) and designates PCPs as the owners of patient care by requiring patients to get a referral from their PCP before seeing a specialist.	Increases power and influence of managed care organizations, which limits PCP autonomy, drawing ownership of patient care away from PCPs. Increase in overall number of health care plans available to patients creates uncertainty about reimbursement for services, and uncertainty limits the knowledge and investment that engender PCP ownership.
Mandates implementation of electronic medical record systems	Facilitates the coordination of interdisciplinary care through primary care, giving PCPs more control over each patient's health care.	PCPs may offset increased administrative costs for electronic records by increasing patient panels. Larger patient panels mean less time getting to know, and invest themselves in, each patient—thus inhibiting ownership over care. PCPs may be tempted to stereotype patients more frequently using cut-and-paste templates available in electronic record systems. Stereotyping diminishes a PCP's investment in patient care. Electronic charting may distract from time interacting with the patients, which limits the knowledge and investment needed for PCP ownership of care.

ACA provision	Positive impact on providers' psychological ownership	Negative impact on providers' psychological ownership
Provides financial incentives for implementing PCMH/ACO systems	Facilitates redesign of primary care practices in ways that enhance accountability and control of care.	Uncertainty in incentives may lead many doctors to increase their patient panels to ensure revenue. Larger patient panels means less time getting to know each patient.
Authorizes inclusion of direct primary care plans in health marketplace	Facilitates the growth of direct primary care, which is an alternative to managed care that incentivizes PCP ownership over patient care. The two-party payment system encourages PCPs to own patient care or risk losing direct revenue.	Rapid expansion of direct primary care may exacerbate the primary care shortage, which would either leave many Americans without a PCP or would require PCPs to increase their panel sizes, further limiting their ability to know and invest themselves in patients.

Despite financial resources allocated through the American Recovery and Reinvestment Act of 2009—which offer yearly compensatory funds to medical practices that switch to electronic records systems—many providers are feeling the financial squeeze imposed by the mandate because electronic record-keeping systems can be quite expensive to purchase and require a great deal of training and use before providers and medical staff become proficient with them (Dranove, Forman, Goldfarb, and Greenstein 2012). Additionally, the transfer of existing records to an electronic records system places huge demands on the administrative staff of medical practices, which necessitates additional compensation for staff (Bendix 2013; Dranove, Forman, Goldfarb, and Greenstein 2012). To offset these often unanticipated costs, many providers increased their already crowded panels in order to sufficiently increase revenue (Bendix 2013). While larger panels increase profits, they also typically decrease the ability of PCPs to invest themselves in really getting to know the medical needs of each patient, inhibiting PCP psychological ownership of patient care. As one doctor succinctly stated, "More work to satisfy ACA requirements equals less time with patients" (Bendix 2013: 22). As ownership theory implies (Pierce et al. 2003), the routes of psychological ownership require an investment of time into the target(s).

Recent studies indicate that even after overcoming the initial investments of time, money, and attention in transitioning to electronic medical records, many doctors may be overusing electronic record systems during patient exams (Hoff 2011). This overuse of computers in the exam room has been noted by patients. During an interview, one doctor stated, "I've had patients who have left their previous doctor because they said that in a 15-minute appointment the doctor spent 10 minutes typing" (Bendix 2013: 22). It comes as no surprise, then, that 25% of physicians surveyed in a study felt that mandated electronic records systems, in concert with the pressures to see an increasing number of patients, actually threaten PCP routes to psychological ownership over patient care by minimizing both the time and undivided attention that providers give to their patients (Bendix 2013). Additionally, among the 78 providers whom he interviewed, Hoff (2011) found that reliance on "cut and paste" templates encouraged providers to generalize and stereotype the medical conditions of their patients, which led providers to focus on the disease rather than the patient.

Many of the ACA provisions and mandates designated to strengthen and reinforce primary care in the U.S. health care system incentivize compliance by providing resources and reimbursements to primary care practices that are willing to implement them (Davis, Abrams, and Stremikis 2011). However, the distribution policies attached to these resources may make it difficult for many PCPs to use these otherwise excellent primary care initiatives. Unlike the successful tax credit system created to help Americans who earn lower incomes by subsidizing health insurance premiums—which is already one of the ACA's banner initiatives—many of the funds designed to incentivize the development of higher-quality primary care, such as the creation of PCMHs and ACOs, are retroactively dispersed (Kocher, Emanuel, and DeParle 2010). Aside from the care coordination funds offered by many private insurance companies, which amount to about $2.50 per patient per month (Majette 2009), the incentives for building a practice into a PCMH become available only to those who create cost savings for Medicare (Majette 2009). Thus, providers must take proactive steps and incur initial risk and debt to qualify for federal resources.

As an additional example, primary care organizations that want funds allocated to PCMHs are required to meet interdisciplinary staffing and resource measures in order to receive the funds. While PCMHs have been shown to increase the quality of care tremendously for patients (Calman, Golub, and Shuman 2012), they can also be tremendously costly to establish. We posit that, for some PCPs, the costs and risks associated with radically redesigning their medical practices aren't worth the retroactive funds that they would receive for doing so.

Funding for the ACA is contingent on the annual federal budget, but it also depends on Supreme Court rulings, which have recently had an impact on the reimbursement rates that providers can seek from public programs (Huberfeld 2015). We anticipate that even resource-rich practices may be wary of committing themselves to PCMH redesign and interdisciplinary growth with no guarantee that the federal funds offered by the ACA will still be available to them when the providers finally qualify. Thus, financial uncertainty may prevent many providers from investing themselves more fully into higher-quality patient care.

Promising Innovative Mechanisms in the ACA

While the aforementioned provisions contained in the ACA have arguably had mixed impact on PCP ownership of patient care, there are also exciting and innovative aspects of the ACA which—if expanded and developed—could bring about revolutionary changes in both the quality and cost of primary care. These innovations also have the potential to make primary care a more attractive subspecialty of medicine, which may replenish the PCP workforce and alleviate the current primary care provider shortage. One such innovation, which has the capacity to revolutionize primary care in the U.S. health care system, is the ACA's authorization of direct primary care.

One of the most intriguing yet unheralded aspects of the ACA is its authorization of direct primary care. Direct primary care is a primary care model in which patients pay a small monthly fee (usually between $40 and $100 a month per person) directly to the primary care practice and receive comprehensive primary care at the rate of a typical insurance co-pay (usually $20 a visit). First developed in 2002, direct primary care has grown dramatically and is anticipated to be present in all 50 states by the end of 2016 (Carlson 2015; Huff 2015). Direct PCPs create panels of 600 to 1,500 patients—as opposed to the 2,000 to 4,000 patients on traditional managed care provider panels—and are able to provide more personalized care because of the lower volume of total patients. Patient visits in direct primary care typically last between 30 and 60 minutes (Carlson 2015), which allows PCPs the time to gather thorough medical histories and assessments. Increased autonomy facilitates the PCP's investment in individualized patient care. Also, more time spent conversing with patients provides PCPs with more comprehensive knowledge regarding the health and well-being of patients. Additional provider autonomy, increased provider investment, and more comprehensive knowledge of patients' health and well-being enhance provider ownership over patient care (Pierce, Kostova, and Dirks 2001), while also strengthening the doctor–patient relationship.

Early evidence indicates that the direct primary care model appeals to patients and physicians alike. Carlson (2015) reports that patients are often able to set same-day appointments with their physicians or communicate with their physicians via text, telephone, or telemedicine equipment, which are services that aren't available in the managed care model. For PCPs, direct primary care restores clinical and business autonomy to the doctor, which explains why PCPs under the age of 45 have expressed an overwhelming interest in switching to a direct-pay model for primary care (Lincoff 2015). Applying the ownership perspective to this innovation, we assert that providers practicing direct primary care will likely be more inclined to invest themselves in patient care because dissatisfied patients can more readily choose a new primary care doctor, unencumbered by insurance-related constraints. Direct primary care incentivizes a high-quality doctor–patient relationship which, as research has shown (Garcia, Lima, Gorender, and Badaró 2005; Pooley, Highfield, and Neal 2015; Tarrant, Dixon-Woods, Colman, and Stokes 2010), is vital in terms of medical-intervention quality and patient satisfaction with the overall medical experience.

The creators of the ACA innovatively included provisions in the act that allow direct primary care to be bundled with catastrophic medical insurance and sold in health insurance exchanges in select states (Carlson 2015; Dewey 2015; Huff 2015). This ACA provision has seemingly triggered a cascade of state legislation that removes proposed legislation pertaining to direct patient care from committees and health codes pertaining to insurance, which is anticipated to facilitate the growth of direct primary care significantly (Carlson 2015; Dewey 2015). However, we have identified additional steps by which the ACA could facilitate the transition away from managed primary care toward direct primary care, thereby further incentivizing providers' psychological ownership of patient care.

POLICY RECOMMENDATIONS

First, we propose that the effectiveness of the ACA could be enhanced by expanding this small, state-based provision to the entire United States by creating incentives that will facilitate a mass movement of PCPs away from the managed care model and toward the direct primary care model. For example, the ACA could mandate that all MCOs conducting business on the health marketplace carry catastrophic plans specifically tailored to bundling with direct primary care, which would make direct primary care more readily available to consumers in all states, in turn allowing the government to subsidize comprehensive health care access for all Americans at a much lower cost than the current tax credit subsidies for health insurance premiums (Huff 2015).

The ACA could further enhance the quality of primary care with more proactive incentive structures. As mentioned previously in this chapter, the ACA has already successfully implemented a tax-based incentive system to make insurance premiums affordable for all Americans, and these incentives have made access to health care a reality for millions of citizens. As it is implemented right now, many providers chafe at administrative requirements in the ACA, which they often interpret as unfunded administrative mandates and, to make the required adjustments to their practices, many providers have increased their panels to even more unsustainable sizes (Bendix 2013). Offering proactive tax credits or low-interest business loans to PCPs who have committed to developing their primary care practices into PCMHs would undoubtedly have similar effects to the tax credits made available to health care consumers through the health insurance marketplace, and it would make private practice a reality for many medical students who are naturally inclined toward primary care but who balk at the financial risks associated with the unsustainable managed care model. With proactive incentives available, physicians may see the development of private practices as an opportunity rather than as a government-mandated risk (Miller and Hudson-Thrall 2010).

One major concern with widespread use of the direct primary care model is that smaller panel sizes for PCPs will further exacerbate the primary care shortage (Huff 2015). While this concern is indeed legitimate, there are various ways in which the benefits of direct primary care can be harnessed to addresses the PCP shortage. First, PCPs who engage in direct primary care report that they are more satisfied with their jobs than PCPs practicing in traditional primary care (Carlson 2015). More-satisfied physicians are less likely to transfer mid-career to a different medical specialty and are also less likely to retire early, as many PCPs have done over the past 30 years (U.S. Department of Health and Human Services, Health Resources and Services Administration 2013).

Second, the shift to direct primary care has already started making primary care a more attractive option for medical students choosing their specialty area (Carlson 2015). Aside from expanding direct primary care—which Wanda Filer, the current president of the American Academy of Family Physicians, has stated could make family medicine an attractive option for medical students once again (Huff 2015)—the federal government could further incentivize primary care as a specialization of choice by offering loan remission for new PCPs who set up direct primary care practices in underserved areas or by offering low-interest business loans, tax credits, or grants to new providers who have an immediate plan to build a direct primary care PCMH practice.

Third, federal legislation could make this shift less financially burdensome by allocating resources—in the form of grants or low-interest loans—to PCPs already working in primary care practices who want to transition their existing practices into direct primary care PCMHs (Huff 2015). Facilitating the shift of existing primary care practices to the PCMH model would meet the ACA goals of creating more interdisciplinary, high-quality primary care, while also facilitating a system that limits administrative requirements and allows providers to take more ownership over patient care. Before expanding direct primary care policies, however, government entities must sponsor additional studies regarding the impacts of current direct primary care on the lives of patients now receiving that care, with special attention paid to those who are socially disadvantaged (i.e., those who live in poverty or are members of social groups who remain vulnerable).

DIRECTIONS FOR FUTURE RESEARCH

In recognition of certain limitations—in addition to new and recent developments in the labor relations literature—we highlight certain areas that may be worthy of further investigation to better assess the validity of the claims we make in this chapter. First, we draw attention to the growing labor shortage of PCPs (Schwartz 2012). Projections suggest that the shortage could escalate into a more full-blown crisis by as early as 2020 if the status quo initiated by the ACA is maintained (U.S. Department of Health and Human Services, Health Resources and Services Administration 2013). However, empirical research should better quantify these claims, given the relative "newness" of the ACA. Because some of the provisions have yet to fully take effect, these doomsday-type predictions may be exaggerated. Additionally, future research should consider whether international PCPs may substitute for American PCPs. For example, Kaushal and Kaestner (2015: 1102) concluded that "foreign- and U.S.-trained nurses are equally productive and close substitutes" in regard to training and wage differentials. If American and international PCPs are close substitutes, then focusing only on the shortages associated with students training to become PCPs in American medical education institutions (e.g., Schwartz 2012) may be too myopic if an additional labor pool is potentially available.

Second, the loss of physician job autonomy and perceptions of job quality warrant additional attention. Job quality involves some of the factors referred to earlier, including compensation-related elements and a certain degree of job control (Osterman 2013). Autonomy has long been recognized as an important determinant of well-being, enhanced motivation, and other positive individual-based outcomes (e.g., Cottini and Lucifora 2013; Hackman and Oldham 1976; Karasek 1979). We argued earlier that MCOs reduce physician autonomy in regard to patient care. Based on the well-understood notion that autonomy is good for workers, we implied that the loss of autonomy would result in dissatisfaction or other negative outcomes.

However, Briscoe (2007) offers an interesting counterargument suggesting that less autonomy (created by bureaucratic structures) can result in greater temporal flexibility for physicians, which acts as a buffer against work-related demands. Specifically, he found among a sample of physicians that "in order for workers to achieve the flexibility necessary to vary their schedules on short or long time frames, they require the ability to hand off clients so that windows of time can be fully protected" (2007: 309). On the one hand, passing patients from physician to physician further blocks routes of psychological ownership by limiting the ability to know the target and to invest the self into the target. On the other hand, reduced psychological ownership—which comes as a result of more formalized structure created and imposed by the ACA—can create opportunities for greater schedule flexibility, in line with Briscoe's logic. Although the sentiment in the prevailing literature is tipped heavily in favor of the former idea, future research should determine the extent to which reduced physician autonomy created by the ACA can result in positive outcomes.

Third, the identity-based implications of how the ACA reduce the expression of positive self-identities (in line with psychological ownership) are not entirely clear. When physicians have positive perceptions of the health care system in which they are embedded, they are more likely to evaluate their system positively, self-identify with the system, and engage in more cooperative behaviors (Dukerich, Golden, and Shortell 2002). Yet research demonstrates that various courses of action are possible when self-identities are negative or diminished. For example, individuals may choose to self-enhance by seeking positive feedback or they may self-verify by seeking subjective feedback that is accurate with their self-construal (Swann, Pelham, and Krull 1989). If the ACA diminishes the self-identity of PCPs, how do PCPs respond? Do they seek to self-enhance or self-verify? Do they abandon their PCP-based identity? Do they maintain a health care–related identity but identify with a different type of group, consistent with social identification theory (Tajfel and Turner 1985)? Future research can explore these questions.

Finally, future research might take a more abstract or broader perspective by integrating institutional theory perspectives, viewing the conundrum of PCPs as actors embedded in their institutional field. Fields tend toward isomorphism as a result of coercive, mimetic, and normative pressures (DiMaggio and Powell 1983). The ACA has emerged as one such coercive pressure that is leading the practices of PCPs toward convergence. The ways in which fields can be exposed to conflicting institutional demands have already been documented (Pache and Santos 2010). In this sense, PCPs have always been forced to balance between market demands associated with profitability and care demands associated with the Hippocratic Oath and serving the best interests of their patients (e.g., Dunn and Jones 2010).

Yet in its current form, the ACA appears to have tipped the balance where the market logic has become more important. Nonetheless, the institutional work perspective recognizes that actors are knowledgeable, reflexive agents who can find ways to balance and integrate competing institutional demands and pressures (Creed, DeJordy, and Lok 2010; Smets, Jarzabkowski, Burke, and Spee 2015). Moving forward, it will be interesting to examine the different types of micro-processes in which PCPs engage to try to restore the balance between the institutional demands associated with profit and care, in addition to whether those micro-processes result in institutional maintenance or change.

CONCLUSION

Applying the tenets of ownership theory and the principal–agent problem, we have articulated how the managed care model may have negatively impacted the quality of primary care in the U.S. health care system. Managed care organizations limit physician autonomy and information, while also de-prioritizing physicians' investment in the care of patients—thereby blocking the routes of PCPs to ownership of patient care, while also severing physicians' roots of psychological ownership. Although the ACA has shifted primary care incentives from serviced-based to outcomes-based compensation, the act's reliance on the managed care model limits its potential for improving the quality of primary care in the United States. Despite this weakness in the act, the ACA also contains a number of innovative provisions that, if further developed and expanded, could revolutionize the way in which primary care is conducted in the U.S. health care system.

One such provision is the ACA's authorization of health marketplace plans that bundle direct primary care fees with high-deductible insurance required for treatment received at hospitals. Direct primary care is especially attractive to PCPs because it removes the constraints of managed care from primary care interventions, restoring autonomy and information to the physician, facilitating the physician's self-investment into care for each individual patient. While direct primary care has been successful in a number of states over the past decade, further research is required to assess the effectiveness of direct primary care in producing high-quality primary care at a sustainable cost to consumers and physicians alike.

REFERENCES

Ancane, G., B. Palmowski, and A. Ancans. 2015. "Lost in Translation? The Doctor–Patient Relationship Revisited." *World Medical Journal* 61, no. 1: 28–30.

Anderson, G. F., K. Davis, and S. Guterman. 2015. "Medicare Payment Reform: Aligning Incentives for Better Care." Issue brief. New York, NY: Commonwealth Fund.

Arnold, L., and D. T. Stern. 2006. "What Is Medical Professionalism?" In *Measuring Medical Professionalism*, edited by D. T. Stern, 15–37. New York, NY: Oxford University Press.

Avey, J. B., B. J. Avolio, C. D. Crossley, and F. Luthans. 2009. "Psychological Ownership: Theoretical Extensions, Measurement and Relation to Work Outcomes." *Journal of Organizational Behavior* 30, no. 2: 173–91. doi:10.1002/job.583.

Bakan, I., Y. Suseno, A. Pinnington, and A. Money. 2004. "The Influence of Financial Participation and Participation in Decision-Making on Employee Job Attitudes." *International Journal of Human Resource Management* 15, no. 3: 587–616. doi:10.1 080/09585192.2004.10057654.

Baker, L. C. 1997. "The Effect of HMOs on Fee-for-Service Health Care Expenditures: Evidence from Medicare." *Journal of Health Economics* 16, no. 4: 453–81. doi:10.1016/ s0167-6296(96)00535-8.

Bartol, K. M., E. A. Locke, S. L. Rynes, and B. Gerhart. 2000. "Incentives and Motivation." In *Compensation in Organizations: Current Research and Practice*, edited by S. L. Rynes and B. Gerhart, 104–47. San Francisco, CA: Jossey-Bass.

Benartzi, S., R. H. Thaler, S. P. Utkus, and C. R. Sunstein. 2007. "Company Stock, Market Rationality, and Legal Reform." *Journal of Law and Economics*, 50, no. 1: 45–79.

Bendix, J. 2013. "Can the Doctor–Patient Relationship Survive?" *Medical Economics* 90, no. 23: 12–23.

Blumenthal, D., M. Abrams, and R. Nuzum. 2015. "The Affordable Care Act at 5 Years." *New England Journal of Medicine* 372, no. 25: 2451–458. doi:10.1056/ NEJMhpr1503614.

Brennan, T. A., D. J. Rothman, L. Blank, D. Blumenthal, S. C. Chimonas, J. J. Cohen, J. Goldman. 2006. "Health Industry Practices That Create Conflicts of Interest." *Journal of the American Medical Association* 295, no. 4: 429–33. doi:10.1001/ jama.295.4.429.

Briscoe, F. 2007. "From Iron Cage to Iron Shield? How Bureaucracy Enables Temporal Flexibility for Professional Service Workers." *Organization Science* 18, no. 2: 297–314. doi:10.1287/orsc.1060.0226.

Burdi, M. D., and L. C. Baker. 1999. "Physicians' Perceptions of Autonomy and Satisfaction in California." *Health Affairs* 18, no. 4: 134-45. doi:10.1377/hlthaff.18.4.134.

Calman, N. S., M. Golub, and S. Shuman. 2012. "Primary Care and Health Reform." *Mount Sinai Journal of Medicine: A Journal of Translational and Personalized Medicine* 79, no. 5: 527–34. doi:10.1002/msj.21335.

Carlson, R. P. 2015. "Direct Primary Care Practice Model Drops Insurance and Gains Providers and Consumers." *Physician Leadership Journal* 2, no. 2: 20–26.

Chi, N.-W., and T.-S. Han. 2008. "Exploring the Linkages between Formal Ownership and Psychological Ownership for the Organization: The Mediating Role of Organizational Justice." *Journal of Occupational and Organizational Psychology* 81, no. 4: 691–711. doi:10.1348/096317907x262314.

Claxton, G., M. Rae, M. Long, N. Panchal, A. Damico, K. Kenward, and H. Whitmore. 2015 (Sep. 22). "2015 Employer Health Benefits Survey." http://kaiserf.am/2cHLoCv.

Cottini, E., and C. Lucifora. 2013. "Mental Health and Working Conditions in Europe." *Industrial and Labor Relations Review* 66, no. 4: 958–88. doi:10.1177/001979391306600409.

Creed, W. E. D., R. DeJordy, and J. Lok. 2010. "Being the Change: Resolving Institutional Contradiction through Identity Work." *Academy of Management Journal* 53, no. 6: 1336–64. doi:10.5465/amj.2010.57318357.

Davis, K., M. Abrams, and K. Stremikis. 2011. "How the Affordable Care Act Will Strengthen the Nation's Primary Care Foundation." *Journal of General Internal Medicine* 26, no. 10: 1201–203. doi:10.1007/s11606-011-1720-y.

Dawkins, S., A. W. Tian, A. Newman, and A. Martin. 2015. "Psychological Ownership: A Review and Research Agenda." *Journal of Organizational Behavior* (e-pub). doi:10.1002/job.2057.

Deom, M., T. Agoritsas, P. A. Bovier, and T. V. Perneger. 2010. "What Doctors Think About the Impact of Managed Care Tools on Quality of Care, Costs, Autonomy, and Relations with Patients." *BMC Health Services Research* 10, no. 1: 331. doi:10.1186/1472-6963-10-331.

Dewey, C. 2015. "Direct-Pay Medicine Presents Alternative Health Care Model." *Grand Rapids Business Journal* 33, no. 9: 11.

Dharamsi, S., A. Ho, S. M. Spadafora, and R. Woollard. 2011. "The Physician as Health Advocate: Translating the Quest for Social Responsibility into Medical Education and Practice." *Academic Medicine* 86, no. 9: 1108–13. doi:10.1097/acm.0b013e318226b43b.

DiMaggio, P. J., and W. W. Powell. 1983. "The Iron Cage Revisited: Institutional Isomorphism and Collective Rationality in Organizational Fields." *American Sociological Review* 48, no. 2: 147. doi:10.2307/2095101.

Dranove, D. 2000. *The Economic Evolution of American Health Care: From Marcus Welby to Managed Care.* Princeton, NJ: Princeton University Press.

Dranove, D., C. Forman, A. Goldfarb, and S. Greenstein. 2012. *The Trillion Dollar Conundrum: Complementarities and Health Information Technology.* NBER working paper. Cambridge, MA: National Bureau of Economic Research. http://www.nber.org/papers/w18281.

Dukerich, J. M., B. R. Golden, and S. M. Shortell. 2002. "Beauty Is in the Eye of the Beholder: The Impact of Organizational Identification, Identity, and Image on the Cooperative Behaviors of Physicians." *Administrative Science Quarterly* 47, no. 3: 507. doi:10.2307/3094849.

Dunford, B. B., D. J. Schleicher, and L. Zhu. 2009. "The Relative Importance of Psychological versus Pecuniary Approaches to Establishing an Ownership Culture." *Advances in Industrial and Labor Relations* 16: 1–21. doi:10.1108/s0742-6186(2009)0000016004.

Dunn, M. B., and C. Jones. 2010. "Institutional Logics and Institutional Pluralism: The Contestation of Care and Science Logics in Medical Education, 1967–2005." *Administrative Science Quarterly* 55, no. 1: 114–49. doi:10.2189/asqu.2010.55.1.114.

Dworkin, R. W. 2000. "The Cultural Revolution in Health Care." *The Public Interest* 139: 35–49.

Eisenhardt, K. M. 1989. "Agency Theory: An Assessment and Review." *The Academy of Management Review* 14, no. 1: 57–74. doi:10.2307/258191.

Garcia, R., M. G. Lima, M. Gorender, and R. Badaró. 2005. "The Importance of the Doctor–Patient Relationship in Adherence to HIV/AIDS Treatment: A Case Report." *Brazilian Journal of Infectious Diseases* 9, no. 3: 251–56. doi:10.1590/s1413-86702005000300008.

Golden, A. G., J. Ortiz, and T. T. Wan. 2013. "Transitional Care: Looking for the Right Shoes to Fit Older Adult Patients." *Care Management Journal* 14, no. 2: 78–83. doi:10.1891/1521-0987.14.2.78.

Gray, V., D. Lowery, and J. K. Benz. 2013. *Interest Groups and Health Care Reform Across the United States*. Washington, DC: Georgetown University Press.

Grumbach, K., D. Keane, and A. Bindman. 1993. "Primary Care and Public Emergency Department Overcrowding." *American Journal of Public Health* 83, no. 3: 372–78. doi:10.2105/ajph.83.3.372.

Hackman, J. R., and G. R. Oldham. 1976. "Motivation through the Design of Work: Test of a Theory." *Organizational Behavior and Human Performance* 16, no. 2: 250–79. doi:10.1016/0030-5073(76)90016-7.

Hall, B. J., and J. B. Liebman. 1998. "Are CEOs Really Paid Like Bureaucrats?" *Quarterly Journal of Economics* 113, no. 3: 653–91. doi:10.1162/003355398555702.

Hall, B. J., and K. J. Murphy. 2002. "Stock Options for Undiversified Executives." *Journal of Accounting and Economics* 33, no. 1: 3–42. doi:10.1016/s0165-4101(01)00050-7.

Hall, M. A., and R. Lord. 2014 (Oct. 22). "Obamacare: What the Affordable Care Act Means for Patients and Physicians." *British Medical Journal* 349: G5376. doi:10.1136/bmj.g5376.

Hoff, T. 2011. "Deskilling and Adaptation Among Primary Care Physicians Using Two Work Innovations." *Health Care Management Review* 36, no. 4: 338–48. doi:10.1097/hmr.0b013e31821826a1.

Huberfeld, N. 2015. "The Supreme Court Ruling That Blocked Providers from Seeking Higher Medicaid Payments Also Undercut the Entire Program." *Health Affairs* 34, no. 7: 1156–1161. doi:10.1377/hlthaff.2015.0138.

Huff, C. 2015. "Direct Primary Care: Concierge Care for the Masses." *Health Affairs* 34, no. 12: 2016–19. doi:10.1377/hlthaff.2015.1281.

Iglehart, J. K. 1994. "The Struggle Between Managed Care and Fee-for-Service Practice." *New England Journal of Medicine*, 331: 63–67. doi:10.1056/nejm199407073310129.

Jensen, M. C., and W. H. Meckling. 1976. "Theory of the Firm: Managerial Behavior, Agency Costs and Ownership Structure." *Journal of Financial Economics* 3, no. 4: 305–60. doi:10.1016/0304-405x(76)90026-x.

Karasek, R. A. 1979. "Job Demands, Job Decision Latitude, and Mental Strain: Implications for Job Redesign." *Administrative Science Quarterly* 24, no. 2: 285. doi:10.2307/2392498.

Katz, J. 2002. *The Silent World of Doctor and Patient.* Baltimore, MD: Johns Hopkins University.

Kaushal, N., and R. J. Kaestner. 2015. "Are Foreign-Trained Nurses Perfect Substitutes for U.S.-Trained Nurses?" *Industrial and Labor Relations Review* 68, no. 5: 1102–125. doi:10.1177/0019793915592624.

Khushf, G., and R. Gifford. 1998. "'Understanding, Assessing, and Managing Conflicts of Interest. Surgical Ethics." In *Surgical Ethics*, edited by L. B. McCullough, J. W. Jones, and B. A. Brody, 342–66. New York: Oxford University Press.

Klein, K. J. 1987. "Employee Stock Ownership and Employee Attitudes: A Test of Three Models." *Journal of Applied Psychology* 72, no. 2: 319–32. doi:10.1037/0021-9010.72.2.319.

Kocher, R., E. J. Emanuel, and N. M. DeParle. 2010. "The Affordable Care Act and the Future of Clinical Medicine: The Opportunities and Challenges." *Annals of Internal Medicine* 153, no. 8: 536. doi:10.7326/0003-4819-153-8-201010190-00274.

Koh, H. K., and K. G. Sebelius. 2010. "Promoting Prevention Through the Affordable Care Act." *New England Journal of Medicine* 363, no. 14: 1296–99. doi:10.1056/nejmp1008560.

Lasagna, L. 1995. "Modern Hippocratic Oath." *Medical Economics* 72, no. 11: 202.

Lathrop, B., and D. R. Hodnicki. 2014. "The Affordable Care Act: Primary Care and the Doctor of Nursing Practice Nurse." *Online Journal of Issues in Nursing* 19, no. 2. doi:10.3912/OJIN.Vol198No02PPT02.

Lincoff, N. 2015 (Jun. 30). "The Future of Healthcare Could Be in Concierge Medicine." *Healthlines RSS News.* http://bit.ly/2cnwyo5.

Luquis, R. R., and H. L. Paz. 2015. "Attitudes About and Practices of Health Promotion and Prevention Among Primary Care Providers." *Health Promotion Practice* 16, no. 5: 745–55. doi:10.1177/1524839914561516.

Majette, G. R. 2009. "From Concierge Medicine to Patient-Centered Medical Homes: International Lessons and the Search for a Better Way to Deliver Primary Health Care in the U.S." *American Journal of Law and Medicine* 35, no. 4: 585–619.

Marcotte, L., C. Moriates, and A. Milstein. 2014. "Professional Organizations' Role in Supporting Physicians to Improve Value in Health Care." *Journal of the American Medical Association* 312, no. 3: 231. doi:10.1001/jama.2014.6762.

McKinlay, J., and L. Marceau. 2008. "When There Is No Doctor: Reasons for the Disappearance of Primary Care Physicians in the US During the Early 21st Century." *Social Science and Medicine* 67, no. 10: 1481–491. doi:10.1016/j.socscimed.2008.06.034.

McKinlay, J. B., and J. D. Stoeckle. 1988. "Corporatization and the Social Transformation of Doctoring." *International Journal of Health Services* 18, no. 2: 191–205. doi: 10.2190/YEVW-6C44-YCYE-CGEU.

McMurray, J. E. 1998. "Heartsick." *Annals of Internal Medicine* 129, no. 10: 838. doi:10.7326/0003-4819-129-10-199811150-00024.

Mechanic, D. 2000. "Managed Care and the Imperative for a New Professional Ethic." *Health Affairs* 19, no. 5: 100–11. doi:10.1377/hlthaff.19.5.100.

Miller, P., and T. Hudson-Thrall. 2010. *Health Reform and the Decline of Physician Private Practice: A White Paper Examining the Effects of the Patient Protection and Affordable Care Act on Physician Practices in the United States.* White paper. 2010. http://bit.ly/28O728x.

Osterman, P. 2013. "Introduction to the Special Issue on Job Quality: What Does It Mean and How Might We Think About It?" *Industrial and Labor Relations Review* 66, no. 4: 739–52. doi:10.1177/001979391306600401.

Pache, A. C., and F. Santos. 2010. "When Worlds Collide: The Internal Dynamics of Organizational Responses to Conflicting Institutional Demands." *Academy of Management Review* 35, no. 3: 455–76. doi:10.5465/amr.2010.51142368.

Petersen, L. A., L. D. Woodard, T. Urech, C. Daw, and S. Sookanan. 2006. "Does Pay-for-Performance Improve the Quality of Health Care?" *Annals of Internal Medicine* 145, no. 4: 265–72. doi:10.7326/0003-4819-145-4-200608150-00006.

Pierce, J. L., T. Kostova, and K. T. Dirks. 2001. "Toward a Theory of Psychological Ownership in Organizations." *Academy of Management Review* 26, no. 2: 298–310. doi:10.5465/amr.2001.4378028.

Pierce, J. L., T. Kostova, and K. T. Dirks. 2003. "The State of Psychological Ownership: Integrating and Extending a Century of Research." *Review of General Psychology* 7, no. 1: 84–107. doi:10.1037/1089-2680.7.1.84.

Pontes, M. C. 1995. "Agency Theory: A Framework for Analyzing Physician Services." *Health Care Management Review* 20, no. 4: 57–67. doi:10.1097/00004010-199502040-00010.

Pooley, H. M., J. Highfield, and A. Neal. 2015. "The Experience of the Long-Term Doctor–Patient Relationship in Consultant Nephrologists." *Journal of Renal Care*, 41, no. 2: 88–95. doi: 10.1111/jorc.12092.

Ransom, S. B., S. G. McNeeley, M. L. Kruger, G. Root, and D. B. Cotton. 1996. "The Effect of Capitated and Fee-for-Service Remuneration on Physician Decision Making in Gynecology." *Obstetrics and Gynecology* 87, no. 5, part 1: 707–10.

Rosen, C., J. Case, and M. Staubus. 2005. "Every Employee an Owner. Really." *Harvard Business Review* 83, no. 6: 122–30.

Rosen, C., and M. Quarrey. 1987. "How Well Is Employee Ownership Working?" *Harvard Business Review* 65, no. 5: 126–32.

Rosenthal, M. B., R. G. Frank, Z. Li, and A. M. Epstein. 2005. "Early Experience with Pay-for-Performance: From Concept to Practice." *Journal of the American Medical Association* 294, no. 14: 1788–93. doi:10.1001/jama.294.14.1788.

Rosenthal, M. B. 2008. "Beyond Pay for Performance—Emerging Models of Provider-Payment Reform." *New England Journal of Medicine* 359, no. 12: 1197–1200. doi:10.1056/nejmp0804658.

Rousseau, D. M., and Z. Shperling. 2003. "Pieces of the Action: Ownership and the Changing Employment Relationship." *Academy of Management Review* 28, no. 4: 553–70. doi:10.5465/amr.2003.10899368.

Safran, D. G., A. R. Tarlov, and W. H. Rogers. 1994. "Primary Care Performance in Fee-for-Service and Prepaid Health Care Systems. Results from the Medical Outcomes Study." *Journal of the American Medical Association* 271, no. 20: 1579–86. doi:10.1001/jama.271.20.1579.

Schwartz, M. D. 2012. "The US Primary Care Workforce and Graduate Medical Education Policy." *Journal of the American Medical Association* 308, no. 2: 2252. doi:10.1001/jama.2012.77034.

Silver, G. 1997. "Editorial: The Road from Managed Care." *American Journal of Public Health* 87, no. 1: 8–9. doi:10.2105/ajph.87.1.8.

Simon, S. R., R. J. D. Pan, A. M. Sullivan, N. Clark-Chiarelli, M. T. Connelly, A. S. Peters, J. D. Singer, T. S. Inui, and S. D. Block. 1999. "Views of Managed Care—A Survey of Students, Residents, Faculty, and Deans at Medical Schools in the United States." *New England Journal of Medicine* 340, no. 12: 928–36. doi:10.1056/nejm199903253401206.

Smets, M., P. Jarzabkowski, G. T. Burke, and P. Spee. 2015. "Reinsurance Trading in Lloyd's of London: Balancing Conflicting-Yet-Complementary Logics in Practice." *Academy of Management Journal* 58, no. 3: 932–70.

Smith, P. C., A. Stepan, V. Valdmanis, and P. Verheyen. 1997. "Principal–Agent Problems in Health Care Systems: An International Perspective." *Health Policy* 41, no. 1: 37–60. doi:10.1016/s0168-8510(97)00012-2.

Stavropoulou, C. 2011. "Non-Adherence to Medication and Doctor–Patient Relationship: Evidence from a European Survey." *Patient Education and Counseling* 83, no. 1: 7–13. doi:10.1016/j.pec.2010.04.039.

Stoddard, J. J., J. L. Hargraves, M. Reed, and A. Vratil. 2001. "Managed Care, Professional Autonomy, and Income. Effects on Physician Career Satisfaction." *Journal of General Internal Medicine* 16, no. 10: 675–84. doi:10.1046/j.1525-1497.2001.01206.x.

Swann, W. B., B. W. Pelham, and D. S. Krull. 1989. "Agreeable Fancy or Disagreeable Truth? Reconciling Self-Enhancement and Self-Verification." *Journal of Personality and Social Psychology* 57, no. 5: 782–91. doi:10.1037/0022-3514.57.5.782.

Tajfel, H., and J. C. Turner. 1985. "The Social Identity Theory of Intergroup Behavior." In *Psychology of Intergroup Relations* (2nd edition), edited by S. Worchel and W. G. Austin, 7–24. Chicago: Nelson-Hall.

Tarrant, C., M. Dixon-Woods, A. M. Colman, and T. Stokes. 2010. "Continuity and Trust in Primary Care: A Qualitative Study Informed by Game Theory." *The Annals of Family Medicine* 8, no. 5: 440–46. doi:10.1370/afm.1160.

Thompson, D. F. 1993. "Understanding Financial Conflicts of Interest." *New England Journal of Medicine* 329, no. 8: 573–76. doi:10.1056/nejm199308193290812.

Tozzi, J. 2014. "The Doctor Is Out of Network." *Business Week* 4372: 39.

U.S. Department of Health and Human Services, Health Resources and Services Administration. 2013. "Projecting the Supply and Demand for Primary Care Practitioners Through 2020." Bureau of Health Professions. http://1.usa.gov/28NvUs8.

Van Dyne, L., and J. L. Pierce. 2004. "Psychological Ownership and Feelings of Possession: Three Field Studies Predicting Employee Attitudes and Organizational Citizenship Behavior." *Journal of Organizational Behavior* 25, no. 4: 439–59. doi:10.1002/job.249.

Chapter 2

New Models of Care and Workforce Change in the NHS in England

Stephen Bach
School of Management
King's College London

INTRODUCTION

Delivering high-quality health care in a context in which resources are growing more slowly than at any other time in the history of the United Kingdom's National Health Service (NHS) is a daunting challenge facing policy makers and health care professions in the NHS (NHS England 2014). Many of the issues confronting the health system are similar to those in other advanced economies (Carter 2016; NHS England 2014):

- the growth of an aging population, often presenting with multiple health conditions
- the escalating cost of health care, especially hospital care
- the legacy of the economic crisis that has prompted successive governments to shrink the state and curtail the rate of growth of health care expenditure
- a jaded workforce that is under intense strain, exacerbating recruitment and retention problems
- an increasingly vocal clientele that is more questioning of the service delivered

These difficulties confront many health care systems in advanced countries, but they are shaped by the specific political and institutional context of health care provision in England. Health care remains dominated by the publicly funded NHS, which offers universal coverage and health care but not social care—and is delivered free at the point of use. In 2013, UK expenditure on health care comprised 8.5% of GDP, which was below the Organisation for Economic Co-operation and Development average of 8.9%. Public expenditure, mainly on the NHS, accounted for 83% of expenditure (Organisation for Economic Co-operation and Development 2015b).

The NHS is predominantly financed from general taxation, and its budget is allocated by Parliament and channeled through the Department of Health. The largest component of the NHS budget is transferred to NHS England, which delivers its mandate for the Department of Health. The secretary of state for health has the ultimate responsibility for the management of the health system and is accountable to Parliament.

This centralized system of financing and accountability results in NHS policy being influenced strongly by shifting government political priorities and makes NHS budgets especially susceptible to the overall state of the economy. The secretary of state of health has a legal responsibility to provide a comprehensive health care system, and the NHS constitution formalizes what patients can expect from the NHS. These services are not defined in great detail and relate to matters such as receiving care without discrimination, standards of service required (e.g., maximum waiting times), and access to drugs that have been approved by the National Institute of Clinical Excellence (NICE).

Primary health care is delivered mainly through neighborhood-based general practitioners who act as gatekeepers to secondary care. Hospital care is dominated by public hospitals that are organized either as public hospitals, directly accountable to the Department of Health, or as foundation trusts. Foundation trusts are public benefit corporations with a board of governors and members drawn from the constituencies they serve. They have enhanced financial and operational autonomy, with scope to borrow commercially; the ability to generate a surplus to be reinvested in services; and additional pay flexibilities. Two thirds of secondary care providers in the acute sector have gained foundation trust status but fewer mental health, community, and ambulance trusts have done so.

Monitor, the economic regulating agency, now oversees all providers (previously it regulated foundation trusts only), and it works alongside the quality and safety regulator, the Care Quality Commission. All hospitals contract with local authorities who commission the majority of NHS services, with trusts reimbursed by nationally determined diagnosis-related group rates.

By 2016, the NHS confronted a critical moment in its evolution because, in addition to being ranked as the best value and most effective health care system compared with systems in other leading industrial countries (Davis, Stremikis, Squires, and Schoen 2014) and having overwhelming public support for a tax-funded and comprehensive NHS (Gerschlick, Charlesworth, and Taylor 2015), a sense of uncertainty was emerging about its future shape and sustainability in a prolonged period of austerity. These doubts related mainly to funding, but they also reflected some unease about quality and outcomes following highly critical reports about care quality, patient safety, and unacceptable variations in standards (Francis 2013; National Advisory Group on the Safety of Patients in England 2013). A deteriorating recruitment and retention position, especially in relation to nursing staff, reinforced these trends (NHS Employers 2015; Royal College of Nursing 2015a).

The basic conundrum faced by the NHS is that a sickness service designed in 1948 and centered on acute hospital provision has not evolved sufficiently to address the complex and changing health and social needs of the population. These difficulties have encouraged a focus on system change and the use of "vanguards" to pilot new models of care delivery (Dalton 2014; NHS England 2014, 2015). There has been more engagement with NHS decision makers, which contrasts with previous NHS reorganizations that were formulated by the government in office with little prior consultation with key NHS stakeholders (Timmins 2012).

The main elements of the ambition to achieve system transformation coalesce around an emphasis on service integration and on building services around the end user, accompanied by new models of care, an enhanced role for community provision, and early intervention to keep people healthy and out of hospital. The government also envisages a shift from a centralized health care system, directed and monitored from the center of government (but accompanied in practice by fragmentation and substantial variation in local practice) toward more devolved but locally cohesive systems of care. Policy documents are replete with the language of transformation and innovation, and this reflects a heightened sense of urgency that far-reaching changes in models of care are required to ensure the sustainability of the NHS (NHS England 2014, 2015).

New models of care have major implications for professional roles and ways of working, but limited attention has been directed at these consequences. Altering organizational models and working practices within a health care system under sustained financial and service pressure is difficult. NHS trust finance directors cite staff morale as the aspect of organizational performance that gives them most cause for concern, ahead of delayed transfers of care and waiting time targets (King's Fund 2015).

This chapter outlines the NHS model of care; how it has been restructured; and the evolving financial, organizational, and workforce challenges it confronts. Marketization has contributed to the fragmentation of the health care system, and policy has become centered on increased integration and the development of new models of care. Attempts at system transformation have major implications for the workforce and have encouraged new ways of working and the development of new roles. The consequences of these developments and the barriers to workforce and system change are assessed in this chapter.

The Conservative government is committed to reducing public expenditure as a share of national income and has implemented far-reaching austerity measures. The case of health care restructuring in England therefore illustrates the extent to which budgetary restrictions and austerity measures facilitate or hinder system change.

THE NHS UNDER PRESSURE: RESTRUCTURING AND SYSTEM FRAGMENTATION

The NHS confronts four main challenges that shape the government's transformation agenda: system fragmentation in a more diverse health care landscape, patient safety, funding, and workforce capacity and engagement.

Structural Reform

The NHS has shifted from an integrated to a more fragmented system over recent decades. Although an emphasis on joined-up (i.e., integrated) services has been a feature of health policy for many decades, it is only recently that integration has become *the* priority of policy makers. From the 1980s onward, NHS reforms led to disaggregation and disintegration as the precepts of the new public management emphasized the separation of "steering" from "rowing" and the establishment of more-autonomous providers—because a hierarchically integrated NHS was viewed as over-centralized and unresponsive to local needs (Ferlie, Pettigrew, Ashburn, and Fitzgerald 1996; Osborne and Gaebler 1992).

In the 1980s, general managers were introduced, and they transitioned into CEO roles, increasing in importance with the establishment of the internal market in the 1990s. The division between purchasers and providers was intended to inject an element of competition into the health care system by enabling purchasers to commission health care services from NHS trusts but also from private providers. As NHS trusts developed, they tended to coalesce around the main areas of service provision, with acute hospital trusts being the most numerous and other services organized into separate mental health, community, and ambulance trusts.

Over recent decades there has been an incremental but accelerating involvement of the private sector in delivering nonclinical and increasingly clinical (nonemergency) services (Givan and Bach 2007; NHS Support Federation 2016). Under the Labour government, the share of expenditure devoted to health increased from 6.6% of GDP to 9.6% of GDP, staff shortages were addressed, waiting times were reduced, and hospital infrastructure was modernized. A period of Conservative-led coalition government between 2010 and 2015 was accompanied by austerity measures and an ill-conceived and controversial reorganization of the NHS. Public satisfaction with the NHS tracked this policy evolution. In 2010, the British social attitudes survey reported 70% satisfaction with the NHS (it was 39% in 2001), but it declined to 60% overall satisfaction by 2015 (Appleby and Robertson 2016).

The coalition government's 2012 Health and Social Care Act proved very contentious because it strengthened competitive requirements by mandating that clinical commissioning groups (CCGs) use competitive tendering for clinical services based on a national tariff. In contrast to previous attempts at marketization, the 2012 act provided the NHS regulator, Monitor, with powers to investigate and remedy anti-competitive behavior, encouraging further growth in private and voluntary sector providers (Pownall 2013; Tailby 2012). Long-standing divisions between primary and secondary care and within secondary care were reinforced by the increase in foundation trusts, the opening up of the NHS to a range of providers, and the establishment of a large number (more than 200) of new and relatively small commissioning authorities.

The 2012 act removed strategic direction of the health care system below the national level by abolishing strategic health authorities, thereby inhibiting change in local health economies (Glennerster 2015: 301). Foundation trusts contributed to the fragmentation of the health system and encouraged a "silo mentality" because trusts are preoccupied with their independence, generating financial incentives to maintain hospital activity levels.

Competition rules make hospital and service reorganization more difficult; there have been referrals to the competition authorities about the awarding of contracts and with respect to trust mergers—a necessary corollary of system integration. The former NHS chief executive expressed his frustration and suggested that the competition law might need to be amended to enable system change (Health Committee 2014: 37–38). Moreover, providers have to deal with many CCGs that have differing reporting requirements and expectations, and these relationships are often low trust and adversarial.

A major challenge, therefore, is that within an ostensibly highly centralized health system, there has been an absence of system leadership to bring about more integrated and patient-centered services (Ham et al. 2015: 38; Timmins 2015). General practitioners (GPs) provide an important source of coordination and prevent multiple patient-initiated visits to different specialists. However, as independent, self-employed practitioners, GPs have sometimes proved reluctant to participate fully in plans to integrate care.

Patient Safety

In addition to system fragmentation, a second major challenge relates to patient safety and has been center stage since the discovery of appalling standards of care at Mid Staffordshire NHS Foundation Trust that contributed to an unknown number of avoidable deaths at Stafford General Hospital. This scandal and other subsequent cases raised many difficult questions about the capacity of the NHS to oversee and deliver safe and high-quality care; about the efficacy of existing managerial, professional, and regulatory systems; and about the effective recruitment and training of staff (Department of Health 2012, 2015).

Between 2005 and 2008, the abysmal standards at Stafford General Hospital, a small district general hospital, contributed to much patient suffering. The first inquiry (Francis 2010) examined care at the hospital and gathered testimony from more than 900 patients and their families. It detailed a litany of failures in basic care that included inadequate and delayed pain relief that resulted in many elderly patients crying out for pain relief; inadequate provision of food and water, leaving patients severely dehydrated and without proper nutrition; and poor standards of hygiene, exacerbated by the failure to take patients to the toilet in a timely manner and by forcing patients to remove used bandages and dressings from public areas.

These failures were attributed to a chronic shortage of staff and an inappropriate mix of staff, including inadequate provision of senior (consultant) medical staff; inadequate training and supervision of staff; failure to take patient complaints seriously; and a bullying culture in which staff were fearful of blowing the whistle. These shortcomings stemmed from a managerial culture in which achieving NHS targets was the dominant concern, and it led to junior doctors leaving seriously ill patients to treat minor cases that might breach the government's maximum four-hour wait in casualty. Underpinning this behavior was the trust board and its senior managers' preoccupation with obtaining foundation trust status.

A subsequent public inquiry produced a 1,700-page report and 290 recommendations that built on the first report and pointed to wider failings in the NHS (Francis 2013). It led to an apology by the prime minister in the House of Commons, as well as wide-ranging deliberation about the specific failings at Stafford Hospital, systemic failings in the regulatory and supervisory system, and broader aspects of staff management, including the training and values of support staff (Cavendish 2013). Robert Francis, who led the inquiry, noted that the inquiry team heard about "unhealthy cultures, poor leadership and an acceptance of poor standards" in other settings and concluded that "Stafford was not an event of such rarity or improbability that it would be safe to assume that it has not been and will not be repeated" (Francis 2013: 25).

The 2013 report identified a series of interlinked areas for action. These areas included the need for a system of fundamental standards that provide clarity on what patients can expect and make it easy for patients and staff to identify when these standards are breached. Francis emphasized the importance of an open and transparent culture in which staff and patient concerns are taken seriously rather than ignored or repressed and that ensure that whistleblowing policies can actually be used (Francis 2013).

A number of changes are being implemented to enhance openness, governance, and accountability. There has been a complete overhaul of provider inspection regimes, directors have to demonstrate that they meet a "fit and proper person test," and a new duty of candor has been introduced for all staff. Much more attention is being directed at the appropriate training and mix of staff required in a changing health system.

Despite important measures to alter organizational practice, responses in the NHS staff survey indicate that staff remain equivocal about their ability to report incidents. In response to the question, "My organisation encourages us to report errors, near misses or incidents," 27% of respondents agreed and 2% strongly agreed, with most responses being neutral (NHS England 2016: question 12b).

These attempts to shift organizational policy and practice are occurring in a context in which the NHS is under renewed pressure to curb expenditure and accommodate increased demand.

NHS Expenditure

A major preoccupation relates to funding and the squeeze on resources faced by the NHS in the aftermath of the economic crisis. Since 2010, successive governments have drawn on the crisis to implement austerity policies as part of a larger ambition to reduce the scope and scale of the state (Bach 2016; Grimshaw and Rubery 2012). The government plans to reduce the share of public expenditure from 40% of national income in 2008–09 to around 36% and eliminate the deficit by 2019–20. This would constitute the lowest level of public spending for 60 years (excluding 1999 through 2001) (Institute of Fiscal Studies 2016).

The NHS has been identified as a relative government priority, but increases in funding of around 3.8% in real terms per annum since 1948 were replaced by around 1% real growth between 2010 and 2015. In the *Five Year Forward View*, NHS chief executive Simon Stevens projected a £30 billion funding gap by 2020–21 (NHS England 2014). The NHS is required to generate annual efficiencies of 2% to 3%, in addition to recent cost reduction programs. During 2015–16, the financial performance of NHS providers declined sharply. The year-end deficit of £2.45 billion, the biggest overspend in its history, is almost three times greater than in 2014–15, with most trusts posting a deficit. The deficit stemmed from rising levels of emergency admissions that translated into a high use of agency and contract staff, delays in transfers of care, and financial sanctions for missing targets (NHS Improvement 2016).

One response is to reduce variations in practice with large differences in cost and performance in relation to the price paid by trusts for hip prosthesis and pathology tests, the stocks of medicines held, and aspects of estate management. Although variations in performance must take account of case mix, it has been concluded that significant unwarranted variations in resource utilization continue to exist (Carter 2016).

Moving beyond incremental change in quality and efficiency toward service redesign is therefore integral to developing sustainable plans for NHS providers (Dalton 2014; Health Committee 2014).

Staff Engagement and Workforce Shortages

Attempts to transform health care are underpinned by the efforts of the workforce, but the NHS confronts recruitment and retention difficulties among clinical staff and uneven levels of staff engagement. For health care providers, around half of their costs are accounted for by the employment of clinical staff. The NHS employs 1.2 million staff in England (excluding primary care staff) of which 824,000 full-time equivalents are clinical staff, including 141,000 doctors and 329,000 nurses, health visitors, and midwives. NHS clinical staffing has been increasing in recent years by an average of 1.4% per year between 2004 and 2014, with variations between staff groups. This upturn in clinical staffing reflects both increased demand and managerial responses to the Francis report (2013), which focused on increased employment of registered nurses. This goal has not been easy to accomplish because nurse training programs have declined by 19% over the past decade.

There is a disconnect between the current trajectory of the health and social care systems and the workforce in place to service those needs (Addicott, Maquire, Honeyman, and Jabbal 2015). These difficulties are exacerbated by the shortcomings of workforce planning in the NHS. There is a degree of ambiguity about who is responsible for planning the future workforce, and the plans of NHS trusts are shaped as much by affordability concerns as by service needs (National Audit Office 2016).

The NHS confronts recruitment and retention difficulties and as the Carter report observed:

> We were struck by the extraordinary commitment and loyalty NHS staff have to their occupations and the service overall. They have high resilience but we have observed they are feeling jaded from the constant pressure to do more with less and the relentless scrutiny of their performance. Coupled with

this, their pay has remained relatively flat for some time and is set to do so for the foreseeable future. (2016: 18)

The NHS staff survey is undertaken annually in England, and 299,000 staff employed by the NHS in 2015 responded, with variations in scores between trust types and staff group. The overall staff engagement score is based on staff members' perceived ability to contribute to improvements at work, their willingness to recommend the organization as a place to work or receive treatment, and the extent to which they feel motivated and engaged with their work. The NHS engagement score has been improving slightly, from 3.68 out of 5 (2012) to 3.74 (2013) to 3.76 (2014) to 3.78 (2015) (NHS England 2016), and more than half of staff reported that they often or always look forward to going to work. These encouraging signs, however, sat alongside almost half of staff disagreeing or disagreeing strongly with the statement: "There are enough staff at this organisation for me to do my job properly" (NHS England 2016: question 4g). This workplace environment may have contributed to 14% of staff reporting that they experienced harassment or bullying from their manager, frequently more than once, and 18% received it from colleagues (NHS England 2016: questions 15c and 15d).

Only 37% of staff were satisfied or very satisfied with their pay, and the workforce has been subject to a prolonged and continuous period of pay restraint, with a two-year pay freeze between 2011 and 2013. Subsequently, the government's public sector pay policy set out an average 1% annual pay increase for the NHS that is planned to continue until the end of the Parliament in 2019–20. Pay restraint has made an important contribution to budgetary savings in the NHS. For the first time in its history, however, the professional trade union representing midwives took strike action in protest of the 1% pay increases, and during 2015–16, the government was in a protracted and increasingly bitter dispute with hospital doctors (excluding the most senior grades, which have a separate employment contract).

NHS staff also have strong misgivings about the government's ambition to downgrade "unsocial hours payments" (enhanced payments for working specific shifts), justified by the goal of moving further toward a seven-day workweek. NHS staff also have concerns about further steps toward progression-based pay in which increments are awarded on a strictly performance-related basis.

One consequence of these varied pressures is that NHS trusts are becoming more reliant on temporary nursing and medical staff, bringing a sharp increase in expenditure on agency staff. This increase in expenditure not only reflects staff shortages but also has been interpreted as staff exiting full-time NHS employment and seeking more flexible and better-paid agency work, a pattern that has occurred in the past among nurses (Tailby 2005).

In summary, these structural challenges relate to the legacy of continuous, market-biased restructuring; shortcomings in patient safety; financial concerns; and disquiet about workforce engagement and capacity. The result is a complex and fragmented health system with unclear system leadership and—not surprisingly—a managerial culture that is relatively risk averse (Quilter-Pinner and Muir 2015). This scenario represents a difficult context in which to move to new models of care and alter working practices, but it has also increased the urgency of the transformation agenda among key NHS stakeholders.

The immediate need to address increased demand with fewer resources and to maintain service quality has therefore directed attention toward a focus on innovation (Department of Health 2011). An underlying premise of government policy is that financial restraint provides a sense of urgency and a catalyst for service transformation.

HEALTH CARE INNOVATION AND SYSTEM TRANSFORMATION: WORKFORCE IMPLICATIONS

Innovation in services is less straightforward to define than in manufacturing because outputs are less tangible, and the worker and end user are simultaneously involved in the production and consumption of services (Gallouj and Savona 2009). Innovation in manufacturing has been preoccupied with technological innovation, but in the service sector, interest in technological change has been supplemented by an emphasis on organizational innovation and the type of structures and incentives that produce high-quality services.

In England, competition and choice mechanisms have been forcibly advocated (Le Grand 2007), resulting in extensive outsourcing and moves toward shared services despite misgivings about their efficacy and consequences for staff when implemented within public services (Seddon 2014; Smith Institute 2014). Many of these measures are legitimated in terms of improving service delivery and being responsive to service users, but paradoxically, it is frequently the failure to take into account the requirements and responses of staff and users that lies behind failed information technology and other major innovations in the NHS.

This situation highlights the extent to which service quality in health care is based on the process and outcomes of the direct interaction between the producer and the consumer. The workforce therefore comprises an integral element of effective health care innovation and is central to system transformation. The NHS has embraced the importance of innovation, defining it as

> an idea, service or product, new to the NHS or applied in a way that is new to the NHS, which significantly improves the quality of health and care whenever it is applied ... innovation is as much about applying an idea, service or product in a new context, or in a new organisation, as it is about creating something entirely new. Copying is good. (Department of Health 2011: 9)

This definition is similar to Kessler's (2016), which focuses on human resource (HR) innovation in health care and defines it as an idea or program that is new to the adopting organization. This leaves open the question of the forms that HR innovation takes, and it may comprise new ways of managing (i.e., new approaches to recruitment and selection or training), new ways of working (i.e., new routines and ways to deliver services by those in established roles), and new roles (i.e., the assignment of tasks to a completely new job role) (Kessler, Heron, and Dopson 2016).

It is recognized that innovation in human resource management (HRM) in health care is difficult because strong occupations with well-established professional identities and systems of regulation are often resistant to changes in working practices that may threaten professional status (Bach, Kessler, and Heron 2009; Herzlinger 2006). Moreover, the extent to which these different forms of workplace change exist in isolation is an open question.

New ways of working in response to a particular organizational requirement may highlight the need for further change, in terms of a new role, to fully adjust working practices to altered circumstances. At the same time, a new role can be expected to be accompanied by new ways of working. New ways of managing, such as recruiting on values, may coexist and be equally applicable to new ways of working and new roles. For these reasons, the distinction between new roles and new ways of working is useful, but they are considered in tandem—reflecting the realities of workplace practice.

New Ways of Working and New Roles

Despite criticisms of NHS HRM practice, trust managers have sought to encourage the development of new ways of working and new roles. Particular attention has focused on the health care support workforce that comprises around a third of the caregiving workforce and provides around 60% of direct care (Cavendish 2013). Despite concerns about the training and accountability of the health care support workforce identified by the Francis report (2013), NHS trusts confronted with cost and capacity pressures have continued to develop the health care support worker role and establish more structured training pathways.

Increased focus on support roles has been bolstered by several national initiatives to formalize those roles, as well as training and development opportunities for support workers (Cavendish 2013). Wide variations in practice exist between NHS trusts because local managers retain more discretion than do regulated staff over how support roles are used, but some support workers are carrying out a wider range of more complex nursing work than in the past (Cavendish 2013; Kessler et al. 2012). More attention (from a very low level) is being directed at the training requirements of the health care support workforce, with more precise mapping of the requirements of those roles and a 12-week mandatory induction program—measures that are raising the profile and attention directed at this component of the workforce. NHS trust managers, reinforced by commissioner monitoring, are much stricter about ensuring that staff fulfill their mandatory training requirements in a timely fashion.

NHS trusts are also looking to develop new roles, and it is instructive to examine two roles that have received considerable attention: the assistant practitioner (AP) and the physician associate (PA). The experience with both innovations indicates that the establishment of new roles remains problematic, and many barriers exist that constrain their uptake in the NHS.

Assistant practitioners sit between registered nurses and traditional support workers. They deliver health and social care, with knowledge and skills that extend beyond the traditional support worker role; may transcend traditional boundaries; and often deliver more specialist protocol–led care. Assistant practitioners are not confined to nursing; they are also present in the scientific workforce and are found among allied health professionals, such as radiographers.

Despite the interest within the NHS in AP roles, their development has been limited. Precise numbers are difficult to gauge because trusts use other job titles and use grades (Band 4 in the NHS grading structure) as a proxy for job role, but this is misleading: if no Band 4 roles are available, APs might not be banded according to the skills and knowledge they have acquired. Although studies point to the positive role of APs in providing additional capacity when registered nurses are not able to be recruited and have shown that APs are more responsive to patients and can work more flexibly, many barriers to their acceptance and diffusion across the NHS have been identified (Bungay, Jackson, Lord, and Smyth 2013). NHS providers rarely take a strategic overview of their workforce, and AP posts are often established in response to targeted funding opportunities or because specific individuals, usually support workers, have demonstrated particular aptitudes to develop their role and can fulfill a specific organizational need (Miller, Williams, Marvell, and Tassinari 2015). It is very rare for trusts to advertise and recruit to these roles, and existing studies point to small numbers of APs (fewer than 50) being employed, even by the most innovative trusts.

These findings also indicate some blurring in the distinction between new roles and new ways of working because existing staff often migrate into such roles. The main barriers that have been identified in the establishment of APs relate to uncertainties and confusion about their role and competencies, making registered nurses understandably wary of delegating tasks because of supervision and accountability issues in relation to an unregulated workforce.

Registered nurses also often have an uncertain gendered professional identity (Bach, Kessler, and Heron 2009), and APs are perceived as a threat to this professional identity. The most established AP role exists in radiography, reflecting the crucial role of the Society and College of Radiographers in setting out a scope of practice document for APs that clearly identifies activities that are within and also out-with the APs scope of professional practice (Miller, Williams, Marvell, and Tassinari 2015).

Reinforcing these conclusions are PAs, who have been much discussed but little used to date. There are only around 200 UK-trained PAs, and approximately 35 were newly qualified in 2014, although more training programs are being established (NHS Wales 2015). There remains considerable conservatism and uneven acceptance of new roles; acceptance often depends on the clear establishment of need, the use of champions to promote the new roles, and having trust in the individual identified to fill the role (Kessler 2016).

The path dependency of the NHS in terms of its workforce requirements and how it responds to these challenges can be illustrated further by the case of international recruitment for registered nurses. Internationally recruited nurses (IRNs) have been a long-standing feature of NHS workforce practice, but there has been a noticeable change in their utilization. In 2000–01, around 15% of practicing nurses in the United Kingdom were foreign born, and that percentage increased to almost 22% by 2011–12 (Organisation for Economic Co-operation and Development 2015a: 114). This increased reliance on IRNs has coincided with a more measured and cautious appraisal of their contribution. Not only has the NHS been criticized for poaching overseas staff, leading to erroneous claims from the former NHS chief executive that the NHS was self-sufficient by 2007 (Crisp 2011: 110), but nurse managers have also expressed reservations about the cost effectiveness of international recruitment. Moreover, an association has been reported between the use of non-UK–educated nurses and lower patient satisfaction (Germack et al. 2015). Nonetheless, HR and nurse managers invariably turn toward the quick fix of international recruitment, and in 2015–16, international recruitment was on a very marked upward trajectory, with registered nurses temporarily included on the government's shortage occupation list during 2015 (Royal College of Nursing 2015b).

Although trust managers in the short term have limited options to rapidly scale up the registered nursing workforce when shortages occur, given the three-year time lag to train a nurse, the continuing dependence of the NHS on IRNs indicates the continuing failure of workforce planning and suggests that NHS managers find it more straightforward to use established workforce solutions than embrace new roles and new ways of working.

Health Care Integration: New Models of Care Workforce Implications

A different source of workforce innovation stems from the agenda relating to new models of care, highlighted by Herzlinger (2006) in relation to her review of health care innovation in the United States. The development of models of integrated care draws on a variety of past initiatives to join up health and social care and to create a more seamless service. These past measures often involved joint commissioning of services for specific groups, such as older people, and some pooled their resources to encourage joint or partnership working. In 2008, 16 care trusts were established in which local authorities delegated some of their social care responsibilities to the NHS, but whole system shifts toward integrated care remained elusive.

This ambition has become more prominent in current NHS chief executive Simon Stevens' roadmap for change set forth in the *Five Year Forward View* (NHS England 2014). That report outlined the need to remove "artificial barriers between hospitals and primary care, between health and social care, between generalists and specialists—all of which get in the way of care that is genuinely coordinated around what people need and want" (NHS England 2014: 6). It set out seven new models of care, but they were not of equal significance, with some concentrating on specific services (maternity services, care homes) while most attention has focused on two models.

The first model is Multi-Specialty Community Providers (MCPs), which involves the expansion of primary care networks or federations to incorporate a wider range of professionals, including hospital specialists, to deliver a range of community-based services. The main aim is to move specialist care out of hospitals. The second model, Primary and Acute Care Systems (PACS), is similar to accountable care organizations (ACOs) in the United States. PACS envisage "vertical" integration—joining up primary, community, and mental health services with hospitals that manage primary cares services and, possibly over time, being accountable for a whole population and paid on a capitation basis. These models potentially represent a major departure from the emphasis on the purchaser–provider split that has been the bedrock of health policy for a quarter of a century, and they signal more emphasis on the evolution of local solutions (Jupp 2015).

Although the two care models are the main focus of attention, there is also interest in enhancing health care in care homes and developing approaches that reduce pressure on casualty departments (NHS England 2015). The variety of models indicates there is often a lack of precision about the organizational forms and the consequences of integration that is regarded uncritically as a universal application that is beneficial for all stakeholders (Glasby and Dickinson 2014).

Reflecting a long-standing focus with structural change of the NHS, one dimension of integration relates to organizational forms. Glasby and Dickinson (2014) differentiate between vertical integration, a hierarchical form bringing together primary, community, and acute services, and horizontal integration, a network form of organization that links similar organizations (e.g., alliances and partnerships between hospitals) or networks of community and social care services that cross NHS and local government boundaries.

Joining up different parts of the NHS is challenging, but even more complex are the boundaries and barriers that exist between the NHS, which provides medical care, and local government, which provides social care (Goodwin et al. 2012). This divide is reinforced because local government and the NHS are funded and organized differently: the NHS is tax funded and free at the point of use; social care is funded by specific grants, is means tested, and charges apply. Social care has a much higher proportion of private provision than the NHS, and distinctive professional cultures exist that are reinforced by different pay and grading systems. In addition, the NHS generally provides better employment terms and conditions (Trades Union Congress 2015).

A second dimension relates to the purpose of integration. Although there is a consistent theme of being person centered, to improve coordination and reduce service duplication, this integration disguises differences of emphasis. In a period of austerity, large acute hospitals and the government are primarily concerned with financial considerations, and the main purpose of integration is to reduce hospital admissions, ensure rapid discharge of patients, and encourage less costly community-based provision. The voluntary sector and service users, with support from many health and social work professionals, consider the main purpose of integration to be focused on developing services built around the individual and based on values of independence, choice, and user control that is captured in individual care plans and reinforced by the use of personal budgets. The influential voluntary sector organization, National Voices, has been pivotal in developing a narrative of person-centered and empowered care.

Third, a variety of instruments and approaches that include a strong workforce dimension are prominent in the provision of integrated care (Johnson 2014; Jupp 2015):

- joint commissioning arrangements
- emphasis on care pathways to ensure that different professions (even if working in separate organizations) adopt a consistent approach to specific conditions
- use of multidisciplinary teams in which team members may be employed by different organizations but share responsibility and data
- use of technological innovation to support care closer to home
- employment of care coordinators and navigators who ensure a single point of referral
- signposting of services for users, with an emphasis on providing care closer to home
- co-location of professionals to break down barriers between services
- the pooling of resources to reduce financial incentives that encourage separatism and a silo mentality
- an emphasis on early intervention and prevention that draws on risk analysis of particular populations

In recent years, further steps have been taken to encourage integration: the Better Care Fund was established to pool £3.8 billion to be spent jointly on social services and community services; personal budgets, intended to enhance responsiveness to users, have been provided; and a variety of legal routes have been created to enable public bodies to cooperate (Jupp 2015). There are many local examples of innovation, and they are being sponsored and evaluated as part of several transformation programs (Erens et al. 2015; NHS England 2015). It is notable, however, that many of the same high-profile cases are referred to in policy-related briefings. These examples of best practices evolved over many years, indicating the painstaking process of building trust and effective working relationships to bring about sustained change in ways of working and the establishment of new roles (Local Government Association 2014).

The Torbay Care Trust exemplifies these developments. The trust was created in 2005 to bring health and social care together in one organization, facilitating the development of integrated teams of health and social care staff that use a single assessment process. Integration was made meaningful to patients and staff by focusing on how delivery would benefit a hypothetical patient, "Mrs. Smith." This philosophy is underpinned by locality-based teams that focus on well-being and support identified by local residents, with the related goals of reducing inappropriate hospital admissions and yielding positive results (Centre for Workforce Intelligence 2013: 13; Goodwin et al. 2012: 5). Acute hospitals are aiming to prevent unnecessary admissions and facilitate effective discharge. Trusts are establishing low-technology step-down facilities within hospitals or close to hospitals to free up acute beds. In one region, a separate specialist emergency facility was established to ensure that emergency admissions do not have consequences for elective work across the region's hospitals.

South Warwickshire NHS Trust developed a community-based, multidisciplinary emergency response team. The Discharge to Assess model involves joint health and social care commissioning to support three distinct pathways, depending on need, to encourage more rapid discharge with appropriate community-based support, including dedicated, short-term care home provision. The approach has reduced hospital lengths of stay by a third and increased discharge rates by 30%. Social workers value the increased autonomy and improvements it has brought to service users (Carter 2014).

Integration: Workforce Implications

These altered care models have significant workforce implications, yet they have garnered limited consideration. The guidance from the NHS Centre for Workforce Intelligence (2013) in its *Think Integration, Think Workforce* report is simplistic. It outlines three steps to integration: "Be clear about the integration agenda," "Address the integrated workforce management challenge," and "Implement successful workforce change with an emphasis on good communication and clear leadership"—an approach endorsed by similar guidance documents (Skills for Care 2013).

The shift toward more community settings and a higher profile for mental health, along with a government commitment to parity of esteem between physical and mental health services, necessitates that the workforce undertakes a wider range of tasks, with more training and expertise in mental health, an ability to work across different care settings, and an ability to work with a range of providers. The community workforce has always been primarily a nurse-led service, but staffing patterns are altering as the proportion of relatively high-cost district nursing staff is reduced and health care support workers become a more integral part of the acute and community workforce (Kessler, Heron, and Dopson 2012). Community settings frequently involve more autonomous work, and support worker roles extend beyond nursing work to incorporate other duties traditionally undertaken by physiotherapists or occupational therapists.

Integrated care has stimulated multidisciplinary working across professional and organizational boundaries—shifting professional roles, challenging existing professional identities, and highlighting training requirements. Joint funding of jobs by the NHS and local government has led to the growth of care navigators (who assist patients in getting well after discharge), care coordinators, and health trainers. Professional staff, such as nurses and social workers, undergo vastly different training and subscribe to separate medical and social models of health, which makes professional staff wary of accepting direction and supervision from staff outside their profession and reluctant to refer patients to services that lie outside their professional norms and values (Erens et al. 2015: 532; Goodwin et al. 2012).

Human resource practices that break down these boundaries—the silo mentality—focus on joint management arrangements and joint training, co-location of different professional groups to establish trust and effective working relationships, and appointment of care coordinators from nursing and social work backgrounds to manage both staff groups (Local Government Association 2014: 19).

The importance of understanding the roles and responsibilities of various professional staff is also frequently highlighted (Skills for Care 2013). Community nurses form the bedrock of community health services, but they are concerned that their role is poorly understood by other members of the community workforce, which leads to unsuitable referrals and work being inappropriately allocated to them. More than two thirds of community nursing staff felt that some activities would be better done by other staff (Ball, Philippou, Pike, and Sethi 2014: 35).

Many studies point to the importance of highlighting the benefits for the end user as a way to encourage a joint vision and commitment to integrated working that redirects attention from organizational needs to the values necessary to provide person-centered care (Local Government Association 2014). The emphasis on values stems from the Francis report (2013), which highlighted a disturbing lack of compassion among the nursing workforce.

The Chief Nursing Officer (2012) reiterated the importance of ensuring that services are delivered with care and compassion, and values-based recruitment has become a means to achieve this goal. Values-based recruitment places less emphasis on formal qualifications and candidates for nursing, and nursing support candidates are assessed to ensure they exhibit the right values to support team-working and excellent patient care. Candidates for support roles are able to self-assess their own values to gauge their fit with NHS values as detailed in the NHS constitution. Reinforcement of these values is also being promoted by the implementation of the Care

Certificate, which comprises a set of standards shared across health and social care that new employees in support roles have to demonstrate within ten weeks of commencing work. What remains uncertain is the extent that staff recruited with these values are able to maintain them in highly pressured work environments in which staff shortages and bullying remain prominent concerns (NHS England 2016).

The emphasis on values that reflect the needs of end users for integrated care is also being reinforced by the increased involvement of end users in recruitment and selection of health and social care staff and, more generally, the increased involvement of end users in shaping service delivery (Bach 2015). Emphasizing responsiveness to end users, however, may increase challenges for staff who increasingly have to deal with a complex landscape of public and patient involvement in which there is much duplication of voice (i.e., involvement) mechanisms (Sensier 2015: 30).

In addition, 83% of nurses working in district community teams agreed that "public expectations are difficult to meet" (Ball, Philippou, Pike, and Sethi 2014: 43). Trained professional staff not only have to adapt to an environment in which the opinions of "experts by experience" carry more weight, but they also have to adjust to a context in which the composition of the workforce is more diverse. In particular, the shrinking of the state and the government's emphasis on creating a big society of empowered volunteers means that professional staff are working more often alongside volunteers who are not bound by the same norms and performance expectations as employees.

Difficult issues also arise in balancing the requirement to be responsive to service users and to maintain reasonable working conditions and work–life balance. Tensions frequently arise in relation to the seven-day workweek—in particular, the expectation within government that weekend and evening work should be regarded as a normal part of the workweek and should not attract any premium payment. This issue became a prominent feature of a bitter and long-running contract dispute between the government and hospital doctors during 2015–16.

A strong commitment to user voice has not always been matched by a similar emphasis on staff voice within moves toward integrated care. Staff face considerable uncertainty as new models of care redraw the organizational boundaries of health and social care organizations. Staff seconded from the NHS to local government lack clarity about their pension position and how to gain appropriate HR advice (Johnson 2014). When staff are transferred to another employer, their terms and conditions are protected for two years by Transfer of Undertakings Protection of Employment (TUPE) regulations, but the situation is complex and case law is constantly evolving.

A major issue arises when staff are transferred from NHS to local government employment or when NHS and local government staff, such as social workers, work together. NHS staff generally receive higher pay and better terms and conditions than their counterparts in local government, which is a factor that militates against joint working (Trades Union Congress 2015). Innovative attempts to address these barriers to integrated working are taking place in Manchester, which is pioneering a distinctive form of health and social care integration as part of a more ambitious plan to devolve power to the English regions (Communities and Local Government Committee 2016). Trade unions are concerned that devolution may be a way of delegating cuts, but the unions are working in partnership with all parties, and a Workforce Engagement Board has been established to prevent worsening terms and conditions of employment and unnecessary employment transfers unless there is a clear service or legal basis for such a transfer (Greater Manchester Combined Authority 2015).

CONCLUSION

In common with the majority of health care systems, the NHS in England confronts a range of structural, financial, demographic, and workforce challenges—but the challenges have unique forms because of the institutional character and evolution of NHS restructuring in recent decades. These challenges have been intensified by recent government austerity policies that create much unease about the state of the NHS and uncertainty about its future trajectory.

Among the NHS policy community, a dominant response has been to focus more on transforming models of care, which includes encouraging new ways of managing the workforce, elaborating and formalizing values of compassion and dignity, emphasizing competencies and skills rather than formal qualifications and professional regulation, and stimulating new roles that exemplify and embed new models of care.

Health care is a complex industry that traditionally has been reluctant to challenge professional interests and established ways of working. The combination of the financial crisis, recognition of the limitations of existing care models, concerns about quality of service, and staff shortages have stimulated more concerted efforts to bring about shifts in health care delivery. In the past, the NHS has relied on top-down, centrally driven change, but that approach has only sporadically brought about sustained changes in ways of working. The use of pilots, vanguards, and forms of regional devolution has encouraged more local ownership of changes in working practices within a more explicit national framework, but that localism is jeopardized by the financial context in which the NHS operates—which encourages a return to centralized control from Whitehall.

Austerity measures therefore are having contradictory effects on the pursuit of system transformation. The state of health care in England illustrates that curtailing the resources advanced to the NHS and intensifying pressure on staff has major consequences for service quality, waiting times, financial sustainability, and workforce capacity. New models of care and the integration agenda are at the center of new ways of working and new roles, but the uneven progress to date indicates that many barriers remain in place. Austerity measures direct an employer's attention toward innovation and change but also severely inhibit system reform. NHS providers focus on short-term financial performance and curtailing demand and have limited scope to focus on system change, encouraging the adoption of familiar managerial recipes such as the use of agency staff, the turn to international recruitment, and the limitation of access to services.

Without increased investment accompanied by efforts to improve staff well-being and engagement, the goals of new models of care remain only partially accomplished as the NHS policy community focuses on short-term solutions, inhibiting the development and implementation of more sustained system transformation.

REFERENCES

Addicott, R., D. Maquire, M. Honeyman, and J. Jabbal. 2015. *Workforce Planning in the NHS*. London, UK: King's Fund.

Appleby, J., and R. Robertson. 2016. *Public Satisfaction with NHS in 2015. Results and Trends from the British Social Attitudes Survey*. London, UK: King's Fund.

Bach, S. 2015. *New Challenges for Public Services Social Dialogue: Integrating Service User and Workforce Involvement: Comparative Report*. London, UK: King's College.

Bach, S. 2016. "Deprivileging the Public Sector Workforce: Austerity, Fragmentation and Service Withdrawal in Britain." *The Economic and Labour Relations Review* 27, no. 1: 11–28.

Bach, S., I. Kessler, and P. Heron. 2009. "Nursing a Grievance? The Role of Healthcare Assistants in a Modernized National Health Service." *Gender, Work and Organization* 19, no. 2: 205–24. doi:10.1111/j.1468-0432.2009.00502.x.

Ball, J., J. Philippou, G. Pike, and J. Sethi. 2014. *Survey of District and Community Nurses in 2013. Report to the Royal College of Nursing*. London, UK: Royal College of Nursing.

Bungay, H., J. Jackson, S. Lord, and T. Smyth. 2013. *What Are the Key Factors in the Successful Implementation of Assistant Practitioner Roles in a Healthcare Setting?* Derby, UK: NHS Midlands and East.

Carter, P. 2016. *Operational Productivity and Performance in English NHS Acute Hospitals: Unwarranted Variations*. London, UK: NHS England.

Carter, R. 2014 (Oct. 29). "Social Work on an Innovative Multidisciplinary Team: "It's Been Empowering." *Community Care*.

Cavendish, C. 2013. *The Cavendish Review: An Independent Review into Healthcare Assistants and Support Workers in the NHS and Social Care Settings*. London, UK: Department of Health.

Centre for Workforce Intelligence. 2013. *Think Integration, Think Workforce*. London, UK: Centre for Workforce Intelligence.

Chief Nursing Officer. 2012. *Compassion in Practice*. London, UK: Department of Health.

Communities and Local Government Committee. 2016. *Devolution: The Next Five Years and Beyond, First Report of Session 2015–16*. London, UK: The Stationery Office.

Crisp, N. 2011. *24 Hours to Save the NHS: The Chief Executive's Account of Reform 2000–2006*. Oxford, UK: Oxford University Press.

Dalton, D. 2014. *Examining New Options and Opportunities for Providers of NHS Care: The Dalton Review*. London, UK: NHS England.

Davis, K., K. Stremikis, D. Squires, and C. Schoen. 2014. *Mirror, Mirror on the Wall: How the Performance of the US Health Care System Compares Internationally*. New York, NY: The Commonwealth Fund.

Department of Health. 2011. *Innovation, Health and Wealth*. London, UK: Department of Health.

Department of Health. 2012. *Transforming Care: A National Response to Winterbourne View Hospital*. London, UK: Department of Health.

Department of Health. 2015. *Winterbourne View: Transforming Care Two Years On*. London, UK: Department of Health.

Erens, B., G. Wistow, S. Mounier-Jack, N. Douglas, L. Jones, L. Mancorda, and N. Mays. 2015. *Early Evaluation of the Integrated Care and Support Pioneers Programme: Interim Report*. London, UK: Policy Innovation Research Unit.

Ferlie, E., A. Pettigrew, L. Ashburn, and L. Fitzgerald. 1996. *The New Public Management in Action*. Oxford, UK: Oxford University Press.

Francis, R. 2010. *Independent Inquiry into Care Provided by Mid Staffordshire NHS Foundation Trust January 2005–March 2009: Volume 1*. London, UK: The Stationery Office.

Francis, R. 2013. *Report of the Mid Staffordshire NHS Foundation Trust Public Inquiry*. London, UK: The Stationery Office.

Gallouj, F., and M. Savona. 2009. "Innovation in Services: A Review of the Debate and a Research Agenda." *Journal of Evolutionary Economics* 19, no. 2: 149–72. doi:10.1007/s00191-008-0126-4.

Germack, H., P. Griffiths, D. Sloane, A.-M. Rafferty, J. Ball, and L. Aiken. 2015 (Dec. 2). "Patient Satisfaction and Non-UK Educated Nurses: A Cross-Sectional Observational Study of English National Health Service Hospitals." *BMJ Open*. http://bit.ly/2csjxbX.

Gerschlick, B., A. Charlesworth, and E. Taylor. 2015. *Public Attitudes to the NHS*. London, UK: The Health Foundation.

Givan, R. K., and S. Bach. 2007. "Workforce Responses to the Creeping Privatization of the UK National Health Service." *International Labor and Working-Class History* 71, no. 1: 1–21. doi:10.1017/s0147547907000373.

Glasby, J., and H. Dickinson. 2014. *Partnership Working in Health and Social Care* (2nd edition). Bristol, UK: Policy Press.

Glennerster, H. 2015. "The Coalition and Society (iii): Health and Long Term Care." In *The Coalition Effect, 2010–2015*, edited by A. Seldon and M. Finn. Cambridge, UK: Cambridge University Press.

Goodwin, N., J. Smith, A. Davies, C. Perry, R. Rosen, A. Dixon, J. Dixon, and C. Ham. 2012. *Integrated Care for Patients and Populations: Improving Outcomes by Working Together*. London, UK: King's Fund/Nuffield Trust.

Greater Manchester Combined Authority. 2015. *Protocols with Trade Unions*. Manchester, UK: Greater Manchester Combined Authority.

Grimshaw, D., and J. Rubery. 2012. "The End of the UK's Liberal Collectivist Social Model? The Implications of the Coalition Government's Policy During the Austerity Crisis." *Cambridge Journal of Economics* 36, no. 1: 105–26. doi:10.1093/cje/ber033.

Ham, C., B. Baird, S. Gregory, J. Jabbal, and H. Alderwick. 2015. *The NHS Under the Coalition Government*. London, UK: King's Fund.

Health Committee. 2014. *Public Expenditure on Health and Social Care, Seventh Report of Session 2013–2014*. London, UK: The Stationery Office.

Herzlinger, R. 2006 (May). "Why Innovation in Health Care Is So Hard." *Harvard Business Review*.

Institute of Fiscal Studies. 2016. *IFS Green Budget*. London, UK: Institute of Fiscal Studies.

Johnson, M. 2014. *Tackling Barriers to Integration in Health and Social Care, Viewpoint 69*. London, UK: Housing Learning and Improvement Network.

Jupp, B. 2015. *Reconsidering Accountability in an Age of Integrated Care*. London, UK: Nuffield Trust.

Kessler, I. 2016. "Innovation and New Work Roles in the NHS." *Human Resource Management Journal*. In press.

Kessler, I., P. Heron, and S. Dopson. 2012. *The Modernization of the Nursing Workforce: Valuing the Healthcare Assistant*. Oxford, UK: Oxford University Press.

King's Fund. 2015. *Quarterly Monitoring Report*, 17. London, UK: King's Fund.

Le Grand, J. 2007. *The Other Invisible Hand: Delivering Public Services Through Choice and Competition*. Princeton, NJ: Princeton University Press.

Local Government Association. 2014. *Service Integration and the Workforce*. London, UK: Local Government Association.

Miller, L., J. Williams, R. Marvell, and A. Tassinari. 2015. *Assistant Practitioners in the NHS in England*. London, UK: Skills for Health.

National Advisory Group on the Safety of Patients in England. 2013. *A Promise to Learn—A Commitment to Act: Improving the Safety of Patients in England*. London, UK: Department of Health.

National Audit Office. 2016. *Managing the Supply of NHS Clinical Staff in England*. London, UK: National Audit Office.

NHS Employers. 2015. *NHS Employers' Submission to the NHS Pay Review Body 2016/17*. London, UK: NHS Employers.

NHS England. 2014. *Five Year Forward View*. London, UK: NHS England.

NHS England. 2015. *New Care Models: Vanguards—Developing a Blueprint for the Future of NHS and Care Services*. London, UK: NHS England.

NHS England. 2016. *NHS Staff Survey National Weighted Data*. London, UK: NHS England.

NHS Improvement. 2016. *Performance of the NHS Provider Sector: Year Ended 31 March 2016*. London, UK: NHS Improvement.

NHS Support Federation. 2016. *Contract Alert: Outsourcing in the NHS February 2016*. Brighton, UK: NHS Support Federation.

NHS Wales. 2015. *Developing the Role of the Physician Associate in the Area of the Mid Wales Healthcare Collaborative* (Draft Report). NHS Wales. http://bit.ly/1WzuRCz.

Organisation for Economic Co-operation and Development. 2015a. "Changing Patterns in the International Migration of Doctors and Nurses to OECD Countries." In *International Migration Outlook*. Paris, France: Organisation for Economic Co-operation and Development.

Organisation for Economic Co-operation and Development. 2015b. *Health at a Glance 2015*. Paris, France: Organisation for Economic Co-operation and Development.

Osborne, D., and T. Gaebler. 1992. *Reinventing Government: How the Entrepreneurial Spirit Is Transforming the Public Sector*. New York, NY: Penguin.

Pownall, H. 2013. "Neoliberalism, Austerity and the Health and Social Care Act 2012: The Coalition Government's Programme for the NHS and Its Implications for the Public Sector Workforce." *Industrial Law Journal* 42, no. 4: 422–33. doi:10.1093/indlaw/dwt016.

Quilter-Pinner, H., and R. Muir. 2015. *Improved Circulation: Unleashing Innovation in the NHS*. London, UK: Institute for Public Policy Research.

Royal College of Nursing. 2015a. *A Workforce in Crisis? The UK Nursing Labour Market Review 2015*. London, UK: Royal College of Nursing.

Royal College of Nursing. 2015b. *International Recruitment 2015*. London, UK: Royal College of Nursing.

Seddon, J. 2014. *The Whitehall Effect*. Axminster, UK: Triarchy Press.

Sensier, J. 2015. "Response: The View from Healthwatch." In *Reconsidering Accountability in an Age of Integrated Care*, edited by B. Jupp. London, UK: Nuffield Trust.

Skills for Care. 2013. *Evidence Review—Integrated Health and Social Care*. Leeds, UK: Skills for Care.

Smith Institute. 2014. *Outsourcing the Cuts: Pay and Employment Effects of Contracting Out*. London, UK: Smith Institute.

Tailby, S. 2005. "Agency and Bank Nursing in the UK National Health Service." *Work, Employment and Society* 19, no. 2: 369–89. doi:10.1177/0950017005053178.

Tailby, S. 2012. "Public Service Restructuring in the UK: The Case of the English National Health Service." *Industrial Relations Journal* 43, no. 5: 448–64. doi:10.1111/j.1468-2338.2012.00695.x.

Timmins, N. 2012. *Never Again? The Story of the Health and Social Care Act 2012*. London, UK: King's Fund/Institute for Government.

Timmins, N. 2015. *The Practice of System Leadership*. London, UK: King's Fund.

Trades Union Congress. 2015. *Outsourcing Public Services*. London, UK: Trades Union Congress.

Chapter 3

Building the Infrastructures of Accountable Care: Early Lessons from Four Commercial ACOs

Brian Hilligoss
College of Public Health
The Ohio State University

Ann Scheck McAlearney
College of Medicine
The Ohio State University

Paula H. Song
Gillings School of Global Public Health
University of North Carolina at Chapel Hill

INTRODUCTION

In the United States, significant efforts are under way to reform the highly fragmented health care delivery system, rein in the soaring costs of care, and improve the quality of care and the health of the American population. Among these many efforts is the formation of accountable care organizations (ACOs), groups of health care providers that collectively assume financial risk for managing the health outcomes, total costs, and quality of care for defined populations of potential patients. Whereas U.S. health care providers have traditionally been paid on a fee-for-service basis, effectively rewarding them for volumes of services provided, ACOs represent an attempt to shift greater accountability for cost, quality, and health outcomes onto providers, effectively rewarding them for value—outcomes per dollar spent (Porter 2010).

ACOs are frequently referred to as a type of payment reform, and changes to reimbursements and the restructuring of incentives are often foregrounded in discussions of how ACOs are proposed to change behaviors and transform financial and clinical outcomes. There are multiple payment arrangements possible under the ACO model, but they fall broadly into two types: shared savings and full financial risk arrangements. Under shared savings ("upside only") arrangements, providers share with payers (insurance companies, Medicare, etc.) any savings obtained from increased efficiency. Under full financial risk arrangements, providers are paid a set amount for each patient for a given time period: if actual costs are lower than that amount, the provider retains the savings, but if actual costs exceed that amount, the provider incurs a loss. Under both types of arrangement, measures of quality of care are tied to payments, and providers must meet certain thresholds on these measures to qualify for full payments. The measures used vary by payer and contract but tend to include measures of preventive care provision (e.g., colorectal cancer screenings, pediatric immunizations) and patient experience (e.g., perceptions of provider communication). Some ACO contracts include a mix of arrangements, with shared savings tied to some services and full financial risk to others.

This emphasis on payment reform is understandable given that reimbursement arrangements are the primary mechanisms for influencing health care delivery under the control of policy makers and the Centers for Medicare and Medicaid Services (CMS). But payment reform is only one piece of the puzzle. Attendant changes to the organizational structure and in the capabilities of the health care delivery system are also needed to reduce health care expenditures while improving quality (Burns and Pauly 2012; Crosson 2011; Kreindler et al. 2012; McClellan et al. 2010; Rittenhouse, Shortell, and Fisher 2009). Whether framed narrowly as payment reform, or more broadly as system transformation, ACOs have ambitious goals that likely require multiple activities supported by robust infrastructures.

According to proponents, the goal of an ACO is to slow spending growth (Fisher and Shortell 2010; Fisher et al. 2009; McClellan et al. 2010; Shortell and Casalino 2010) while improving quality of care (Fisher and Shortell 2010; Fisher et al. 2009; McClellan et al. 2010) and the health of a defined population (Casalino, Erb, Joshi, and Shortell 2015; National Priorities Partnership 2008). In short, an ACO has the ambitious goal of the triple aim: improving the patient experience, improving the health of populations, and reducing the total costs of care (Berwick, Nolan, and Whittington 2008). Early empirical evidence of the ability of ACOs to achieve this goal is weak or mixed, with some ACOs reducing costs and improving quality and others failing to show improvements (McWilliams, Landon, Chernew, and Zaslavsky 2014; McWilliams, Chernew, Landon, and Schwartz 2015; Salmon et al. 2012; Song et al. 2014). These mixed results suggest an underappreciation for both the complexity of the challenge facing ACOs and the significant changes and investments required.

If ACOs are to achieve their ambitious goals, experts suggest they must engage in a variety of activities. In particular, ACOs must develop and monitor measures (Fisher and Shortell 2010; Fisher et al. 2009; Larson et al. 2012; McClellan et al. 2010; Shortell and Casalino 2010; Singer and Shortell 2011), including total costs of care (National Priorities Partnership 2008) and quality metrics, in order to evaluate performance and support ongoing learning and improvement (Fisher and Shortell 2010; Singer and Shortell 2011). ACOs must also manage and coordinate care effectively across the care continuum (Larson et al. 2012; National Priorities Partnership 2008; Rundall et al. 2016), including better integration of hospital operations and independent physician practices (Singer and Shortell 2011). Furthermore, ACOs may need to engage in practice redesign and process improvement (McClellan et al. 2010; Shortell and Casalino 2010) to enhance efficiencies and eliminate waste (National Priorities Partnership 2008). Finally, ACOs may also need to engage patients more actively in their own care (National Priorities Partnership 2008; Shortell et al. 2015).

The activities ACOs must undertake in pursuit of their ambitious goal in turn require a firm foundation. Discussions of ACOs sometimes use the language of construction. Terms such as "build" (Addicott and Shortell 2014; Crosson 2011; Kreindler et al. 2012), "foundation" (Kreindler et al. 2012; Lowell and Bertko 2010), and "infrastructure" (Addicott and Shortell 2014; Burns and Pauly 2012; Fisher and Shortell 2010; Fisher et al. 2012; Larson et al. 2012; McClellan et al. 2010; Shortell and Casalino 2010; Shortell, Casalino, and Fisher 2010) indicate that each ACO is, to some extent, a new entity that must be assembled, likely requiring considerable planning, effort, and resources.

Among the infrastructural components that experts suggest are needed are payment systems that reward value rather than volume (Fisher et al. 2009; Shortell, Casalino, and Fisher 2010), health information technologies (Fisher and Shortell 2010; Fisher et al. 2012; Larson et al. 2012; Shortell and Casalino 2010); robust data analytic capabilities (Burns and Pauly 2012), and a strong primary care base (Burns and Pauly 2012; McClellan et al. 2010; Rittenhouse et al. 2009). Although they have received much less attention, a number of social structures have also been identified as important for ACOs. Specifically, teamwork and leadership are necessary foundational elements (Shortell and Casalino 2010; Shortell, Casalino, and Fisher 2010), along with governance structures that effectively balance the diverse perspectives and concerns of multiple stakeholders (Kreindler et al. 2014; Larson et al. 2012; Singer and Shortell 2011). While a variety of crucial infrastructural components have been identified in the literature, these have not, to our knowledge, been conceptually organized.

The metaphor of infrastructure is helpful for examining what an ACO consists of and for identifying what foundations the leaders of health services organizations may need to construct if they hope to pursue the goal of accountable care. "Infrastructure" is a collective term for the subordinate parts of a system that give the system its foundation and form.

Importantly, infrastructures enable a great variety of activities—and, without infrastructures, those same activities would be much more difficult, if not impossible. For illustration, one need only think of how challenging the morning commute would be for many if there were no paved roads or bridges. And infrastructures are not only the stuff of civil engineering; any ongoing collective enterprise is supported by infrastructure (Bowker and Star 1999). ACOs are no exception.

As the developers of the ACO concept have argued, it is vital not only that we demonstrate whether or not ACOs achieve their goals but also that we understand how and why they are or are not successful (Fisher and Shortell 2010). The ACO models being developed and tested today likely represent early versions (Fisher et al. 2012) in what will be an ongoing evolution in the effort to transform the health care system to one that is accountable not only for the cost and quality of care but also for optimizing the health of communities (Halfon et al. 2014). Understanding how or why current efforts do or do not produce desired results is critical for informing subsequent initiatives and further advancements. Thus, we need research that identifies the structural foundations, mechanisms, strategies, and assumptions that underlie and drive the various ACOs that are developing around the country. To that end, one important line of investigation is identifying the infrastructures that ACO leaders are building and a theoretical explanation of how these infrastructures are proposed to support transformation—that is, while the literature on ACOs points to a variety of structures to be built, we lack a means of conceptually organizing these structures and of identifying the roles each is presumed to play in efforts to achieve the goal of accountable care. In this chapter, we provide detailed empirical documentation of the efforts of four ACOs to develop infrastructures for accountable care. We present our findings as an inductively developed, empirically grounded framework that identifies core infrastructures of ACOs and posits how these infrastructures are believed to support efforts to pursue the goal of accountable care.

METHODS

Using a holistic multiple case study design (Yin 2003), we conducted qualitative case studies of four ACOs, all of which had both full financial risk and shared savings accountable care contracts (McAlearney, Song, and Hilligoss, forthcoming). We gathered data through site visits, during which we interviewed both administrators and providers involved in the ACOs and collected documents relevant to the organizations. We analyzed these data using an iterative inductive coding process and developed a theoretical framework that categorizes ACO infrastructures and explains how these infrastructures are intended to enable accountable care.

Sample and Data Collection

In choosing organizations to study, we selected those that were assuming full financial risk for at least one defined population under a Medicaid or private insurance contract. We focused on organizations with full financial risk arrangements because such contracts place greater responsibilities on provider organizations than do shared savings arrangements. We therefore expected that ACOs assuming full risk for populations would necessarily have invested greater efforts in building infrastructures and transforming capabilities than would ACOs engaged only in shared savings contracts. We focused on organizations serving populations beyond the Medicare Shared Savings and Pioneer Programs because ACOs of commercially insured populations have received very little attention in the literature.

Qualitative organizational case studies are time and resource intensive, meaning that any research project can investigate only a small sample. To minimize the limitations of a small sample, we maximized variability by selecting a diverse set of ACOs to study. For example, we selected ACOs that serve adult populations and ACOs that serve pediatric ones. We selected ACOs with organizational structures built around large hospital systems, as well as an ACO built around a primary care group practice and involving no hospital partner. We selected ACOs serving populations in five different states (Colorado, Illinois, Kansas, Missouri, Ohio), including a mix of urban, suburban, and rural populations. Finally, the ACOs in our sample ranged from those bearing full risk for relatively small populations (e.g., 15,000 lives) to those bearing risk for very large populations (e.g., 300,000 lives).

During the summer of 2013, we conducted two- to three-day site visits to each of the four ACOs. We categorized our informants in three groups based on their primary role in the ACO as they described it to us in the interview. *Executives* were C-suite leaders (e.g., CEO, CFO, CIO), vice presidents, and medical directors. *Managers* were administrators in all other management positions, including both mid-level managers (e.g., project managers, care coordination managers, IT specialists) and those responsible for physician offices. *Physicians* were health care providers, typically specializing in primary care, who were affiliated with the ACO. Most interviews lasted one hour and were digitally recorded. Informants were asked general questions about the history, development, structure, implementation, measurement, and performance of the ACO. In addition, informants were also asked targeted questions relevant to their specific responsibilities. While most interviews were conducted face to face, a few were conducted over the telephone either during the visit or soon afterward. We interviewed a total of 68 individuals. The number of informants per site varied from 12 to 22 owing to variations in the sizes of the organizations. Documents such as annual reports, strategic plans, progress reports, marketing materials, and handouts from presentations were also gathered during site visits.

Analysis

All recordings of interviews were transcribed and then coded using Atlas.ti (Scientific Software Development 2008). The initial round of coding was deductive. Transcripts were coded using a priori categories pertaining to broad topics of interest such as "ACO structure and organization," "contracts and risk arrangements," "care management," "quality," and "physician engagement," among others.

The second round of coding was inductive. In vivo codes were developed from terms and phrasing used by informants (Charmaz 2006). These codes indexed references to the structures that ACO leaders were putting into place, as well as the activities in which they were engaging or which they indicated perceiving as crucial to achieving their goals. More than 100 codes were created during this round, including "incentives," "buy-in," "coordinating care," "reporting," "ongoing efforts to build the network," "trust," and "culture change." These codes were then gathered into categories, representing four different infrastructures of the ACOs. Within each of these categories, codes were subdivided based on whether they characterized the infrastructure itself or explained why the infrastructure was perceived to be important, including what activities it supported. Finally, a number of codes captured themes that cut across multiple infrastructures. These were further analyzed to develop findings about the interdependencies of the four infrastructures. Throughout the process, brief memos were written to explore excerpts of transcripts, to compare and contrast codes, and to outline categories and themes.

FINDINGS

We found that in all four ACOs we studied, the infrastructures were built on existing foundations. None had begun from scratch. All four had considerable experience managing risk for a defined population, and all had some experience integrating and coordinating care. In the following subsections, we first briefly describe each ACO we studied then present our findings about core ACO infrastructures based on our synthesis of evidence across the four cases.

Four Commercial ACOs

New West Physicians

New West Physicians (New West) is a primary care group practice and medical management company with multiple locations in the Denver metropolitan area. The organization was formed in 1994 and entered its first risk-based contract the following year. As of mid-2013, New West had a full-risk contract with a Medicare Advantage plan covering 15,000 lives, as well as incentive-based arrangements (upside only) with three commercial managed care payers covering 33,000 lives. Structurally, New West was unique in that it included neither a hospital nor any medical specialists in the organization. Instead, New West contracted with a network, which it developed, consisting of roughly 500 preferred specialists. New West also used contracts held by the insurer for hospitals and other ancillary (nonphysician) providers in the market.

AdvocateCare

AdvocateCare (Advocate) is an ACO associated with Advocate Health Care system and launched in 2010 through Advocate Physician Partners as part of a landmark full-risk contract with Blue Cross Blue Shield of Illinois. Advocate Physician Partners is a not-for-profit "super PHO" (physician hospital organization) that coordinates contracting between the Advocate Health Care system (including ten acute care hospitals) and a network of 1,000 employed and 3,000 independent physicians who participate in the ACO. Advocate grounded its ACO model in its renowned Clinical Integration Program. At the time of our visit, the AdvocateCare ACO served more than 575,000 lives, including approximately 106,000 Medicare recipients under the Medicare Shared Savings program, 32,000 under full-risk Medicare Advantage contracts, and more than 280,000 privately insured lives. Advocate Health System had experience managing full-risk contracts dating back to the health maintenance organization (HMO) arrangements of the mid-1990s.

Partners For Kids

Partners For Kids (PFK), established in 1994, is a not-for-profit PHO, jointly owned by Nationwide Children's Hospital, in Columbus, Ohio, and by its network of 350 primary care physicians and 420 specialists. This physician network represented a mix of both employed and independent providers. Informants referred to PFK as the nation's first and largest pediatric ACO, assuming full risk for more than 300,000 children through capitated arrangements with five Medicaid managed care plans. PFK had been managing full risk for defined populations since shortly after it was established.

Children's Mercy Pediatric Care Network

Children's Mercy Pediatric Care Network (CMPCN) is an integrated pediatric delivery network comprising hospitals and clinics, employed physicians, independent community pediatricians, and other health care providers in Kansas City, Missouri, and Kansas City, Kansas. CMPCN was established in 2012 as a taxable, not-for-profit, sole member corporation of Children's Mercy Hospitals and Clinics. The ACO evolved out of a Medicaid managed care plan owned by Children's Mercy and sold in 2010 in response to state policy changes. At the time of our visit, CMPCN managed the care of 110,000 Medicaid-eligible children in western Missouri through a global risk model. In addition, the ACO managed the care of 60,000 Medicaid-eligible children in eastern Kansas through a shared savings arrangement.

Infrastructures

Our analysis revealed core infrastructures common to all four ACOs: an economic infrastructure, a sociocultural infrastructure, an information infrastructure, and a care continuum infrastructure. Figure 1 provides a visual representation of the framework. We discuss each infrastructure separately below and then examine their interdependencies.

Economic Infrastructure

Through contracts with payers and other providers (e.g., independent community-based physician practices, hospitals, or specialty practices), the four ACOs we studied were developing economic infrastructures that provided financial incentives to both the organization and individual providers or practices. The terms of these contracts and the details of the

FIGURE 1
Core Infrastructures Common to All Four ACOs

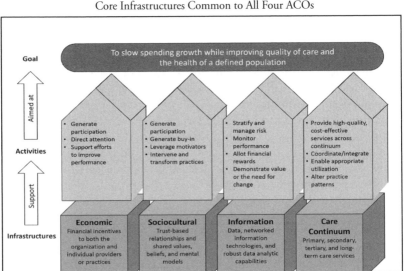

incentives varied among the organizations, but they all had some form of economic infrastructure that attempted to support the goal of accountable care through the provision of financial incentives, including shared savings, premium payments, downside risk bearing, and ownership. These economic infrastructures were being developed to enhance the appeal of value-driven care to both individual providers and entire organizations, such as hospitals and health systems.

We identified three activities supported by the economic infrastructures. First, these infrastructures supported efforts to generate participation in the ACO model. Financial rewards induced key parties to participate by making it more appealing economically than the alternative. For example, one of the ACOs pointed to the premium rates or per-member per-month (PMPM) payments that they provide to independent physician practices as instrumental in getting those practices to join or otherwise cooperate with the ACO:

> I think it's been very interesting about how [the ACO has] gotten, for the most part, really all of the [primary care] providers—definitely in this community—to be a part of the organization. And they've been able to do that [by] being able to pay them a little bit extra I think for the work that they do. (Manager)

Moreover, in some instances, financial incentives provided an inducement to participate in various ACO initiatives. For example, one ACO offered an "engagement cap," a modest PMPM payment to encourage practices to participate in efforts to enhance primary care through the establishment of patient-centered medical homes (PCMHs), a comprehensive care delivery model in which all care is oriented around the whole person and coordinated through the primary care setting:

> The engagement cap basically says you will let us come into your practice and help turn you into a medical home. You know, you'll be receptive, and we'll work together. And it also says that you will share data with us—whatever data you have anyway—you will share it with us. That's the engagement cap. Pretty easy to get at this point. (Executive)

Similarly, the financial terms of the contracts the ACOs negotiated with payers made participation in risk-bearing ACO arrangements appealing. For example, leaders at one ACO viewed the full financial risk model as attractive because it allowed them to "get closer to the dollar" and ensure their own financial stability in a time when there were "some serious liquidity issues" with one of their largest payers.

Second, the economic infrastructure supported efforts to direct attention toward the goal of accountable care in general and toward specific performance or quality targets in particular. As one ACO executive stated, "When you put a little bit of money—it doesn't have to be a tremendous amount of money, … it gets people to pay attention." Another ACO leader at the same site explained how that organization used financial rewards to focus provider attention on quality metrics as part of its long-standing quality improvement program:

> So [in 1996], it sort of wasn't on anybody's horizons, but we put a quality program in place and started setting aside a portion of physician reimbursement and distributing it back to them based on performance in quality studies. (Executive)

The other three ACOs also tied a portion of provider reimbursement to quality targets as a means of increasing attention to quality. However, in contrast to the sentiment described above, the amount of the incentive does impact the ability of that incentive to capture attention—for at least some physicians. As one physician said, "[U]nless it's a boatload of money, it's not going to attract my attention."

Third, the economic infrastructure was intended to support efforts to improve performance. In addition to directing attention toward certain quality or performance targets, the promise of financial rewards for achieving those targets was perceived as leading to improved performance. One leader explained:

> And we also have a structure where one of the keys is … that we don't distribute all of the dollars in the incentive group. So each physician has an amount they can earn, but they only get sort of the percent they actually … earn out of that, and any that they don't earn just gets [put back] into the big incentive pool for next year, for all physicians to be funded. So, there is some real incentive to actually [improve] your performance. (Executive)

Sociocultural Infrastructure

ACOs require new ways of working, including increased cooperation and coordination among health care providers and the incorporation of cost and quality considerations into decisions. These new ways of working appear to rely on a well-developed sociocultural infrastructure. Thus, each of the four ACOs exerted considerable time and effort to build sociocultural infrastructures—that is, to establish, maintain, and enhance relationships and to develop shared beliefs and values. ACO leaders spoke of their efforts to gain the trust of various stakeholders, from providers to staff to payers to policy makers. They emphasized the crucial role that effective communication and repeated interactions played in these efforts to build relationships and to generate understanding of and commitment to the ACO model and goals.

Informants at all four ACOs spoke of the challenge involved in shifting from mental models associated with traditional care delivery approaches to new mental models required for accountable care. In particular, informants suggested that many stakeholders had difficulty shifting from a focus on volume and individual patients to a focus on value, prevention, populations, and the careful management of risk. This shift in thinking, however, was perceived as critical to success of the ACO model. One leader explained:

> You definitely have to have engaged providers or seek a way to engage the providers or else it doesn't work. And you've got to have medical staff that's fully on board with the concept. I mean it's a pretty big change even for medical people to kind of go to this value proposition and manage in population health instead of just managing specific episodes or something. You need a pretty committed medical staff to make it work. (Executive)

Changes in financial incentives, while necessary, were not sufficient to generate this shift, perhaps in part because some changes in behaviors, structures, and ways of thinking needed to happen before the new financial models were fully implemented or results were available. In addition, the amount of financial incentives was not always sufficient in and of itself to support change. Rather, as one ACO manager explained, it took "a lot of hand holding, a lot of communication, a lot of involvement in building this whole thing." This same manager emphasized the importance of

> really good communication over and over and over and over again. This is difficult to understand. You know, even our [hospital leadership], I'd say to date, there's still some of them that don't—this isn't quite gelling yet.... but it takes a lot of time. It's not easy stuff, you know. (Manager)

Consequently, ACO leaders stressed that constructing the necessary sociocultural infrastructure takes considerable time and effort:

> We like to say we were an overnight success nine years in the making. We could see this coming down the pike. ... [We] first did the [commercial] shared savings. I was a hospital president at the time. It took no less than four times for us to really, to hear it, to absorb it, and to appreciate what this was beginning to do. (Executive)

Importantly, none of these organizations built this sociocultural infrastructure from scratch with the launch of the ACO. Instead, they leveraged existing relationships and values. They then worked to enhance and add to them over time.

Constructing the sociocultural infrastructure entailed not only building relationships and mental models *within* the ACO but also with key external entities. Leaders at all four ACOs stated that good working relationships with payers (insurance companies, Medicare, etc.) provided foundations on which to have fruitful contract negotiations. At the two pediatric ACOs, for example, leaders stressed the importance of good relationships with Medicaid managed care organizations, and one pediatric ACO pointed to strong positive relationships with state government as crucial to their success.

ACO sociocultural infrastructures also included mechanisms for involving physicians in governance or otherwise ensuring that provider perspectives and concerns were considered in key decision-making processes. One ACO executive said, "You need to have very strong governance partnership with physicians, both employed and independent. That's a foundational piece." Physicians were included on the governing boards of Advocate, New West, and PFK. CMPCN did not include independent physicians on its governance board, but it did solicit input from those practitioners regularly through an advisory council. These approaches to governance and decision making are sociocultural in the sense that they infuse the values and perspectives of providers into the actions and structures of the organization and help to generate commitment and a sense of identity with the organization on the part of independent practitioners.

The sociocultural infrastructures support efforts to change behaviors and practice patterns in ways that appear to be crucial for ACO success. First, having established shared values around population health, quality metrics, and accountable care goals more generally, ACO leaders were then able to use this sociocultural infrastructure as a foundation on which to leverage motivators to drive provider behavior changes. For example, all four ACOs used comparative reporting to show individual providers or practices how their performance on certain key ACO measures compared with those of their peers in the organization. This comparative reporting then stimulated the motivation of providers to meet or exceed group performance levels, as one manager explained:

> We've been able to—over time—just kind of compare that data from office to office. So, we may say, "[T]his is where you are," and then compare them to other offices. So, [compared to] other offices, you're doing really well in your asthma action plans. ... So, we've seen value in that too, because in general, providers are very competitive, and they like to see where they fall. (Manager)

One of the ACOs took this comparative reporting one step farther, displaying unblinded rankings of providers on various quality measures at quarterly stakeholder meetings. Several informants suggested that this practice regularly motivated those individuals ranked near the bottom to improve their performances in subsequent reports.

Second, the sociocultural infrastructure enabled ACO efforts to intervene and transform practices directly for those matters that could not be addressed by simply stimulating motivation. ACO leaders perceived that the trust-based relationships, shared values, and mental models that they worked to build subsequently made it easier for them to intervene and transform practice patterns, as one ACO executive explained:

> And once you've got the physicians' buy-in, really, the training or the education associated with managing risk was really very simple. Prescribe generic drugs, try an ultrasound before you order a CAT scan: just do the right thing the first time, but make sure that it is the right thing, that you haven't jumped from A to Z without … yeah. It's a mindset. It really is a mindset. (Executive)

All four ACOs had programs of varying kinds aimed at practice improvement, such as providing care coordination services, implementing electronic health records, building patient-centered medical homes (PCMHs), and providing training in quality improvement methods (a matter we discuss later in this chapter). While established trust-based relationships opened the way for these interventions, in some instances these interventions were nevertheless met with resistance. Moreover, as the following account demonstrates, the sociocultural infrastructure continues to develop over time, with each subsequent action and interaction either weakening or strengthening the foundation:

> We have the benefit of a culture with independent physicians which is based in some trust, but trust has a limit. And the trust is built up over time, … delivering on our promise to reimburse them for quality results. And, yet, when we wanted to put care managers in their offices, that pushed up against that limit of our trust that we had with them. And in fact, it was one physician that even said, you know, "I don't trust anybody I don't pay." So they thought maybe we'd be spies. … A couple of weeks ago … we met with him and his care manager, and he said, "Please don't ever take this resource away from me. I can't afford it, and it's delivering so much great value." (Manager)

Finally, as with the economic infrastructure, the sociocultural foundations also appear to encourage parties to participate in the ACO. Informants suggested that a sense of trust in the organization or an identification with its mission motivated some independent providers to join:

> [T]hat trust factor as a partner was there with the independent physicians, and I felt like the physicians understood, most of them, that [the ACO] is the place that I want to practice, and [the ACO] is the place that I know is going to be successful in this venture or this journey. (Executive)

Information Infrastructure

While economic and sociocultural infrastructures support participation and are crucial foundations for changing behaviors, ACOs also need the practical capabilities to monitor, measure, and manage the performance of the organization, the health of populations, and the care provided to individual patients. Leaders at all four ACOs emphasized the importance that data, information technologies, and reporting play in achieving the goal of accountable care. Sufficient access to reliable data was perceived as crucial by all four ACOs. For example, leaders at one ACO explained how a lack of access to historical data on a particular population led the organization to pursue a shared savings model rather than the full-risk model they were simultaneously pursuing with another population for which they had extensive historical data. All four ACOs had developed or were developing information processing capabilities, harnessing electronic health record (EHR) data, utilizing patient registries, and in some cases, constructing data warehouses. Although all four sites noted problems with payer claims data, including delays in availability, they all stressed the importance of obtaining and using these data to track performance and drive improvement.

Given the limitations of claims data, however, all four sites recognized the value of producing and analyzing internally generated data. In most cases, this meant investments in EHRs. One ACO adopted a single EHR system for all practices and obtained agreement from local hospitals that were not directly affiliated with the ACO to access those hospitals' EHRs in order to monitor ACO patients who were hospitalized. Another ACO instituted an EHR mandate for all independent practices involved in the ACO. Where EHRs were less common and financial resources to obtain them were limited, ACO leaders built alternative information infrastructures to enable data sharing and reporting needed for population health management activities, as one ACO manager explained:

> In our market, the practices that we deal with, most do not have [EHRs]—can't financially afford the EMRs. So that's a challenge. So, we have a portal that we're setting up so that they can go in and start pulling their data, but we just started

that, and it's really kind of a basic site. Here's your panel listing, here's your gaps in care report, ... and actually a couple of weeks ago [we] just released a new feature on the portal where, if their patients are seen at any of our ... hospitals, they get live data feeds. (Manager)

Developing robust information infrastructures was a significant challenge identified by leaders at all four ACOs. Information infrastructures to support population health management require timely, reliable, complete datasets. Informants identified the incompleteness of data as a significant source of challenge:

I think the most difficult—well, again, this [is] from my point of view—probably the most difficult thing we've faced is really data. Getting the data that we need to really be able to perform what we need for population management. And that's seeing all of the data on the patients, not only the data that's for care provided [by ACO providers]. So, you really see the whole spectrum of the patient. So you can do your risk assessment, so you can help the patients, help the doctors understand, get focused, I guess, on the care that's really needed.... [O]nce they go out of—I don't want to say out of network, but where we can't see the data, we're blind, basically. So, ... it's been a struggle. (Executive)

At one ACO, most of the affiliated independent primary care providers lacked EHRs. This lack, in turn, made it difficult for that ACO to build a fully robust information infrastructure. Similarly, informants at another ACO reported that data on care provided outside of the ACO typically came in paper format and required scanning. This format limited the analytic capabilities of the ACO.

Information infrastructure supported key activities related to population health management. For example, information infrastructure was crucial to efforts to stratify and manage the downside risk associated with the populations for which they were responsible. Information infrastructure also enabled monitoring of performance, including patient outcomes, utilization of services (both preventive and acute), and various measures of quality and costs. All ACOs produced a variety of reports that allowed them to monitor performance along different dimensions and at various levels of the organization. For example, as one ACO manager explained:

We have a monthly report that we produce.... We came up with five measures that allow us to understand how we're managing the population. So, we look at admits per 1000, readmissions overall for the population, ER visits per 1000, and then a measure of care coordination, which we've defined as admissions at [our] hospitals.... And then we have reports

that drill down even further, down to the individual practice
level. And we distribute data to those physicians monthly.
(Manager)

This monitoring, in turn, provided information necessary to identify
areas for improvement, to allot financial rewards, and to demonstrate
value or the need for change.

Care Continuum Infrastructure

To effectively manage population health, ACOs need to be able to ensure
the availability and coordination of cost-effective, high-quality services
across the care continuum, either by directly providing those services or
by contracting with outside providers. None of the ACOs we studied were
fully vertically integrated across all types of services. One ACO manager
explained what this meant:

> If it's not a big group like this, then you do have to find
> those partners who can provide some of those other services.
> It makes it a lot easier if it's all right here in one place, but
> otherwise you're going to have to make sure that you get all of
> the other pieces. So you've got to bring many more people to
> the table and many more contractual relationships. (Manager)

Consequently, all four organizations had to engage in developing contractual arrangements with other providers, including in some cases those
who were technically outside of the ACO. For example, one ACO we
studied did not have long-term care facilities, including skilled nursing
facilities (SNFs) in its system. Nevertheless, when setting up the ACO,
post-acute care was identified as a significant expense and an area requiring careful management. One executive explained the strategy:

> We have thirty SNFs that we partnered [with] in an
> arrangement where we put our providers in their facilities every
> day. So I have now thirty advanced practice nurses that report
> up to me that partner and collaborate with [our] physicians to
> manage all the patients discharged to the thirty facilities. . . .
> Our goal is to follow that patient, transition them well from
> hospital to SNF, to prevent any readmissions, and to manage
> their length of stay appropriately in the SNF, and then make
> sure they're discharged back to [our] services. (Executive)

Advocate used 5 full-time and 15 part-time "SNFists," physicians who
practice in an SNF (similar to hospitalists) to manage the care of ACO
patients discharged to the 30 facilities that were technically outside of the
ACO. In a similar manner, another ACO, comprised entirely of primary

care providers, developed contractual arrangements with area hospitals and employed eight hospitalists to oversee the care of patients during hospitalizations. That organization also diligently managed its specialist referral network to ensure it was referring patients only to specialists who practiced in ways that aligned with the ACO's mission of providing cost-effective, high-quality care:

> So over a long period of time, literally, five, ten, fifteen years, in some cases, you get a fairly good subjective gestalt about both the quality and cost efficiency of specialist practices, and so far, that's what we've used to make our decisions. We can also tell based on which specialists come to us to embrace us as partners. So we have a cardiology group, for example, that routinely meets with us and brings to us new initiatives on how to improve cost and quality. And, you know, that's a no-brainer. The other cardiology practices in town don't do that.... [O]ver time, we've honed what we believe to be a good balance of cost-effective, quality [specialist] physicians. (Executive)

Both of the pediatric ACOs owned nearly all pediatric specialty and hospital services within their respective regions, and so these ACOs built their care continuum infrastructure by contracting with local independent pediatricians to include them within the ACOs. Buying practices was another strategy that leaders acknowledged having considered, but none of the ACOs we studied had actively pursued this approach.

Another feature of the care continuum infrastructure pertained to structures that bridged the transitions between care settings and reduced fragmentation. One ACO identified transitions as one of its eight strategic domains and developed information sharing processes to improve transitions between institutions and from institutions to the outpatient setting. Other ACOs hired staff, such as physician assistants, to contact and counsel all ACO patients discharged from hospitals. In addition, all four ACOs included some form of care coordinator or case management program, typically aimed at coordinating the care of the most complex, high-utilization patients. For example, one informant explained that case management was used for patients who were high utilizers of emergency departments or who have certain diagnoses associated with high costs:

> [W]e have certain disease processes that just automatically flag and are sent to the case managers, you know, terminal illnesses, again chronic comorbidities, different things that trigger kind of a response to the case manager. Ideally the case manager should outreach back to the [primary care provider] and then just kind of collaborate care. (Manager)

Finally, robust care continuum infrastructures also involved programs to enhance the capabilities of independent primary care practices. All four ACOs had programs in place to help individual practices improve their abilities to manage their attributed patient panels. Two ACOs had dedicated teams that were helping practices set up PCMHs. Similar efforts at a third ACO resulted in all practices achieving Level 3 PCMH certification, the highest level available from the National Committee for Quality Assurance accreditation program. All four ACOs also had programs to help practices improve their processes. Three ACOs had teams that conducted or trained practices in conducting PDSA (plan–do–study–act) quality improvement cycles to enhance efficiency and improve utilization of preventive care services. At the fourth ACO, a medical management committee reviewed the relevant research literature and set practice guidelines, which were then disseminated to all practices in the organization.

The care continuum infrastructure supported key activities related to population health management. For example, this infrastructure enabled the ACOs to provide high-quality cost-effective services across the care continuum, either directly from providers who adhered to the mission of the ACO or through contractual arrangements with external providers. In addition, the care continuum infrastructure provided ACOs the capabilities to control, to some extent, the utilization, integration, coordination, and ongoing improvement of health care services. This infrastructure was pivotal to efforts to improve the utilization of preventive services and to decrease the utilization of high-cost services, such as emergency department (ED) visits, often associated with the lack of primary care or the undermanagement of chronic conditions. Finally, some of the mechanisms built into this infrastructure enabled the organizations to drive desired behavior changes by altering processes through practice improvement interventions.

Interdependencies of the Four Infrastructures

The four infrastructures can interrelate in intricate ways such that changes to one may necessitate adjustments to another. One instance of this can be seen in the following story in which an advisory committee, comprising community primary care physicians, reacted to proposed changes to the economic infrastructure (i.e., physician compensation), citing deficiencies in the information infrastructure:

> One of the things that [affects physician] compensation is ED utilization, and it's a visit per thousands type of measure. And when we sort of introduced the overall compensation model, we said, this'll be one of the measurements. And the docs were sort of, okay. There wasn't a lot of pushback there. But they said, "If we're going to do that, we need sort of real-

time data when it comes to our patients and when they're in the ED, 'cause what we get now is, we get sort of a quarterly profile report that shows what our metrics are. That doesn't really help us. That's claims data. There's a six-month lag." You know, all that stuff.... So, we built basically a data feed into our data warehouse from the hospital that says when John Doe ... is in our ED or Urgent Care, ... the community PCP will get a notice of that the next morning.... So, it was the community docs on that [committee] that said, ... "[W]e'll be measured and paid according to that, ... but give us some real-time data." (Executive)

In this example, a proposed change to the economic infrastructure prompted the community PCPs to request an enhancement of the information infrastructure. The belief implied is that both infrastructures had to be adjusted—mutually adjusted—if there was to be any chance of achieving the goal of reducing ED utilization. Moreover, the sociocultural infrastructure is also at play in this story. The existence of the physician advisory committee and, more important, the fact that administrators listened to that committee, would indicate the influence of a culture that values the perspective of the community physician. In short, the work of achieving, maintaining, and improving alignment may often involve interactions among the different infrastructures as each one has potentially an enabling and constraining effect on the others.

Similarly, getting access to data needed to construct the information infrastructure often involved leveraging the relationships and trust of the sociocultural infrastructure. For example, in preparing to assume full risk for a particular defined population, one ACO needed access to historical data—which only the payer had—on that population. When explaining how they were able to obtain these data, informants pointed to their positive relationships with the payer. Building and executing economic infrastructures that are fair and motivating requires access to data on cost and quality performance trends. One ACO noted that its initial financial incentive structure proved too complicated to execute given limitations of the existing information infrastructure. These examples are illustrative, but not exhaustive, of the interdependencies among the different infrastructures. These interdependencies suggest that the initial work of constructing and the ongoing activities of maintaining and enhancing an ACO are highly complex and challenging endeavors.

DISCUSSION

Accountable care organizations are far more than payment reforms. While significant changes to reimbursement and incentive arrangements were key aspects of the ACOs we studied, these economic elements represent only a portion of the complex, interdependent infrastructures that the organizations were constructing. Our findings suggest that ACOs require new ways of working together, with a greater focus on collaboration and interpersonal skills. Thus, extensive resources must also be devoted to building infrastructures that would support the social and operational aspects of reorganized work. ACOs need strong economic models that give providers a greater stake in performance and incent them to pursue the goal of providing high-quality, cost-effective care (Fisher and Shortell 2010; Lowell and Bertko 2010; Shortell and Casalino 2008). But ACO stakeholders also need trust-based relationships, shared values, and common mental models to help them negotiate mutually beneficial arrangements, align their efforts, and make difficult changes. In addition, to deliver accountable care, ACOs need extensive, dependable, robust data; sophisticated information technology systems; and advanced analytic and informative dissemination capabilities. They also need the means to provide care across the continuum; to oversee, improve, and ensure the quality of that care; and to coordinate it effectively. In short, ACOs require a complex set of infrastructures to undergird and support their efforts to achieve the goal of accountable care.

Importantly, these infrastructures *enable* actions. They are not sufficient in themselves. Rather, they are the foundation on which changes may be enacted. Our goal in this chapter has been to develop a framework that highlights the infrastructures that form the foundation of an ACO and to draw attention to the considerable complexity of that foundation. In separate analyses, we explored the actions that these ACOs are taking to change behaviors and create alignment (Hilligoss, Song, and McAlearney, forthcoming).

Some ACO activities are supported by more than one infrastructure. For example, all four infrastructures appear to be important for transforming practice patterns and motivating provider behavior changes. Financial incentives (economic infrastructure); relationships and social motivators (sociocultural infrastructure); data, analytics, and reports (information infrastructure); and process improvements (care continuum infrastructure) together provide the foundation on which such transformations may be pursued. In addition, our findings indicate that the infrastructures interrelate in complex ways, such that changes to one may necessitate corresponding changes to another. This would suggest that, although it may be convenient for analytic purposes to conceptualize and discuss the infrastructures separately, in practice they must be constructed and managed simultaneously and interdependently.

This interdependency highlights yet another implication: an ACO is not a one-time build. Rather, it is an ongoing construction that must be tended to, enhanced, and adjusted over time. Indeed, in spite of having had many years of experience assuming risk and managing the health of populations, all four of the ACOs in our study represent evolving models. The continuous state of change that characterizes the health care sector necessitates this. Health care organizations are still learning how to leverage the power of the data they have and of information technologies. They are still experimenting with different reimbursement and financial incentive arrangements. They are still exploring what new relationships might be forged among entities that were previously independent, and they are still developing new mental models of what it means to be accountable for the health of populations (Halfon et al. 2014). As these experimentations and explorations continue, the interrelationships between and among the infrastructures must be re-examined, and the infrastructures themselves must be mutually adjusted and realigned.

The interdependencies of the infrastructures also have implications for efforts to measure the impact of specific mechanisms, such as particular incentive arrangements. Because multiple infrastructures are likely contributing to outcomes, teasing apart their impacts may be difficult at best. A robust evaluation of an ACO will, therefore, likely need to include measures of multiple infrastructures (Fisher et al. 2012; Shortell, Casalino, and Fisher 2010). Further research might examine in greater detail how different infrastructures interact and influence one another, whether certain combinations of infrastructural arrangements are more useful for attaining the goal of accountable care than others, and how ACO leaders use these infrastructures to drive changes in behaviors and outcomes.

Strengths and Limitations

We confined our analysis here to identifying the core infrastructures that constitute the foundations of four commercial ACOs operating in the private sector. While we cannot assert the generalizability of our findings, the fact that these infrastructures are common to four rather significantly different organizations seems to suggest some degree of transferability of the findings. Furthermore, many aspects of our framework relate to findings from other empirical studies (Colla, Lewis, Shortell, and Fisher 2014; Fisher et al. 2012; Kreindler et al. 2012) and to assertions of expert opinions (Burns and Pauly 2012; McClellan et al. 2010; Shortell, Casalino, and Fisher 2010; Singer and Shortell 2011) expressed in the literature. Our work adds to this existing literature by drawing together a variety of ideas into a unifying framework of ACO infrastructure. In so doing, we highlighted the complex interdependent nature of the foundation that appears to be required for delivering accountable care. Our framework was inductively developed from and grounded in four in-depth empirical case studies. As with any theoretical framework, it provides but one way to view the phenomenon. Other framings are surely possible.

ACKNOWLEDGMENTS

The authors are extremely grateful to the organizations and informants who participated in this study and to the members of our project advisory team. We also thank our research team members who assisted at various stages of this project: Dr. Julie Robbins, Dr. Jennifer Hefner, Daniel Gaines, Pamela Beavers, Alexandra Moss, Megan Sinclair, Kendall Haas, Mary Frances Gardner, and Jessica Stewart. This research was funded by the Robert Wood Johnson Foundation; however, the study sponsors had no involvement in the collection, analysis, or interpretation of data; in the writing of this manuscript; or in the decision to submit the manuscript for publication.

REFERENCES

Addicott, R., and S. M. Shortell. 2014. "How 'Accountable' Are Accountable Care Organizations?" *Health Care Management Review* 39, no. 4: 270–78. doi:10.1097/hmr.0000000000000002.

Berwick, D. M., T. W. Nolan, and J. Whittington. 2008. "The Triple Aim: Care, Health, and Cost." *Health Affairs* 27, no. 3: 759–69. doi:10.1377/hlthaff.27.3.759.

Bowker, G. C., and S. L. Star. 1999. *Sorting Things Out: Classification and Its Consequences.* Cambridge, MA: MIT Press.

Burns, L. R., and M. V. Pauly. 2012. "Accountable Care Organizations May Have Difficulty Avoiding the Failures of Integrated Delivery Networks of the 1990s." *Health Affairs* 31, no. 11: 2407–416. doi:10.1377/hlthaff.2011.0675.

Casalino, L. P., N. Erb, M. S. Joshi, and S. M. Shortell. 2015. "Accountable Care Organizations and Population Health Organizations." *Journal of Health Politics, Policy and Law* 40, no. 4: 821–37. doi:10.1215/03616878-3150074.

Charmaz, K. 2006. *Constructing Grounded Theory: A Practical Guide Through Qualitative Analysis.* London, UK: Sage.

Colla, C. H., V. A. Lewis, S. M. Shortell, and E. S. Fisher. 2014. "First National Survey of ACOs Finds That Physicians Are Playing Strong Leadership and Ownership Roles." *Health Affairs* 33, no. 6: 964–71. doi:10.1377/hlthaff.2013.1463.

Crosson, F. J. 2011. "The Accountable Care Organization: Whatever Its Growing Pains, the Concept Is Too Vitally Important to Fail." *Health Affairs* 30, no. 7: 1250–55. doi:10.1377/hlthaff.2011.0272.

Fisher, E. S., M. B. McClellan, J. Bertko, S. M. Lieberman, J. J. Lee, J. L. Lewis, and J. S. Skinner. 2009. "Fostering Accountable Health Care: Moving Forward in Medicare." *Health Affairs* 28, no. 2. doi:10.1377/hlthaff.28.2.w219.

Fisher, E. S., and S. M. Shortell. 2010. "Accountable Care Organizations: Accountable for What, to Whom, and How." *Journal of the American Medical Association* 304, no. 15: 1715–16. doi:10.1001/jama.2010.1513.

Fisher, E. S., S. M. Shortell, S. A. Kreindler, A. D. Van Citters, and B. K. Larson. 2012. "A Framework for Evaluating the Formation, Implementation, and Performance of Accountable Care Organizations." *Health Affairs* 31, no. 11: 2368–78. doi:10.1377/hlthaff.2012.0544.

Halfon, N., P. Long, D. I. Chang, J. Hester, M. Inkelas, and A. Rodgers. 2014. "Applying a 3.0 Transformation Framework to Guide Large-Scale Health System Reform." *Health Affairs* 33, no. 11: 2003–11. doi:10.1377/hlthaff.2014.0485.

Hilligoss, B., P. H. Song, and A. S. McAlearney. Forthcoming. "Aligning for Accountable Care: Strategic Practices for Change in Accountable Care Organizations." *Health Care Management Review*.

Kreindler, S. A., B. K. Larson, F. M. Wu, K. L. Carluzzo, J. N. Gbemudu, A. Struthers, A. D. Van Citters, S. M. Shortell, E. C. Nelson, and E. S. Fisher. 2012. "Interpretations of Integration in Early Accountable Care Organizations." *Milbank Quarterly* 90, no. 3: 457–83. doi:10.1111/j.1468-0009.2012.00671.x.

Kreindler, S. A., B. K. Larson, F. M. Wu, J. N. Gbemudu, K. L. Carluzzo, A. Struthers, A. D. Van Citters, S. M. Shortell, E. C. Nelson, and E. S. Fisher. 2014. "The Rules of Engagement: Physician Engagement Strategies in Intergroup Contexts." *Journal of Health Organization and Management* 28, no. 1: 41–61. doi:10.1108/jhom-02-2013-0024.

Larson, B. K., A. D. Van Citters, S. A. Kreindler, K. L. Carluzzo, J. N. Gbemudu, F. M. Wu, E. C. Nelson, S. M. Shortell, and E. S. Fisher. 2012. "Insights from Transformations Under Way at Four Brookings-Dartmouth Accountable Care Organization Pilot Sites." *Health Affairs* 31, no. 11: 2395–406. doi:10.1377/hlthaff.2011.1219.

Lowell, K. H., and J. Bertko. 2010. "The Accountable Care Organization (ACO) Model." *Journal of Ambulatory Care Management* 33, no. 1: 81–88. doi:10.1097/jac.0b013e3181c9fb12.

McAlearney, A. S., P. H. Song, and B. Hilligoss. Forthcoming. "Accountable Care Organization Development in the Private Sector: A Qualitative Study of Four Organizations." *American Journal of Managed Care*.

McClellan, M., A. N. McKethan, J. L. Lewis, J. Roski, and E. S. Fisher. 2010. "A National Strategy to Put Accountable Care into Practice." *Health Affairs* 29, no. 5: 982–90. doi:10.1377/hlthaff.2010.0194.

McWilliams, J. M., M. E. Chernew, B. E. Landon, and A. L. Schwartz. 2015. "Performance Differences in Year 1 of Pioneer Accountable Care Organizations." *New England Journal of Medicine* 372, no. 20: 1927–36. doi:10.1056/nejmsa1414929.

McWilliams, J. M., B. E. Landon, M. E. Chernew, and A. M. Zaslavsky. 2014. "Changes in Patients' Experiences in Medicare Accountable Care Organizations." *New England Journal of Medicine* 371, no. 18: 1715–24. doi:10.1056/nejmsa1406552.

National Priorities Partnership. 2008. "National Priorities and Goals: Aligning Our Efforts to Transform America's Healthcare." Report. Washington, DC: National Quality Forum.

Porter, M. E. "What Is Value in Health Care?" 2010. *New England Journal of Medicine* 363, no. 26: 2477–81. doi:10.1056/nejmp1011024.

Rittenhouse, D. R., S. M. Shortell, and E. S. Fisher. 2009. "Primary Care and Accountable Care—Two Essential Elements of Delivery-System Reform." *New England Journal of Medicine* 361, no. 24: 2301–03. doi:10.1056/nejmp0909327.

Rundall, T. G., F. M. Wu, V. A. Lewis, K. E. Schoenherr, and S. M. Shortell. 2016. "Relational Coordination in Accountable Care Organizations: Potential Key to Strengthening Patient Care Management." *Health Care Management Review* 41, no. 2: 88–100. doi:10.1097/HMR.0000000000000064.

Salmon, R. B., M. I. Sanderson, B. A. Walters, K. Kennedy, R. C. Flores, and A. M. Muney. 2012. "A Collaborative Accountable Care Model in Three Practices Showed Promising Early Results on Costs and Quality of Care." *Health Affairs* 31, no. 11: 2379–87. doi:10.1377/hlthaff.2012.0354.

Shortell, S. M., and L. P. Casalino. 2008. "Health Care Reform Requires Accountable Care Systems." *Journal of the American Medical Association* 300, no. 1: 95–97. doi:10.1001/jama.300.1.95.

Shortell, S. M., and L. P. Casalino. 2010. "Implementing Qualifications Criteria and Technical Assistance for Accountable Care Organizations." *Journal of the American Medical Association* 303, no. 17: 1747–48. doi:10.1001/jama.2010.575.

Shortell, S. M., L. P. Casalino, and E. S. Fisher. 2010. "How the Center for Medicare and Medicaid Innovation Should Test Accountable Care Organizations." *Health Affairs* 29, no. 7: 1293–98. doi:10.1377/hlthaff.2010.0453.

Shortell, S. M., N. J. Sehgal, S. Bibi, P. P. Ramsay, L. Neuhauser, C. H. Colla, and V. A. Lewis. 2015. "An Early Assessment of Accountable Care Organizations' Efforts to Engage Patients and Their Families." *Medical Care Research and Review* 72, no. 5: 580–604. doi:10.1177/1077558715588874.

Singer, S. J., and S. M. Shortell. 2011. "Implementing Accountable Care Organizations." *Journal of the American Medical Association* 306, no. 7: 758–59. doi:10.1001/jama.2011.1180.

Song, Z., S. Rose, D. G. Safran, B. E. Landon, M. P. Day, and M. E. Chernew. 2014. "Changes in Health Care Spending and Quality 4 Years into Global Payment." *New England Journal of Medicine* 371, no. 18: 1704–14. doi:10.1056/nejmsa1404026.

Yin, R. K. *Case Study Research: Design and Methods* (3rd edition). 2003. Thousand Oaks, CA: Sage.

CHAPTER 4

Who Regulates? Physicians and the Regulation of Health Care

REBECCA KOLINS GIVAN
School of Management and Labor Relations
Rutgers University

INTRODUCTION

All health care systems must be regulated by someone or something. Whether publicly or privately funded, health care is a high-risk service, and all aspects of its provision are subject to a high degree of monitoring and control. The regulation of health care includes the regulation of health care professionals, health care facilities, payment mechanisms, care protocols, allowable drugs and devices, and more (Field 2008). In practice, this regulation is truly a patchwork quilt of public and private organizations, professional associations, credentialing agencies, accreditors, commissions, and other entities (Moncrieff and Lee 2012). This set of rules, laws, and certifications structures the delivery of care, regulating who can provide care and which organizations can operate in the health care sector (see, for example, Dixon and Ham 2010).

Health care systems are governed by a broad array of regulations, created and enforced by a series of different public and private agencies (Jost 1995). In this chapter, I examine the role of public and private interests in regulating health care. I find that in the United States, regulation is dominated by the organized interests of physicians, through their professional associations. (There are more licensed nurses than physicians in the United States, but their professional associations and unions have never achieved influence beyond the narrow, more traditional areas of professional self-regulation. Nurses simply do not influence broad areas such as payment systems and care protocols.) I argue that the dominant doctors group behaves like owners, controlling the means of health care delivery, even as the interests of most practicing physicians are not well represented.

This chapter presents an analysis of the role of physicians in health care regulation in the United States. The latter part of the chapter introduces a comparison with the United Kingdom to illuminate the striking features of the U.S. system. Comparative research, particularly regarding national institutions, provides important analytic leverage in understanding the key similarities and differences in specific contexts (Dutton 2007; Giaimo and Manow 1999; Hall and Soskice 2001). The key question here is how and whether professionals influence the regulation of health care. The evidence presented shows that in the United States, the dominant professional association in health care, the American Medical Association (AMA), has broad and deep influence over the regulation of health care, while uncovering the paradox that the association does not represent the interests of most physicians. Rather, most physicians have lost their professional autonomy—to the very regulatory web to which the AMA has contributed—and become more like standard employees with a diminished capacity to exercise professional judgment.

Through this analysis of the role of physicians in health care regulation, we see the ways that professional associations in the United States have become closely aligned with employers (and, conversely, that professional associations in the United Kingdom are behaving more like pure trade unions, representing the members of the profession as employees). The relationship between physician associations and bureaucratic regulators is complex—in the United States, the associations have become deeply entwined with the regulators.

This chapter presents several key aspects of health care regulation, including the regulation of professional education and credentialing; the regulation of health care facilities; and the regulation of care protocols and payments. While not comprehensive, those areas cover most of the key bureaucratic interventions in the provision of health care in both countries—reflecting who can deliver care, where they can deliver it, and how they can deliver it.

Regulation in health care is outsourced or delegated by the government. To some degree, this delegation makes sense because it shields regulators from pressures from lobbyists or party political interests. In the United States, the outsourced regulators are heavily linked to (and in some cases controlled by) organized physician interests. Chief among these organizations ostensibly giving voice to professionals is the AMA, which has control over the specialist billing system and significant influence over the Joint Commission (formerly the Joint Commission on the Accreditation of Healthcare Organizations), which has control over hospital accreditation.

A key issue here is the relationship between individual physicians and the AMA. There are numerous rank-and-file physicians who do not support the actions of their de facto singular professional association, such as the members of Physicians for a National Health Program, and the physicians whose professional judgment has been ousted by a profit-seeking managerial class seeking to cut costs and improve "efficiency" (see, for example, Scheiber 2016). It is essential to note that while for most professional groups, "organizational communities may be comprised of subcommunities whose interests stubbornly do not align," in the case of physicians in the United States, this lack of alignment is particularly stark (Greenwood, Suddaby, and Hinings 2002: 76).

In the United States, there are requirements that are putatively voluntary (but de facto mandatory) that are controlled by private entities with little government oversight. In addition, there are numerous sources of overlap between the regulatory agencies, which run the risk of giving some professions outsized power and privatizing the regulation and control of public service and public spending. This creates an additional paradox. While the organized professional associations have consolidated their power and influence over the regulatory system, doctors on the ground are feeling increasingly squeezed. Cost pressures, increased accountability and monitoring, and expanding bureaucratic requirements all contribute to the pressure on front-line, rank-and-file doctors.

Increasingly, physicians feel that the AMA does not represent their interests: less than one quarter of physicians belong to the association. While polling shows that doctors largely favor single payer health care, the AMA has continued its staunch opposition, which has been its hallmark since the days of Franklin Roosevelt (Bybee 2008).

On the front lines of health care, the complex set of rules and regulations diminishes the autonomy and professional judgment of doctors, leading some to unionize (Scheiber 2016). In the past, doctors identified more strongly as producers, or at least professionals without a strong employee interest and distinct from management interests (for much more on that topic, see Starr 1982). There exists, then, a dichotomy in which the organized professional interests of physicians continue to be strong, well resourced, and influential, but many front-line doctors are left without a voice in their profession or their industry (Jackson & Coker 2011). Physicians as a whole, then, are in the paradoxical position of exercising powerful control over regulatory institutions while losing their voice on the front line. In this sense, physicians have become divided into powerful, influential leaders who control the professional associations and regulatory agencies, and the vast majority of rank-and-file physicians who have lost their professional voice and are saddled with the policies of these regulators, controlled by their sometimes professional allies (Physicians Foundation 2012).

PROFESSIONAL REGULATION IN MEDICINE

One key aspect of health care regulation is regulating a labor market dominated by licensed professionals. Traditionally, professionals regulate themselves, determining the education, training, and licensing necessary to use the title and the designated, codified, professional privileges. In this sense then, professionals are different from typical employees because their professional standards mediate the relationship between employer and employee. In other words, an employer cannot hire someone for an available professional job unless that person has met the professional standards, which are neither controlled nor administered by the employer. A professional who loses his or her license will lose his or her job regardless of the employer's preferences. Having control over their labor supply historically allowed these professionals to behave as a monopoly, keeping supply well regulated and wages high (Perkin 1990).

Physicians may seem to be the paradigmatic example of professionals, with the attendant control over education, licensing, and scope of practice. However, professionals do not simply attain this authority. They form powerful associations and leverage their power in the labor market to consolidate and expand their power (see also Greenwood, Suddaby, and Hinings 2002). In some cases, they use this power to protect their professional autonomy, while in others, such as the U.S. health care system, they begin to exert control over not only their own profession but the entire industry.

Self-regulating professional communities ideally keep standards high and provide the right balance of rewards and punishments to maintain high-quality practice. As Sir Donald Irvine, physician and onetime president of the General Medical Council, the licensing body for physicians in the United Kingdom, put it:

> Professionally led regulation is predicated on the fact that the practice of medicine still involves a considerable degree of judgment in the fundamental functions of diagnosis and decisions about treatment. Consequently patients, in the privacy of the consulting room, are still critically dependent on their doctors' getting it right the first time, knowing the limits of their competence and their honesty and integrity. Doctors practicing within a regulatory framework of professional values and standards—professional conscience—are more likely to give of their best for their patients than doctors who are not, because there is peer pressure to do so. (Irvine 2001: 166)

Thus, doctors in the United Kingdom regulate the profession quite narrowly. This is in sharp contrast to the key professional association in the United States, which exerts influence in all aspects of the health care industry, far beyond determining or protecting the role of doctors. The AMA is deeply influential in the United States, with some authority over billing and payment systems and entry to the profession, yet it represents a minority of practicing physicians and, indeed, many rank-and-file doctors feel deeply alienated by its positions. As one observer put it, "The institutional representatives of society do not always represent those that they claim to represent, just as the AMA does not represent all doctors" (Palmer 1999).

In addition to regulating their own professions, doctors tend to head other health care–related regulatory agencies. In both countries discussed in this chapter, there are a series of entities with responsibility for regulating different aspects of health care delivery, from licensing and credentialing professionals to accrediting facilities (Table 1). Many of these agencies and organizations are physician dominated, but in the American case, the AMA has institutionalized power within most of the key organizations and agencies.

PHYSICIAN CONTROL OF REGULATION

The key regulators of health care in the United States are dominated by physicians, with the AMA and specialty medical boards having essential roles. The AMA plays the public role of the voice of the medical profession, although it has only about one quarter of practicing physicians in membership. It has institutional influence in several other organizations, giving it deep influence throughout this regulatory web. The AMA has a fairly conservative history, including opposition to managed care and

TABLE 1
Major Health Care Regulatory Agencies

	United States	United Kingdom
Doctors	State licensing boards and jointly sponsored United States Medical Licensing Exam	General Medical Council
Medical Education	Accreditation Council for Graduate Medical Education* Liaison Committee on Medical Education*	General Medical Council
Facilities/Organizations	Joint Commission*	Care Quality Commission
Billing	Centers for Medicare and Medicaid Services American Medical Association*	N/A
Best Practice and Protocols	Centers for Medicare and Medicaid Services; also see the Patient-Centered Outcomes Research Institute	National Institute for Health and Care Excellence
Drugs and Devices	Food and Drug Administration	Medicine and Healthcare Products Regulatory Agency

*Indicates privately operated and controlled organization.

single-payer health care; in its early days it opposed all health insurance, but in the 1930s declared that voluntary health insurance was acceptable (Starr 1982: 273).

In 1940, about two thirds of doctors were AMA members—the high point for its membership (for the definitive account of the organized professional power of physicians in the United States before the early 1980s, see Starr 1982). Only 14% of the association's more than $280 million annual revenue comes from membership dues, while over 80% of its revenue comes from the sales of its publications and services, including its highly profitable journals and its lucrative billing and coding system, which is essentially required for all health care providers (American Medical Association 2015: 11).

It's clear, then, that the association is not financially dependent on its members to operate and that the bulk of its revenue is secure, regardless of the ebbs and flows of membership. Consequently, there is a disconnect between the organization's claim to speak for doctors and the reality that its material position requires it to behave like a corporation with a product to sell. The AMA, then, has a vested interest in protecting the status quo rather than improving the professional lives of working physicians, most of whom are not members.

One British observer has referred to the practice of medicine in the United States, specifically managed care, as "clinical micromanagement by contract and protocol" (Irvine 2001: 166). While this may be true, and indeed has profound effects on the day-to-day work of physicians, these contracts and protocols are substantially created by physician-dominated regulators—the alphabet soup of CMS, CPT, DRGs, and the Joint Commission. As DiMaggio and Powell point out, "In many cases, professional power is as much assigned by the state as it is created by the activities of the professions" (1983: 152).

As the regulatory network outlined in the following sections shows, much of the professional power of physicians in the United States derives from the power assigned to their associations by the state. Professional lives are made more difficult, and professional judgment is diminished by the regulatory web in which the AMA freely and profitably participates. This observation returns us to the crucial paradox that the key professional association has become intertwined with the interests of employers, leaving rank-and-file members of the profession in the position of employees with little authority or autonomy.

REGULATION OF CARE (PROTOCOLS AND PAYMENTS)

Most health care in the United States is covered by payment systems using current procedural terminology (CPT) codes for physician services and diagnosis-related groups (DRGs) for hospital charges. While the DRG categories are controlled by a government agency (the Centers for Medicare and Medicaid Services, or CMS), the CPT categories are controlled by the AMA, which profits greatly from its control and distribution of the database of categories. The prices for these services vary dramatically across the country, whether they are billed to Medicare/Medicaid (i.e., governmental) payers or to private insurers (Cooper, Craig, Gaynor, and Van Reenen 2015).

The billing system, but not the pricing system, is controlled by centralized regulators. One of these billing system regulators is a government agency, CMS, and the other, the AMA, is not. The pricing system, on the other hand is subject to the foibles of the market where, for example, hospitals with local monopolies charge more than hospitals in competitive geographic areas (Cooper, Craig, Gaynor, and Van Reenen 2015). We see, then, that while one key aspect of the health care landscape is left to the market, another is nationally regulated, albeit by a combination of government and private (professionally controlled) agencies.

Public health care spending in the United States falls primarily into the categories of Medicaid for the poor and Medicare, which is primarily for adults age 65 and older. While there are some other public programs (including the single payer, single provider programs of the Indian Health Service and the Veterans' Health Administration), these two programs make up the bulk of public health care spending. The main regulator of these programs is CMS, which is part of the federal Department of Health and Human Services. CMS authority affects health care provision far beyond the federal programs it officially administers. Put most simply, private insurers and state-level health care administrators use the CMS standards to set requirements for all health care provision. Because virtually all health care providers serve Medicare patients (and most also serve Medicaid patients), they must comply with the CMS systems and tend to use them for all of their patients, including the privately insured. In other words, CMS is the de facto regulator of health care, whether or not the care is provided by one of its programs.

Medicare and Medicaid are funded through a mechanism that reimburses providers partially based on the diagnosis of the patient rather than only on the specifics of the treatment administered. The reimbursement is determined by a DRG, which categorizes every allowable diagnosis and determines the appropriate expenditure. The DRG system was adopted nationally in 1983, after its creation by Yale University researchers and its initial adoption in New Jersey (Goldfield 2010). One physician described it as "Revolutionary. … [T]he federal government gained the upper hand in its financial relationship with the hospital industry" (Goldfield 2010: 13). The DRGs are controlled by CMS. Any updates to the codes, for example, because of changes in medical understandings of particular conditions, are approved by a committee with members from CMS as well as the Centers for Disease Control and the National Center for Health Statistics (Centers for Medicare and Medicaid Services 2015). In this way, then, the DRGs are actually controlled by the government itself rather than being outsourced or delegated to private organizations. However, the system was independently developed by researchers who had not been contracted by the government. In this case, the delegated regulation of an aspect of Medicare payment was not exactly outsourced but rather was developed by academics and then adopted by the government.

The DRG system has far-reaching influence—beyond those who are covered by Medicare. As one insurance reform advocate put it:

> Medicare's procedure and diagnosis-based fee structure for physicians and institutional providers greatly refined the state of the art. However, there is little doubt this has contributed heavily to a physician and provider culture where the codes that are recorded and perhaps sometimes the services that are provided are influenced by what Medicare will pay for. (Jones 1996: 157).

In other words, the DRG system has a profound impact on decisions about what care to provide to a patient.

Medicaid is a federally funded program that is administered by states. Most states now use the Medicare DRG system to determine payments. Many private insurers, including Humana and some of the state "Blues" (i.e., Blue Cross/Blue Shield) also use the codes as the basis for their pricing. The dominance of this system demonstrates that CMS processes are the standard across health care, far beyond only government-purchased care. As one scholar puts it, "Medicare's vast enrollment and the high proportion of physician, hospital, and other revenues represented by its population, have made its payment systems and licensure requirements into de facto standards for private industry" (Jones 1996: 155). Economic analysis indicates that the price of privately purchased health care is largely determined by the level of Medicare payments (see, for example, Clemens and Gottlieb 2013 on physician payments). Medicare, then, is a de facto national regulator, even for privately purchased health care.

REGULATION OF FACILITIES

In the United States, hospitals and clinics are accredited by the Joint Commission, which is technically a voluntary accreditor. It is an independent, nonprofit organization that provides accreditation to health care organizations. The Joint Commission is controlled by its corporate members: the American Hospital Association (the trade and lobbying association for hospitals); the American Medical Association; the American College of

Physicians (the specialist board for internal medicine); the American College of Surgeons; and the American Dental Association (Joint Commission 2016).

Almost all health care payers (whether government entities or private insurers) require facilities to be Joint Commission accredited in order to be eligible for reimbursement. For example, for a health care provider to be eligible for Medicare reimbursement, it must meet the CMS-defined conditions of participation. CMS maintains a relationship with the Joint Commission such that any organization that meets Joint Commission standards is deemed to have met the conditions of participation, which gives the Joint Commission the de facto regulatory power to approve providers. Because few facilities want to operate (or could survive financially) without treating Medicare patients, most hospitals opt for Joint Commission accreditation. All states rely on Joint Commission accreditation for additional eligibility, although the specifics vary—in some states, the accreditation is required for a facility to operate, while in others accreditation is technically required only for Medicaid reimbursement (as noted earlier, Medicaid is federally funded but administered by the states).

The power of this private regulator has become cause for concern among those paying close attention. The question becomes "Who regulates the regulator?" Or as Timothy Jost, a long-standing scholar of the commission puts it, the Joint Commission "is a private institution governed by representatives of hospitals and physicians, the participants in the health care industry who have the most to lose from competition" (1983: 839). Even without any concern about whether this system stifles competition (or indeed any notion of whether competition is a desirable objective in health care), one can see other possible problems when the government abdicates regulatory authority to a private entity controlled by interested parties (Dame and Wolfe 1996). The influence of the Joint Commission can be summarized as "the JCAHO is one of those obscure, private organizations that wield enormous influence in the medical community. It is the Moody's, Standard & Poor and Good Housekeeping of hospital ratings" (Schrage 1995).

The governing body of the Joint Commission is its Board of Commissioners, which includes representatives of the organizations who pay for their membership (for example, industry and physician associations). The organization is clear that its customers are the hospitals and health care institutions it inspects (for a fee), not the patients who use these facilities or the government agencies who rely on these standards. Accredited organizations pay an annual fee to the commission, as well as a higher fee approximately every three years when the commission conducts its intensive onsite survey. The industry and provider representatives therefore control the Joint Commission and determine the regulatory standards, with no scope for scrutiny or oversight.

The Joint Commission has retained its "deeming authority" (i.e., the CMS acceptance of its standards as fulfilling conditions of participation) since the creation of Medicare in 1965. This was partially an expeditious strategy: because many health care providers already used this accreditation system, it was easy to launch Medicare with a large number or participating providers if they did not need to seek further regulatory approval (Jost 1983: 853).

For the first few decades of Medicare, there was no mechanism to regulate or manage the Joint Commission's work: it was a de facto regulator, and it was run by the industry it was putatively regulating. The commission's authority was permanent, and there was no provision in the Medicare law for oversight or a renewal process. In 2008, following a slight change in Medicare law and some political challenges to the role of the Joint Commission, the commission lost its automatic deeming authority (Stark 1998). It must now periodically apply to CMS for this authority to be renewed, and it achieved successful renewal in 2010 and 2014 (Joint Commission 2012: 3). This rule theoretically takes away the Joint Commission's privileged status and gives it a degree of scrutiny and a level playing field with the few other accrediting entities. This change shows an acknowledgment by legislators that the physician-controlled Joint Commission dominates the organization of the health care delivery system, affirming the contention in this chapter that organized physicians control the regulation of health care.

REGULATION OF PROFESSIONALS

One of the key roles of a professional association is to "represent the profession to outsiders" (Greenwood, Suddaby, and Hinings 2002: 73). In the United States, doctors (as well as nurses and most other licensed professions and occupations) are regulated by state-level licensing as well as some national policies. The result, unsurprisingly, is a patchwork quilt of requirements, with a common underpinning—the backing of the quilt, if you will. To practice medicine, physicians must comply with state regulations. Physicians must pass the United States Medical Licensing Examination (USMLE), a national exam operated by a federation of state licensing boards. However, licensure is administered by state boards, which use the USMLE as one of their requirements. State boards are also responsible for background checks, disciplinary and professional issues, and any continuing education requirements. Specialty certification tends to be optional rather than required and is administered by specialty physician boards.

Medical education is more standardized, perhaps on the assumption that physicians are training to practice medicine nationally rather than locally. Post-bachelor's medical education is regulated by the Liaison Committee on Medical Education (LCME), which is sponsored (i.e., jointly controlled) by the AMA and the American Association of Medical Colleges. Residency programs are accredited by the Accreditation Council for Graduate Medical Education (ACGME). The ACGME comprises member organizations, including the AMA and the American Hospital Association. The AMA (along with specialty boards) appoints the committees that in turn accredit specialty residencies. The influence of the AMA, then, covers all aspects of entry to the profession. However, the AMA influences not only access to the profession but also the ability for any organization to be paid for providing health care, because of its control over the protocols used in the billing system.

The AMA generates a massive amount of income by selling products. In 2014, the association reported revenue of $229 million from selling its "publishing and business services" compared with $40 million in membership revenue (American Medical Association 2015: 11). This includes access to the CPT system that is required for billing within all medical specialties, which is owned and controlled by the AMA. As one critical article described the situation:

> The CPT code system is copyrighted to the AMA, and in 1983, the federal government stipulated that it would be the sole system used to reimburse providers under Medicare and Medicaid. This move inevitably prompted private insurers to follow suit, thereby granting the AMA monopoly over the reimbursement process for most procedures and services. (Wolfe 2012: 2)

While the AMA no longer retains this statutory monopoly, all public and private purchasers still currently use these codes (Wolfe 2012)—to the great enrichment of the AMA.

What emerges from the picture of licensing and accreditation in the United States is the outsized role of physicians and their professional organizations. While, by definition, professionals control access to their own profession, in the political economy of health care in the United States, physicians control so much more than that. As discussed earlier in this chapter, the AMA is also responsible for the ability of hospitals to operate (through its influence over the Joint Commission) and for the ability of hospitals and insurance companies to charge and process payments (through its control of the CPT system). Professionals are not only regulating themselves, as is standard, but are controlling all the key aspects of the industry, with the ability to prioritize their own interests (and profits) while minimizing the goals and needs of other stakeholders, including patients, payers, and nonphysician providers.

There is a crucial twist to this argument that physicians' organizations in the United States have outsized power in the health care landscape. As one scholar points out:

> Doctors working in the major cities have with few exceptions become well-paid functionaries in bureaucracies driven as much by the profit motive as by therapeutic considerations. Fear that doctors control too much has been displaced by fear that they control too little. (Haskell 1997)

However, there is still a split—between rank-and-file doctors who work for health care organizations and doctors who own health care organizations. As Paul Starr put it several decades ago, "Since some of [the AMA's] members are likely to be the owners and managers, ... the AMA will find it difficult to represent both sides in labor negotiations" (1982: 427).

Doctors' work is undoubtedly micromanaged in the United States and governed by bureaucracy, with a seriously diminished respect for professional judgment. However, these micromanagers, these bureaucrats, are heavily influenced if not controlled by the physicians' professional organizations whose power reaches beyond the AMA and specialist associations into control of the CPT billing system and the Joint Commission hospital accreditation system. Haskell argues that there is "growing conflict between professional and capitalist priorities," but this conflict does not play out within the professional associations (1997). Rather, within the "representative" professional associations, capitalist priorities have defeated professional priorities, and on the front lines of medicine, physicians are left without a voice for their professional priorities.

While as recently as 2000, 57% of physicians were independent (or self-employed), essentially operating as business owners, the comparable figure at the time of this writing is around 33%; most physicians are now employees rather than sole proprietors or business owners, and they are still adjusting to the challenges of the power imbalance between employer and employee (Accenture Consulting 2015). There is no doubt that physicians understand how poorly the AMA represents their professional interests, particularly as they slide into employee status; only about one quarter of practicing physicians are AMA members (Robeznieks 2013).

REGULATION IN THE UNITED KINGDOM

In the United States, health care is fragmented. It is purchased and provided by both public and private entities, and regulation happens at both the federal and state levels. In the United Kingdom, the health care system is probably the most unified in the world. Health care is publicly funded, publicly provided, and nationally regulated. When one digs into the American case, though, one finds a de facto unified regulatory structure. However, this unitary structure does not mimic that of its British counterpart. Rather, the regulatory apparatus in the American system has become deeply entwined with the organized professional voice of physicians, which consistently shores up its role as an owner of the means of health care delivery, giving rank-and-file front-line physicians little professional control over their work. In the early part of the 20th century, organized physicians associations in the United States and United Kingdom played decisive roles in determining the shape of their health care systems and the mechanisms of health care delivery (Givan 2016; Starr 1982). The sharp divergence in the role of physicians, in two countries in which the role and power of doctors were quite similar for many years, provides an illuminating contrast.

In the United Kingdom, doctors have long self-identified as employees as well as professionals. Their largest professional association, the British Medical Association (BMA), is also their union. The BMA collectively bargains the doctors' contracts with their employers, the government (which controls the National Health Service). The BMA's interests and influence have been much more narrowly focused than those of the AMA, and there has been no drift of its power into other areas of regulation or accreditation as we see in the American system.

The regulatory web in the United Kingdom is much simpler than that in the United States. Most regulation is controlled by agencies at arms' length from the government. These entities are created by statute but given broad operational autonomy to regulate hospitals and professionals, as well as appropriate standards and protocols of clinical care. The BMA's power is that of a professional association and union. It represents doctors as professionals and as employees, but it does not have tentacles in other areas of regulation, as does the AMA.

At the time of the founding of the National Health Service (NHS) in the years immediately after World War II, doctors almost thwarted the whole endeavor. The BMA was opposed to the socialization of the health system, primarily because it threatened the income of its members. As a well-organized union whose labor was difficult (likely impossible) to replace, the BMA leveraged its massive power. Nye Bevan, the Labour minister credited with founding the NHS, had to negotiate with this powerful organized interest group and ultimately bought their assent: the founding legislation of the NHS allowed specialists (known as consultants) to continue to see private patients while also working for the NHS, in order to increase their income. Bevan supposedly referred to this deal with the doctors as "stuffing their mouths with gold" (Irvine 2001: 163). This early illustration of the power of doctors as employees set the tone for the role of doctors in the NHS—as both professionals and employees negotiating with the state as their employer.

In the United Kingdom, the market for physicians is essentially a monopsony, with the NHS as the single buyer of physician labor. The BMA plays the role of both a labor union and a professional association. It represents doctors through collective bargaining and advocacy, while also serving as the voice of the profession.

There is an ongoing question of whether identifying as employees (or being treated by the state as employees) diminishes the professional status of doctors, and indeed threatens the maintenance of professional standards. As one observer puts it, in terms that are also illuminating in the American context:

> Professional self-regulation is a privilege granted by Parliament, not a right. Self-regulation has to be earned continuously to sustain public confidence in the profession. For both patients and doctors, the essence of the case for self-regulation rests primarily on the sense of self-respect that flows from doctors' ownership of professional standards. For a professional person, self-respect is a powerful motivator to be conscientious and trustworthy. Moreover, it creates peer pressure for all doctors to behave well. Self-respect could fall away if doctors become "mere employees" of the state. They could reach the point where they keep within government imposed rules but lose sight of the ideals of their profession.... [T]he eventual loser could be the patient. (Irvine 1999: 1177)

The General Medical Council (GMC) is responsible for the licensing and registration of doctors. The GMC is also responsible for medical training. In this sense, then, it performs the functions of both the U.S. state licensing boards and the ACGME. There is no small amount of logic in connecting professional licensing and the accreditation of education in this way rather than the murkier relationship that exists in the United Kingdom. Clearly the two functions are heavily dependent on each other.

In the United Kingdom, health care organizations (such as hospitals and primary care trusts) are regulated and monitored by the Care Quality Commission (Givan 2016). This independent regulator has the statutory power to "monitor, inspect and regulate services to make sure they meet fundamental standards of quality and safety" (Care Quality Commission 2016). The Care Quality Commission is classified as an arms'-length, or nondepartmental, public body—meaning it has operational independence and autonomy from the government. The Care Quality Commission performs work parallel to that of the Joint Commission in the United States, but it is structurally and organizationally quite different—for example, it is not governed by the entities it putatively accredits.

Decisions about the appropriate type of care for any condition, as well as the most effective medication, are made by the National Institute for Clinical Excellence (NICE, now officially known as the National Institute for Health and Care Excellence). NICE is accountable to the Department of Health but it operates independently (National Institute for Health and Care Excellence 2016b). NICE is responsible for clinical guidelines "on the appropriate treatment and care of people with specific diseases or conditions," as well as guidelines for the use of prescription medications and the allowable formulary (National Institute for Health and Care Excellence 2016a). One could say that NICE's work covers much of the work of the CMS in the United States. There is also a Medicines and Healthcare Products Regulatory Agency in the United Kingdom, which is part of the Department of Health. This agency performs some work similar to that of the Food and Drug Administration in the United States. NICE is fully independent and has no formal ties with any of the professional associations (such as the BMA or any of the Royal Colleges, whose members include family practice and specialist physicians). Again, in contrast to the U.S. situation, NICE is not controlled or formally influenced by any representatives of professional or industry associations.

This analysis of the regulatory bureaucracy in the United Kingdom is briefer than the discussion of the United States for the straightforward reason that regulation is simpler in the United Kingdom. The unitary nature of the NHS has created unified regulatory entities (with a modest amount of devolution to Wales, Scotland, and Northern Ireland). It is significant, however, that most of the regulation in the United Kingdom is carried out by independent regulators created by statute, who are not susceptible to either institutional or informal influence by professionals or, indeed, to other stakeholders in the provision and use of health care. The bureaucrats in the regulation of the NHS look much more like traditional Weberian bureaucrats, operating at arms' length from political interests and societal interests.

By looking at these two distinct national cases, we can understand both the similar evolution of professional power and voice in each country and the key points of divergence as professional roles have evolved (see also Perkin 1990 and Starr 1982).

CONCLUSIONS AND COMPARISONS

In the United States, much of the crucial regulatory work in health care is performed by private organizations created and controlled by organized groups of physicians. In contrast, regulation in the United Kingdom is primarily performed by independent entities created and empowered by statute. In the United States, physician associations behave like capitalist trade associations and use cartel-like strategies to control the production of health care. In the United Kingdom, the physicians are workers who use their collective power to leverage their interests. In both cases, they exhibit the classic traits of professions, controlling access to the profession and the certification mechanisms. It is worth noting that in some cases in the United States, physicians are even more traditional capitalists, such as when they own the hospitals or the diagnostic equipment and aggressively try to increase their profits by "prescribing" more and more care (Brownlee 2008; Gawande 2009). However, even when the doctors do not own the hospitals or the MRI machines, they still act more like owners seeking to protect their profits rather than employees seeking to protect their labor market position.

The analysis in this chapter demonstrates that in the United States, there is a growing split between empowered physician regulators who run the professional associations and staff the bureaucracy, and rank-and-file doctors who deliver medical care. The irony, of course, is that the work of the physician regulators is perceived by the rank-and-file doctors as detrimental to their professional judgment and autonomy (Scheiber 2016).

In the United Kingdom, the major professional association has retained its focus on representing its members as professionals. In the face of attacks on quality health care and the working conditions of doctors, the BMA has held on to its role as a union, representing the interests of doctors as employees and showing a willingness to strike in the face of government intransigence (Campbell 2016).

As American doctors' needs become more and more removed from the interests of their still powerful professional association, it remains to be seen whether a new organization will emerge and whether it might take the shape of a union, a professional association, or something else entirely.

REFERENCES

Accenture Consulting. 2015. "Clinical Care: The Independent Doctor Will NOT See You Now." http://bit.ly/1PxZKQp.

American Medical Association. 2015. *2014 Annual Report*. Chicago, IL: American Medical Association.

Brownlee, S. 2008. *Overtreated: Why Too Much Medicine Is Making Us Sicker and Poorer*. New York, NY: Bloomsbury.

Bybee, R. 2008 (Jul. 1). "The Doctors' Revolt." *The American Prospect*. http://prospect.org/article/doctors-revolt.

Campbell, D. 2016 (Jun. 12). "Who Has Come Out on Top After the First Junior Doctors' Strike in 40 Years?" *The Guardian*. http://bit.ly/1Py0Uv2.

Care Quality Commission. 2016. "Who We Are." Care Quality Commission. http://www.cqc.org.uk.

Centers for Medicare and Medicaid Services. 2015 (Dec. 30). "ICD-10 Coordination and Maintenance Committee." http://go.cms.gov/1PxYlta.

Clemens, J., and J. D. Gottlieb. 2013. "In the Shadow of a Giant: Medicare's Influence on Private Physician Payments." NBER Working Paper No. 19503. Cambridge, MA: National Bureau of Economic Research. http://www.nber.org/papers/w19503.

Cooper, Z., S. V. Craig, M. Gaynor, and J. Van Reenen. 2015. *The Price Ain't Right? Hospital Prices and Health Spending on the Privately Insured.* NBER Working Paper No. 21815. Cambridge, MA: National Bureau of Economic Research. http://www.nber.org/papers/w21815.

Dame, L., and S. M. Wolfe. 1996. *The Failure of "Private" Hospital Regulation: An Analysis of the Joint Commission on Accreditation of Healthcare Organizations' Inadequate Oversight of Hospitals.* Washington, DC: Public Citizen Health Research Group.

DiMaggio, P. J., and W. W. Powell. 1983. "The Iron Cage Revisited: Institutional Isomorphism and Collective Rationality in Organizational Fields." *American Sociological Review* 48, no. 2: 147. doi:10.2307/2095101.

Dixon, A., and C. Ham. 2010. "Liberating the NHS: The Right Prescription in a Cold Climate? The King's Fund Response to the 2010 Health White Paper." London, UK: The King's Fund. http://bit.ly/1PxYOLP.

Dutton, P. V. 2007. *Differential Diagnoses: A Comparative History of Health Care Problems and Solutions in the United States and France.* Ithaca, NY: Cornell University Press.

Field, R. L. 2008. "Why Is Health Care Regulation So Complex?" *Pharmacy and Therapeutics* 33, no. 10: 607–08.

Gawande, A. 2009 (Jun. 1). "The Cost Conundrum: What a Texas Town Can Teach Us About Health Care." *The New Yorker.* http://bit.ly/1PxZj8B.

Giaimo, S., and P. Manow. 1999. "Adapting the Welfare State: The Case of Health Care Reform in Britain, Germany, and the United States." *Comparative Political Studies* 32, no. 8: 967–1000. doi:10.1177/0010414099032008003.

Givan, R. K. 2016. *The Challenge of Change: Reforming Health Care on the Front Line in the United States and the United Kingdom.* Ithaca, NY: Cornell University Press.

Goldfield, N. 2010. "The Evolution of Diagnosis-Related Groups (DRGs)." *Quality Management in Health Care* 19, no. 1: 3–16. doi:10.1097/qmh.0b013e3181ccbcc3.

Greenwood, R., R. Suddaby, and C. R. Hinings. 2002. "Theorizing Change: The Role of Professional Associations in the Transformation of Institutionalized Fields." *Academy of Management Journal* 45, no. 1: 58–80. doi:10.2307/3069285.

Hall, P. A., and D. W. Soskice. 2001. Varieties of Capitalism: The Institutional Foundations of Comparative Advantage. Oxford, UK: Oxford University Press.

Haskell, T. L. 1997 (Dec. 4). "The New Aristocracy (Book Review, *Death of the Guilds: Professions, States, and the Advance of Capitalism, 1930 to the Present* by E. A. Krause)." *The New York Review of Books.* http://bit.ly/1PxZwbY.

Irvine, D. 1999. "The Performance of Doctors: The New Professionalism." *The Lancet* 353, no. 9159: 1174–177. doi:10.1016/s0140-6736(99)91160-1.

Irvine, D. 2001. "The Changing Relationship Between the Public and the Medical Profession." *Journal of the Royal Society of Medicine* 94, no. 4: 162–69.

Jackson & Coker. 2011. "Survey: Physician Opinions of the American Medical Association." Presentation. http://bit.ly/1Py0Iw1.

Joint Commission. 2016 (Mar. 10). "Facts About the Board of Commissioners." The Joint Commission. http://bit.ly/1Py1eKi.

Joint Commission and CMS Crosswalk. 2012. *Comparing Hospital Standards and CoPs.* Report. Oakbrook Terrace, IL: Joint Commission.

Jones, S. B. 1996. "Medicare Influence on Private Insurance: Good or Ill?" *Health Care Financing Review* 18, no. 2: 153–61.

Jost, T. S. 1983. "The Joint Commission on Accreditation of Hospitals: Private Regulation of Health Care and the Public Interest." *Boston College Law Review* 24: 835–923.

Jost, T. S. 1995. "Oversight of the Quality of Medical Care: Regulation, Management, or the Market." *Arizona Law Review* 37: 825–68.

Moncrieff, A., and E. Lee. 2012. "The Positive Case for Centralization in Healthcare Regulation: The Federalism Failures of the ACA." *Kansas Journal of Law and Public Policy* 20: 266–94.

National Institute for Health and Care Excellence. 2016a. "Structure of NICE." National Institute for Health and Care Excellence. http://bit.ly/1Py0cxV.

National Institute for Health and Care Excellence. 2016b. "Who We Are." National Institute for Health and Care Excellence. http://bit.ly/1Py0HIh.

Palmer, K. S. 1999. "A Brief History: Universal Health Care Efforts in the US." Speech, Annual Meeting, Physicians for a National Health Program. http://bit.ly/1Py0RQ0.

Perkin, H. 1990. *The Rise of Professional Society: England Since 1880.* Hove, UK: Psychology Press.

Physicians Foundation. 2012 (Sep. 21). "A Survey of America's Physicians: Practice Patterns and Perspectives." http://bit.ly/1Py0jts.

Robeznieks, A. 2013 (May 9). "AMA Saw Membership Rise 3.2% in 2012." *Modern Healthcare.*

Scheiber, N. 2016 (Jan. 9). "Doctors Unionize to Resist the Medical Machine." *New York Times.* http://nyti.ms/1Py0Zil.

Schrage, M. 1995 (Apr. 21). "Accreditation Becomes Battleground for Defining Quality Health Care." *Washington Post.*

Stark, F. P. 1998. "Why the Joint Commission on Accrediting Healthcare Organizations (JCAHO) Must Do Better." *Congressional Record*, E2139–E2140. Washington, DC: U.S. Congress.

Starr, P. 1982. *The Social Transformation of American Medicine.* New York, NY: Basic Books.

Wolfe, S. M. 2012. "The American Medical Association and Its Dubious Revenue Streams." *Public Citizen Health Letter* 28, no. 11: 1–3.

Chapter 5

Nurse Union Strategies for Improving the Quality of Patient Care

Paul F. Clark

School of Labor and Employment Relations
Pennsylvania State University

INTRODUCTION

Unions exist to provide workers with voice in the workplace. Workers use this voice to improve their compensation and benefits and the conditions at their workplace through collective bargaining. They also use it to help ensure that they receive fair treatment and due process by establishing grievance procedures that include arbitration. And, through their unions, workers engage in voice through political action and government lobbying in an effort to influence government in a way that benefits and protect employees. Somewhat less commonly, workers use voice to gain input into decisions regarding the production of the product, or the provision of the service, that the employer produces or provides through labor–management collaboration and partnerships.

Unions of professional workers seek a voice for their members in all of these areas. However, they—more than other types of unions—seek to participate in decisions involving the work process. The fact that professional work is often predominantly intellectual and requires the significant exercise of discretion and judgment is one reason professional workers tend to be more interested than unions in some other sectors in participating in workplace decision making. Professionals are also more invested in the final product or service than nonprofessional employees (Molyneux 2001).

This chapter addresses the efforts of unions representing registered nurses (RNs)—one of the largest groups of professional workers in the nation—to give their members a greater voice in decisions and work practices that directly impact the quality of patient care. In particular, the chapter focuses on three mechanisms nurses unions have employed to impact the quality of care provided in acute care hospitals: contract language established through collective bargaining, union–management collaboration and partnerships, and political and legislative action. The chapter looks at how RN unions have used these mechanisms to address three important issues: safe staffing levels, mandatory overtime, and the "floating" of nurses to cover understaffed units. The chapter also examines additional ways in which nurses and their unions have used greater voice to improve the quality of patient care.

NURSES, NURSES UNIONS, AND VOICE

Registered nurses (RNs) are the largest group of professionals in the American health care system. In hospital settings they play a vital and unique role as the primary direct care providers. Nurses believe that as individuals and as a profession, they have an obligation to do all that they can to ensure their patients receive the best possible care. For this reason, they have long viewed themselves as the primary patient advocate within the health care system. In fact, the American Nurses Association (ANA) Code of Ethics, as well as most state-level nurse practice codes, list patient advocacy as one of the primary responsibilities of RNs. Most definitions of patient advocacy include a common point: advocates must act to ensure that the patient's welfare is paramount in any medical setting, procedure, or treatment (Tate 2005).

At a time when the American health care system is wrestling with myriad problems, including high cost and underperformance, it needs to use every resource at its disposal to address the challenges it faces. The vast majority of health care facilities and systems in the United States employ a variation of traditional, hierarchical, command and control management. This approach overvalues the contributions of managers and greatly undervalues the potential contributions of RNs and other health care professionals. To make the kind of progress necessary for the U.S. health care system to meet its potential requires hospitals and health care systems to use the knowledge and commitment of their entire workforce—not just administrators and managers.

One of the critical groups of health care workers who are ready and able to contribute to improving patient care are nurses. Many RNs, and most nurses unions, recognize the potential contributions the nursing profession can make and are looking for opportunities to participate to a greater degree in decisions involving the delivery of patient care. This is why many unions representing RNs are beginning to aggressively promote labor–management collaboration and partnerships that will give their members a greater voice in patient care decisions and, they believe, will greatly improve the quality of care and reduce costs.

Given the reluctance of managers to give up sole control of decision making in the health care workplace, unions provide nurses with the collective power needed to win a greater voice in how patient care is delivered. This is one of the key reasons that during a period of generally declining union membership, RNs have been one of the few occupations that has not seen a significant decline in union density over the past 20 years. In fact, the percentage of registered nurses belonging to unions has remained among the highest of any occupation. In 2002, union density among nurses was 17%. It increased to 20% in 2012 and remained at 18% in 2014 (Hirsch and Macpherson 2016).

Certainly nurses recognize that an increased voice can be used to increase salaries and benefits, and the unions they formed have used their collective bargaining rights to pursue improvements in those areas. However, the importance nurses place on having a greater voice in patient care is reflected in the degree to which RN unions have stressed that issue in their organizing drives. And it is reflected in the fact that nurses unions, over the past 10 to 15 years, have focused their collective voice on patient care issues (Clark and Clark 2006).

Several unions represent RNs in the U.S. health care industry. This appears to be a function of at least two factors. First, a large segment of the health care workforce did not become eligible to organize a union until 1974, after many national and international unions were already well established. Thus, there was less reason for the formation of entirely new health care unions. Second, during that period, many existing unions suffered significant membership losses. Not surprisingly, many of those unions saw the growing health care industry as fertile ground for organizing.

A significant proportion of RNs belong to unions that largely, or exclusively, represent only nurses. Most of these "craft type" unions trace their origins to the ANA, which was founded in 1896 as a professional organization to advance the nursing profession. In the years following its founding, the ANA created state-level affiliates in every state. As a professional association, the ANA focused on promoting standards of nursing practice, providing professional development opportunities, and advocating for health care issues that impact nurses and the public (American Nurses Association 2016a). When the National Labor Relations Act (NLRA) was expanded to include health care workers in nonprofit hospitals and nursing homes in 1974, ANA leaders at the national and state levels wrestled with the issue of whether to take on the role of collective bargaining agent. Because of differing views, some ANA state associations split into two separate organizations—one that continued to function solely as a professional association and the other functioning as an independent union.

This was the case for the California Nurses Association (CNA), which severed ties with the ANA in 1995 to become the largest union of RNs in the nation. In 2009, the CNA joined with the Massachusetts Nurses

Association (MNA), the Minnesota Nurses Association (MINNA), and an amalgamation of state nursing associations called the United American Nurses (UAN) to become the National Nurses Union (NNU). At its founding, the union reported a combined membership of 150,000 RNs (Association for Union Democracy 2010).

Since its founding, the NNU has been both one of the fastest growing unions in the country and the most influential and dynamic union in the burgeoning nurse labor movement. It now claims 185,000 members from all 50 U.S. states and continues to grow rapidly, in part because of its organizing work in union-hostile states such as Texas and Florida and in other states that had previously seen little nurse organizing (National Nurses Union 2016).

The union representing the second largest number of nurses— the Service Employees International Union (SEIU)—differs from CNA/NNU in that it represents a wide range of professional and nonprofessional employees in the health care industry, rather than just one professional group. SEIU's "industrial union" approach means that in any given hospital the union might represent nurse aides, therapists, custodians, maintenance workers, office staff, and even physicians, as well as RNs. Of its 2.1 million members, 1.1 million work in health care. A subdivision of the union, the Nurse Alliance, represents 80,000 RNs across the country (Service Employees International Union 2016a).

The AFT Nurses and Health Professionals union represents 82,000 RNs in a variety of settings, including acute care hospitals, making it the third largest nurses union in the United States. Another union with a significant number of nurse members is the American Federation of State, County, and Municipal Employees (AFSCME), which represents 60,000 nurses, most of whom work in acute and long-term care facilities operated by state or local government. And the American Federation of Government Employees (AFGE) represents 55,000 RNs working mostly in the federal government's Veterans Administration facilities.

Other unions representing small numbers of nurses include the United Food and Commercial Workers (UFCW), the Communications Workers of America (CWA), the Office and Professional Employees International Union (OPEIU), and the International Union of Operating Engineers (IUOE).

NURSES AND THE CHALLENGE TO PROVIDE QUALITY CARE

The 1970s and 1980s saw the introduction of a new approach to the provision of health care in the United States. Managed care is a market-driven approach to the delivery of health care services that focuses heavily on cost containment. As this approach gained momentum, one of the main ways that administrators sought to cut costs in acute care hospitals was by downsizing the nurse workforce. As the number of RNs was reduced, the remaining nurses were required to take care of more patients. Because managed care's cost-reduction focus called for hospitals to admit only "the sickest patients for the shortest possible stay" (Sochalski and Aiken 1999: 1), nurses were forced to deal with rising patient "acuity" (the measure of how sick a patient is). Thus, in recent decades, nurses have been asked to care for more patients, and those patients are sicker and require greater attention (Sochalski and Aiken 1999).

In a 2001 survey of RNs, approximately 75% of the respondents reported that both their working conditions and the quality of nursing care in their facilities had declined in recent years. Thirty-eight percent of the nurses in the study reported that they felt "exhausted and discouraged" upon leaving work. Thirty-four percent said they were "discouraged and saddened by what they could not provide their patients," and 29% felt they were "powerless to affect change" (Michigan Nurses Association 2001).

Nurses contend that being unable to provide the kind of quality patient care they believe their patients need and deserve leads to anxiety and guilt. This anxiety and guilt reach the point where many RNs voluntarily leave nursing to work in less stressful occupations outside the health care system. And, of course, the inability of the system to stem the exodus of nurses sets a damaging dynamic in motion—as more nurses quit, fewer are available to care for the steady stream of patients that come and go, forcing the remaining nurses to take on a larger number of patients, which inevitably increases their stress and dissatisfaction, causing more nurses to leave, and on and on. Providing adequate, let alone optimal, patient care under these conditions becomes a very challenging task.

From the perspective of nurses, the most detrimental manifestation of managed care's relentless focus on reducing labor costs was three workplace practices related to nursing care: understaffing, mandatory overtime, and floating.

Nurse staffing concerns over the past 20 years led to a significant amount of research on understaffing and its impacts on health care. For example, a study by Rogowski and colleagues (2013) found that understaffing in neonatal intensive care units, relative to national guidelines, was common and widespread and was associated with an increased risk for nosocomial infections in very low birth weight infants. Also, an influential study by Aiken and colleagues (2010) found that nurse understaffing was associated with significantly higher patient mortality levels. Moreover, research by Kane and colleagues (2007) found that increased nurse staffing in hospitals was associated with lower hospital-related mortality, less failure to rescue, and other improved patient outcomes. Greater nurse staffing was also associated with better outcomes in intensive care units and in surgical patients. Overall, the research on this issue strongly indicates that insufficient nurse staffing significantly reduces the quality of care that RNs are able to provide.

Similarly, research has found that mandatory overtime compelling nurses to work beyond their assigned shifts is associated with significant patient care problems (American Association of Critical-Care Nurses 2016). A study by Trinkoff and colleagues (2011), for example, found that excessively long work hours for hospital nurses over a six-month period were significantly related to patient mortality, after controlling for staffing levels and hospital characteristics. Another study found that the risk of medical errors was three times higher when RNs worked shifts lasting 12.5 hours or more (Rogers et al. 2004). Research has also demonstrated that long work hours have adverse impacts on nurses as well as on patients. The use of excessive overtime has been associated with increases in RNs' needle-stick injuries and musculoskeletal problems (Clarke, Rockett, Sloane, and Aiken 2002; Trinkoff, Le, Geiger-Brown, and Lipscomb 2007), as well as other work-related illnesses and injuries (de Castro et al. 2010).

A review of the literature on floating has found that the practice increases stress and dissatisfaction among RNs and can lead to adverse impacts on the quality of patient care generally and on specific problems such as increased bloodstream infections (Dziuba-Ellis 2006; Larson et al. 2012).

As discussed previously in this chapter, many nurses have turned to unionization as a way to gain a greater voice in the workplace. In particular, nurses have used this greater voice to try to address the challenges to patient care posed by understaffing, mandatory overtime, and floating. To do so, most nurses unions have employed some combination of three voice mechanisms—collective bargaining, joint collaboration and partnerships, and lobbying and legislative action. Each of these mechanisms and the manner in which different nurses unions have employed them is examined in the following sections.

Collective Bargaining

As the result of an amendment to the National Labor Relations Act, RNs working in nonprofit or for-profit acute care hospitals have had the right to organize unions, engage in collective bargaining, and strike (after giving ten days' notice) since 1974. To form a union, nurses in a facility must provide evidence to the National Labor Relations Board (NLRB) that at least 30% of eligible RNs would like an election to decide whether to have union representation. If an election is held, a majority of nurses who vote in the election must vote for the union for it to be certified as their official bargaining representative.

Certification means that the management of the facility is obligated to collectively bargain over wages, hours, and other terms and conditions of employment. Patient care issues such as staffing levels, mandatory overtime, and floating are considered "other terms and conditions of employment," and employers must negotiate over those issues if they are brought up by the union. Whether a union can convince management to agree to its proposals concerning staffing levels, mandatory overtime, and floating depends on the strength and skill the union brings to negotiations.

Staffing Levels

In 2015, the New York State Nurses Association (NYSNA) signed what they described as a "historic" contract covering 17,000 RNs working in 12 private sector hospitals in New York City. The central focus of the negotiations leading to the contract was staffing ratios and their enforcement. The new agreement included a commitment on the hospitals' part to hire 1,000 new RNs to meet the need for more nurses created by previously negotiated staffing ratios. To better enforce the agreed-to staffing ratios and other issues, the contract included language creating joint union–management professional practice committees (PPCs) in each hospital. The main purpose of these committees is to monitor and enforce the negotiated nurse-to-patient ratios (New York State Nurses Association 2015).

The NYSNA contract is just one of the latest and most visible efforts by RN unions to win staffing language that enables nurses to provide high-quality care to their patients. Other examples are the contracts the Massachusetts Nurses Association (MNA) negotiated in 2011 with the Tufts Medical Center in Boston and St. Vincent Hospital in Worcester that featured significant improvements in nurse-to-patient ratios. At Tufts, the hospital agreed to limit patient assignments for nurses working on the medical–surgical floors to six patients on the night shift and to no more than two patients in the intensive care units. The hospital also agreed to language in the contract that ensures that the hospital will not move to a six-patient assignment on medical–surgical floors during the day and evening shifts, for the life of the agreement. In addition, the hospital made a commitment to convert a number of temporary travel nurse positions to core staff, which will further improve care on a number of units (Massachusetts Nurses Association 2011).

At St. Vincent's, the new contract reduced medical–surgical nurse-to-patient ratios from up to six patients on days and evenings and up to seven patients on nights to a limit of four to five patients per nurse on days and evenings and no more than five patients on the night shift. The hospital also agreed to improve RN-to-patient ratios in the hospital's maternity unit to bring them in line with established national standards for maternity care. Another feature of the contract was the addition of a "resource nurse" to supplement core staffing on medical–surgical and telemetry floors on day and evening shifts, coordinate the flow of patients in and out of the units, and support RNs caring for patients with complex needs (Massachusetts Nurses Association 2011).

The NYSNA and MNA contracts are emblematic of collective bargaining involving RN unions in recent years. These settlements build on contracts negotiated across the country over the past 10 to 15 years that have established minimum nurse-to-patient staffing ratios in an effort to improve the quality of care in American hospitals.

Some nurses unions have found that including staffing levels in contracts does not ensure that a hospital's administration will always abide by those standards. Sometimes hospitals will choose not to do so; other times, they are unable to abide by the standards because they do not have an adequate number of RNs. For that reason, nurses unions are now negotiating contract language that requires that staffing disputes be resolved by neutral third parties. For instance, many of the contracts negotiated by the CNA contain provisions requiring the parties to submit any dispute over nurse staffing levels, whether it be contractual or legislatively mandated ratios, to a tripartite arbitration panel made up of one member selected by the union, one member selected by the employer, and a third neutral member jointly chosen by the union and the employer (California Nurses Association 2016a). This provision takes the unilateral right to make decisions about staff out of the hands of management and places it in the hands of a neutral arbitrator—and the fact that the union has the option to take such disputes to arbitration serves as an incentive for management to follow the negotiated staffing guidelines.

Finally, some unions have successfully negotiated provisions that give nurses the final say on appropriate staffing levels. The Minnesota Nurses Association (MINNA) has contract language that gives charge nurses authority to determine whether sufficient staffing resources are available to meet patient care needs and to close the unit to further admissions if staffing is not sufficient (Minnesota Nurses Association 2004). This does not appear to be a widespread practice, at least currently, but it does present model language to which RN unions can aspire.

Mandatory Overtime

When hospitals try to cut costs by operating with the absolute minimum nurse workforce possible, problems arise when a nurse calls in sick or a hospital experiences a higher than normal census. When that happens, administrators turn to mandatory overtime to meet their staffing needs.

Not only is mandatory overtime disruptive to an RNs family life by keeping nurses from meeting family commitments and obligations, it also has negative ramifications for patient care because tired nurses are significantly more prone to making medication errors and suffering lapses in judgment.

One way that RN unions protect their members from the dangers of excessively long hours is by negotiating contractual bans on mandatory overtime. Florida's National Nurses United (NNU) won such protection from mandatory overtime in 2012 for 3,100 RNs at ten Florida hospitals that are part of the Hospital Corporation of America (HCA), the nation's largest for-profit hospital chain (Indest 2012).

The single employer contract covering the largest number of nurses (18,000), between Kaiser Permanente (KP) and the CNA, was one of the first to contain contract language prohibiting the employer from assigning mandatory overtime. Dating back to 2002, CNA contracts have had some of the strongest language on this issue of any nurses union in the country (Business Wire 2002).

Another 17,000 to 18,000 RNs work for KP but are represented by unions other than CNA, including the United Nurses Association of California (UNAC), an AFSCME affiliate; the Oregon Federation of Nurses and Health Professionals (OFNHP), an AFT affiliate; and local unions represented by the UFCW and the OPEIU (Pruitt 2016). These nurses are covered by separate agreements with KP. They were able to get KP to discontinue the use of mandatory overtime in 2003 (the only exception to the ban on mandatory overtime being a government-declared state of emergency) (Kaiser Permanente 2010).

The goal of most nurses unions is a complete ban on mandatory overtime, and an increasing number of contracts contain such language. However, when not able to win a complete ban on overtime, many nurses unions have settled for language that limits mandatory overtime. One such approach is to negotiate contract language that limits its use to emergency situations. SEIU has negotiated such language into their contract with the University of Iowa Hospitals and Clinics. While the language does not eliminate forced overtime, the hospital can no longer force nurses to work overtime instead of hiring more staff to fill vacant positions (Service Employees International Union 2016a).

Another approach to reducing mandatory overtime is to place limits on the amount of overtime employees can be forced to work. The Ohio Nurses Association (ONA) has done this at Northside Medical Center in Youngstown, where management cannot require RNs to work more than 33 hours of mandatory overtime during a calendar year (Cotterman 2015).

Floating

Floating is the practice of moving nurses from their regularly assigned areas to parts of the hospital with a greater need. Many RNs believe this is a problematic practice, particularly when an RN is required to work in an area of the hospital in which he or she has insufficient experience or knowledge to deliver the kind of care required. For example, in many hospitals it is not uncommon to float a nurse who works in a general medical–surgical unit to the intensive care unit or the emergency room, where they are unfamiliar with the procedures, equipment, and medical conditions they will face (Eakin 2016).

Floating is an additional issue that nurses unions are trying to address through collective bargaining. Given that a complete ban on floating is, in most cases, unrealistic, unions have worked to place restrictions on the practice. The most common language negotiated on this issue is a prohibition on moving nurses to areas that are outside their areas of expertise. For example, SEIU's contract with hospitals in New York City includes comprehensive floating policies guaranteeing that nurses cannot be floated to areas where they do not have appropriate qualifications and training and where they have not had an up-to-date orientation (Service Employees International Union 2016b).

Another approach is negotiating contract language requiring that nurses be cross-trained to work in multiple areas and limiting floating to those specially trained nurses. Nurses represented by SEIU Healthcare NW and working at Swedish Medical Center in Seattle have a contract provision that requires that cross-trained nurses be floated before other nurses are (Service Employees International Union 2016c).

Where they can, RN unions bargain "float differentials" requiring hospitals to pay floating nurses a wage premium above and beyond their normal rate. And in some hospitals, contract provisions are included that mandate the creation of special "float pools." This arrangement is a part of an agreement negotiated by SEIU at Swedish Health Services Hospital in Seattle. At that facility, floating is handled by a special group of nurses who receive extensive, wide-ranging training. These nurses also receive a $5 per hour wage differential (Service Employees International Union 2016c).

The CNA has also negotiated language that prohibits "double floating" (the practice of moving nurses a second time in mid-shift) (California Nurses Association 2016a).

Collaboration and Partnerships

A second strategy RN unions have employed to increase nurse voice in decisions involving patient care is the formation of collaboration and partnership mechanisms through which nurses have regular opportunities to discuss patient care–related issues with management. These committees are often established in bargaining and operate throughout the life of a contract. They take many forms, including nurse staffing committees, professional practice committees, joint nursing practice councils, patient care committees, and staff ratio oversight committees; on a regular basis (e.g., biweekly, monthly, quarterly); and often include equal numbers of representatives from the union and from hospital administration.

The effectiveness of collaborative efforts in bringing about change in patient care practices appears to vary considerably. The formation of such groups does not guarantee that the union and employer representatives involved will be able to shift from an adversarial mode to a cooperative one. Where they are able to do so, however, significant improvements to the delivery of quality care can result.

The largest—and most extensive—partnership in the health care industry is the Kaiser Permanente Labor Management Partnership (KPLMP). It includes over 86,000 employees and more than 25 local union partners from eight international unions. However, CNA/NNU has chosen not to participate in the KPLMP. The 17,000 CNA/NNU nurses working in 70 of the KP facilities in northern and central California represent the largest group of eligible employees not participating in the partnership. CNA/NNU refuses to be a part of KPLMP because it believes an adversarial approach is the only effective means to address the problems its members face (California Nurses Association 2008; Clark and Clark 2008).

However, as mentioned previously, several other unions representing approximately 17,000 to 18,000 RNs at KP do participate in the partnership. Those unions include UNAC and OFNHP, as well as local unions represented by UFCW and OPEIU (Pruitt 2016).

Staffing

Staffing issues are a primary topic of discussion for these committees. In the absence of established staffing ratios, a nurse staffing committee could be given the responsibility to put together a staffing plan for a hospital that might set staffing guidelines or even specific staffing levels (American Nurses Association 2016b). Where such guidelines or ratios are in place, these committees often monitor compliance and resolve disputes over staffing. Where they are not, the committees can serve to gather data and study staffing patterns and problems as a first step toward developing solutions.

Mandatory Overtime and Floating

Where mandatory overtime or floating is restricted or banned by contract language or legislation, joint committees can serve to monitor compliance.

In the absence of such restrictions, committees can gather information about such practices and begin to work on solutions.

Lobbying/Legislative Action

In addition to addressing patient care and nursing practice concerns through bargaining, nurses unions also use lobbying and the legislative process to bring about change. The quality of patient care is a potent political issue. Moreover, nurses have a very positive public image, which makes them a formidable political force and allows them to effectively lobby for legislation they support (Sachs 2014).

Staffing

Legislation that sets minimum staffing levels has a significant advantage over the negotiation of staffing levels in collective bargaining agreements. Staffing laws can cover every hospital under a legislature's jurisdiction. Thus, legislation would do across the board what might take nurses unions years, or even decades, to achieve on an individual contract-by-contract basis.

The passage of federal legislation would clearly be the most effective way for unions to address patient care and nursing practice issues. A coalition of nurses unions has successfully lobbied to have the Nurse Staffing Standards for Patient Safety and Quality Care Act, a bill establishing minimum staffing levels, introduced in Congress in every legislative session since at least 2004. The bill has been strenuously opposed by the American Hospital Association, the industry's employer group, each time it has been introduced and has little chance of being enacted in the near future. State legislatures, at least in some parts of the country, have been more open to such legislation (McDonagh 2014).

The most significant effort to date in this regard has been in California, where a ten-year campaign by nurses unions resulted in the 1999 passage of a law mandating RN-to-patient ratios in California hospitals. Hospitals in the state fought the legislation, arguing that, because of the ongoing nurse shortage, the law's passage would cost them $500 million annually and might force them to shut down some of their facilities if they were unable to find enough nurses (California Healthcare Association 2003). At the hospitals' behest, then–Governor Schwarzenegger raised legal challenges that delayed the implementation of the mandated ratios.

However, in early 2005 the court challenges were dismissed and hospitals in that state were ordered "to implement ratios of no more than one RN for every five patients in general medical units" and to restore safe staffing in emergency rooms (California Nurses Association 2016b). The ratios required by the act are significantly better than those found in most American hospitals (such ratios vary from 1:6 to 1:10 or even more), and nurses unions expect the law to attract more nurses to California and have a positive impact on patient care (Lafer 2005).

The CNA was a leader in the effort to establish safe staffing through legislatively imposed RN-to-patient ratios. They have since added a second mechanism to ensure that California hospitals fully implement the established ratios. The CNA makes the establishment of professional practice committees (PPCs) a priority in bargaining at each new hospital it organizes. The PPC is an "RN-controlled" committee "with the authority to document unsafe practice issues and the power to make real changes." The committee is composed of elected staff RNs representing each nursing unit. It meets on paid time at the hospital worksite to monitor the implementation of nurse-to-patient ratios established either through legislation or bargaining. The committee also has the authority to address and change any other patient practice issues it deems unsafe (California Nurses Association 2016a). The addition of negotiated PPCs is an example of unions using combinations of strategies, in this case legislation and contract language, to win advances in patient care.

Massachusetts is the only other state to date that has implemented mandatory nurse-to-patient ratios. In contrast to California, its law is limited to intensive care units (ICUs) for which it requires ratios of 1:1 or 1:2 depending on the stability of the patient. The driving force behind the passage of this legislation was the Massachusetts Nurses Association (MNA), which has been lobbying the Massachusetts state legislature to pass a comprehensive staffing bill since at least 2002. The union sees the passage of the ICU staffing law as a stepping stone to more extensive staffing legislation (Massachusetts Nurses Association 2014).

While California's efforts in the area of safe-staffing legislation have not been replicated, seven other states have passed laws requiring hospitals to have staffing committees responsible for plans and staffing policy. Those states are Connecticut, Illinois, Nevada, Ohio, Oregon, Texas, and Washington. As in California and Massachusetts, nurses unions have been among the main advocates for these laws (American Nurses Association 2016b). While unions have worked hard to establish staffing committees via contract language, establishing committees by legislation accomplishes more because all acute care hospitals in a state would be required to create such committees.

Mandatory Overtime

Legislation has also been introduced at the federal level to address the problem of mandatory overtime in health care settings. The Safe Nursing and Patient Care Act "would prohibit the requirement that a nurse work more than 12 hours in a 24 hour period and 80 hours in a consecutive 14 day period, except under certain circumstances" (American Nurses Association 2016c). The act was strongly supported by nurses unions, but it has not become law (GovTrack.US 2016).

At the state level, however, unions representing nurses have made much more progress in addressing the problem of mandatory overtime. To date, 16 states have passed laws restricting mandatory overtime for RNs: Alaska, Connecticut, Illinois, Maine, Maryland, Massachusetts, Minnesota, New Hampshire, New Jersey, New York, Oregon, Pennsylvania, Rhode Island, Texas, Washington, and West Virginia. And two states—California and Missouri—restrict the use of mandatory overtime by regulation (American Nurses Association 2016d; Wood 2012). Most ban compulsory overtime after a nurse has worked 12 hours, although the New Jersey law prohibits it after eight hours, except in the case of an emergency (American Nurses Association 2016c). Again, in virtually all of those states, nurses unions have been the moving force behind the passage of this legislation.

Floating

Floating is an issue on which nurse unions have made little legislative progress. Their efforts to address this issue have focused largely on the negotiation of collective bargaining provisions restricting the practice.

NURSES UNIONS, VOICE, AND ADDITIONAL PATIENT CARE ISSUES

While this chapter has focused on the three patient care issues that have garnered the most attention from nurses unions, there are a number of other patient care issues on which nurses unions have had an impact by giving nurses greater involvement in patient care decisions. In most of those cases, nurses unions have used a combination of two of the mechanisms discussed in this chapter to provide nurses with the opportunity for greater voice. Those mechanisms are collective bargaining and union–management collaboration/partnership. The following case studies provide more details on these approaches.

The California Nurses Association's Registered Nurses Quality Liaison Program

The CNA used one of these mechanisms, collective bargaining, at the Kaiser Permanente (KP) hospitals in California at which they represent RNs to establish the Registered Nurses Quality Liaison (RNQL) program. Part of the contract settlement of 1998, the RNQL program created 18 new positions "focused solely on identifying and solving systemwide Kaiser nursing practice issues (California Nurses Association 2015: 9)." The program's goals included improving the quality of patient care and outcomes and increasing "staff RN/NP participation in the quality assurance and/or performance improvement process within the organization (California Nurses Association 2015: 17)." These new positions were staffed by RNs selected by bargaining unit nurses themselves and resulted in recognition of the fact that nurses, because of their significant experience and knowledge, were qualified to play a more important role in decision making about patient care, safety, and quality (California Nurses Association 2015).

The program caused KP nurses to "really begin to think of themselves as on par with nursing colleagues in administration" and "gave [them] control of their practice and acknowledged that they are the experts in their field of nursing practice" (California Nurses Association 2015: 9). Over the years, the number of RNQL positions has more than doubled, from 18 to 37, and the program has made innumerable contributions to improved care.

The RNQL program is, at its heart, an employee involvement program, but because of CNA's strong opposition to union–management collaboration in general, and the KPLMP in particular, the language of the program downplays any cooperative angle. From CNA's perspective, the program is a union initiative that they bargained for and won to give their members a greater voice in running KP. The RNQLs are elected by their fellow nurses and are independent from the employer, thus distinguishing the program from KPLMP initiatives.

RNs and nurse practitioners (NPs) working as RNQLs represent CNA on quality process/structure committees, KP's acuity staffing system, professional performance committees, the Nurse Practitioner Regional Committee, and home health committees. These opportunities provide RNQLs with much greater information and access to important contacts in the KP system (California Nurses Association 2008).

CNA believes that the RNQL program has been a significant asset to patient care. Examples of initiatives resulting from the program include the creation of protocols at KP's call centers and after-hours clinics for addressing requests for information from pregnant women. Previously, such callers were instructed to either see their primary care provider the next day or to seek care at a nearby emergency room. The new protocols provided increased and immediate access to valuable information and to care opportunities (California Nurses Association 2008).

The RNQL program was also instrumental in developing both a peer review process and a formal mentoring program for NPs. Nurse practitioners who furnish medications are required by California state regulations to participate in peer review processes to ensure that all NPs are aware of standards of patient care. The RNQLs worked with KP to create and implement a peer review program for KP facilities in northern

California that met the legal requirements. CNA also negotiated a contractual agreement to create an NP mentoring program. RNQLs were instrumental in shaping the mentoring program so that it would meet the needs of NPs (California Nurses Association 2008).

The RNQLs also created a Staff Nurse Quality Awareness program. This program was designed to increase awareness and participation among the nurse workforce in KP's various quality structures. For example, RNQLs resolved a problem in the Bariatrics Service Department at KP that involved a confusing insulin order form that had led to medication errors. RNQLs redesigned the form, eliminating the possibility of potentially serious mistakes in administering insulin (California Nurses Association 2008).

SEIU Healthcare Pennsylvania/Allegheny General Hospital Partnership

Another substantial example of nurses and their unions collaborating with management to improve patient care is the partnership SEIU Healthcare Pennsylvania negotiated with Allegheny Health Network (AHN) in Pittsburgh. This initiative has provided RNs at that hospital with opportunities to develop and implement structures that give nurses a greater voice in improving care delivery and actually result in processes to improve patient satisfaction, patient outcomes, and the financial health of the hospital (Zobrist 2016). Lauded by U.S. Secretary of Labor Thomas Perez as a "national model for labor–management partnerships," the initiative centers around teams and training programs that are created to work on specific areas of improvement using methods based on the "lean manufacturing" approach (Labrador 2014).

Established in 2008, the initiative was funded by grants provided by AHN and the Pennsylvania Department of Labor and Industry. In 2013, the union negotiated for additional funding from the hospital's management. In past years, nurses and management at AHN collaborated on a comprehensive, nurse-driven, quality and performance improvement initiative that created and implemented programs to reduce infections, streamline processes, improve reporting accuracy, and cut down on time taken away from care (Zobrist 2016).

In 2014, five registered nurses at AHN's Allegheny General Hospital developed and implemented a work plan to reduce two "hospital-acquired conditions." The team addressed central line–associated bloodstream infections in the surgical intensive care unit and catheter-associated urinary tract infections in the medical intensive care and step-down units at the hospital. The plan resulted in the virtual elimination of those infections in targeted units in the first month of the initiative (Service Employees International Union 2015).

The program has evolved over time. Most recently, the union and the hospital agreed to a structure that includes four newly created positions called quality coaches. These positions are filled by front-line RNs from the bargaining unit who work full time to support the quality improvement projects of unit-based teams, who are the heart of the program. The parties have committed to the creation of 30 quality teams across the AHN. Significant training is provided to all participants in the program. Already these teams have identified a number of problems to focus on. These issues include patient falls, the manner in which patient assignments are distributed, and patient flow in the emergency room (Zobrist 2016). The agreement also provides for the hiring of a quality manager paid for by AHN and a quality coordinator, whose salary is paid partly by the union (65%) and partly by the health network (35%) (Zobrist 2016).

The increased commitment made by the AHN RNs, the union, and the health system's administration is a testament to the positive experience they have had since the partnership began in 2008. The additional investment has the potential to result in significant improvements in patient care in the years ahead.

The Vermont Federation of Nurses and Health Professionals/ University of Vermont Medical Center Model Unit Process

The Vermont Federation of Nurses and Health Professionals (VFNHP) is an affiliate of the American Federation of Teachers. It represents licensed practical nurses (LPNs) and RNs at the University of Vermont Medical Center (UVMC) (formerly Fletcher Allen Healthcare), an academic medical center in Burlington, Vermont. The Model Unit Process (MUP) is a joint problem-solving process designed to improve quality of care and patient safety.

The MUP has its roots in a 2006 dispute between VFNHP and UVMC over the application of contract language about staffing levels. In the process of arbitrating the dispute, the union offered to withdraw its grievance if the hospital would agree to work with the union on developing a collaborative mechanism that, in addition to jointly determining appropriate staffing levels, would work to find solutions to other care-related problems (Lazes, Figueroa, and Katz 2012). The UVMC administration agreed, and the MUP was established in a sidebar agreement. It was not until 2009 that the process formally became a part of the labor agreement.

Like most union–management collaboration programs, the MUP process has changed and adapted as the parties have learned which processes and structures work and which do not. Since 2008, the MUP program has involved four units at a time. MUP teams comprised of managers and bargaining unit members undergo joint training to prepare themselves to work together on projects over a six-month period. The teams are asked to take on four projects. Two of the projects are required to address the systemwide issues of infection prevention and improved communication. The teams have the opportunity to pick two unit-based issues for their other projects. MUP team responsibilities involve coming up with innovative solutions to problems. Once those solutions are conceived and developed, the implementation of the solutions is usually turned over to that unit's professional practice council (PPC). Unlike MUP teams, which operate for a fixed period of time, PPCs are joint bodies that operate on an ongoing basis (Lazes, Figueroa, and Katz 2012).

The MUP initiative has contributed numerous innovative solutions to significant patient care problems. For instance, the UVMC psychiatric unit MUP tackled an unusual, but critically important, problem that psych units nationwide face. A portion of the inpatients in psychiatric units have a much higher rate of exposure to bedbugs than the population at large. When these patients are admitted, there is a risk that they will introduce this problem into the hospital. This was an ongoing concern in the UVMC psych unit (Lazes, Figueroa, and Katz 2012).

To address this problem, the unit's MUP team developed a more systematic protocol for dealing with the means by which bedbugs can be introduced into the ward. This protocol included making sure that "patients' belongings were bagged and stored on the unit, [that] patients were screened for bedbug exposure, [that] social workers alerted those bringing belongings to bring them in plastic bags and to pack no more than three changes of clothes, and [that] belongings were searched in a designated non-carpeted area" (Lazes, Figueroa, and Katz 2012: 39).

The nurses and nurse managers involved in the UVMC Orthopedic and Urology Surgical Unit's (OUSU) MUP choose the reduction of patient falls as one of its projects. At the time the MUP team took on this project, the OUSU's fall rate was 3.07 per 1,000 patient days, which was above UVMC's target fall rate. The OUSU MUP group set 2.00 falls per 1,000 patient days as its goal and proceeded to develop strategies for meeting this target. These strategies included "the use of bed alarms according to policy for all patients, LNA and RN alternating hourly rounds, charge nurse responsibilities to include the printing of a list of fall risk patients and monitoring bed alarm use of fall risk patients, and posting a list of fall free days in the nurses station to keep staff focused on preventing falls" (Lazes, Figueroa, and Katz 2012: 37).

In the months following the implementation of the corrective strategies recommended by the MUP team, the patient fall rate for the OUSU was 2.00 per 1,000 patient days. As a result, the OUSU PPC took steps to ensure that the strategies would remain in place after the MUP project concluded (Lazes, Figueroa, and Katz 2012).

The UVMC Outpatient Surgery MUP team also came up with an innovative plan to improve patient outcomes in its unit. Citing research that indicated "that patients who are warmer during their surgery spend less time in the hospital as sustained normothermia promotes healing and reduces surgical site infections," the MUP team put in place a plan to keep patients' temperatures at or above 98.6°F (36°C) during their time in the Post Anesthesia Care Unit. After investigating various alternatives, the MUP group decided to use Thermolite hats and warming blankets to keep patients at the proper body temperature to maintain normothermia. After implementing the plan, the team put in place a recordkeeping system that would, after substantial time had gone by, allow the effectiveness of the effort to be evaluated (Lazes, Figueroa, and Katz 2012: 37–38).

Maimonides Strategic Alliance

A last example of a labor–management partnership designed to improve the quality of care in a hospital setting is the Maimonides Strategic Alliance (MSA). The MSA differs from the other partnerships discussed in this chapter because it includes multiple unions representing a range of occupations.

Established in the late 1990s, the MSA is a partnership between Maimonides Health Center in Brooklyn, New York, and three unions: the New York State Nurses Association (NYSNA), representing RNs; the Committee of Interns and Residents (CIR), an SEIU affiliate representing physicians (house staff and residents); and 1199SEIU United Healthcare Workers East (1199), representing the support and technical employees. According to the Strategic Alliance Report 2007, the MSA

> is grounded in the belief that fostering respect among employees and supervisors, promoting rank-and-file leadership, encouraging broad workforce participation in problem-solving and decision-making, and developing a true partnership between unionized workers and management are all essential to the Medical Center's success. (Strategic Alliance 2007: 4)

The MSA is overseen by a hospital-wide Labor Management Council (LMC). Most of the work of the partnership is done by Departmental Labor Management Committees (DLMCs) formed "to work on quality of care and patient satisfaction issues, as well as issues related to employee needs of respect and input into decision-making" (Strategic Alliance 2007: 4). All participants are provided with extensive training on problem solving and teamwork.

Over the years, the nurses participating in the MSA have made many significant contributions to improve the quality of nursing care at the hospital, such as a hospital-wide strategy for reducing patient falls. The strategy cut the number of falls by almost half. At the same time, the use of patient restraints was significantly reduced. DLMCs involving RNs also have developed strategies to reduce the prevalence of pressure sores among patients at risk for that complication. They also initiated an immunization program for elderly patients in danger of developing pneumonia and other bacterial infections (Strategic Alliance 2007).

In addition to the contributions that nursing-related DLMCs have made to patient care, the fact that the MSA involves nearly all professional and nonprofessional occupations means that similar quality-related initiatives occur in every department and unit in the hospital. For example, the physicians in the Cardiology DLMC helped assess and improve the way that caregivers respond to cardiac monitor alarms (emergency codes), decreasing average response times to less than one minute. Likewise, the manner in which special dietary meals are prepared and delivered have undergone significant changes as a result of a DLMC initiative that included a workflow analysis and retraining program led by the hospital's food and nutrition staff. The goal of the initiative was to increase the percentage of meals delivered on time. That metric did in fact improve over time and is now in the high 90s.

As another example, the Environmental Services Study Action Team conceived and implemented a hospital-wide cleanliness and orderliness project to improve sanitation across the entire hospital. That project was part of a larger effort to prepare the hospital for scrutiny by the Joint Commission on the Accreditation of Healthcare Organizations (JCAHO) (Strategic Alliance 2007).

An additional, and unusual, aspect of the MSA is that it is the mechanism by which managers and supervisors are hired at Maimonides. This joint hiring process has been in place for years, and while its impact cannot be measured directly, several departments led by managers hired under the MSA approach have seen significant performance improvements. While also hard to quantify, involving employees in hiring their supervisors gives them a stake in their supervisor's success and provides them with an incentive to help the supervisor succeed. It also ensures that the supervisor is going to be supportive of the partnership approach under the MSA (Strategic Alliance 2007).

CONCLUSION

Nurses see each of the issues discussed in this chapter—understaffing, mandatory overtime, and floating—as issues that affect the quality of the patient care they are able to deliver at their workplaces. The strategies nurses unions employ to address those and other issues—collective bargaining, joint consultation, and lobbying/legislative action—provide RNs with direct and substantial opportunities to have a greater voice in shaping the way care is delivered in hospital settings in the United States.

The case studies discussed in this chapter demonstrate how collaboration and employee engagement in particular can expand the opportunity for nurses to have a voice in a wide range of patient care–related issues.

The opportunity for, and expansion of, RN voice in decisions involving patient care in a hospital setting is a development that benefits all of the stakeholders in the health care system—nurses, nurses unions, patients, administrators, and by extension, other health care workers. Nurses are at the heart of the care delivery system. They are better educated than ever before and have a deep commitment to quality care for their patients. The experience and knowledge they develop over time makes them a valuable and unique source of information and ideas.

No other health care professional spends as much time as RNs in actually delivering hands-on care to patients or has the intimate knowledge of patient needs that RNs do. Physicians and administrators are rarely around at 2 a.m. to see how the facility operates at that time of day. Nor do they regularly use the basic equipment required to take care of acutely ill patients on an hourly or daily basis. The combination of nurses' knowledge and commitment to patient care makes them a tremendous resource for ideas and suggestions about how to deliver care, as well as how to keep costs down. While they have much to contribute, nurses clearly also benefit from having a greater voice in patient care decisions. Helping to improve care increases job satisfaction, and having a greater say in decision making causes nurses to feel valued and appreciated.

Nurses unions benefit from the greater commitment of its members that results from the union providing a greater opportunity for them to have more input in their workplace and, as a result, creating a situation where they are able to provide the quality of care they believe they have a responsibility to provide. As a result, patients receive better care and outcomes, as suggested by the research on staffing levels, mandatory overtime, and floating.

Administrators also benefit from the improved outcomes and associated cost savings that result from enhanced RN participation in the patient-care decision-making process (although some administrators might see greater nurse involvement as diminishing their prerogatives, and hence the value and status of managers).

Finally, other health care workers benefit from improved patient care outcomes, as well as from an openness on the part of administrators to the expansion of voice opportunities for all employees that comes from positive experiences with nurse–administrator collaboration and partnership.

The promise of collaboration and partnership as a model for health care workplaces provides reason for optimism concerning the enormous challenges facing the American health care system. The biggest single challenge facing that system is rapidly increasing costs. The cost issue threatens the very viability of health care in our society. The potential that collaboration and partnership has, if put in place across our health care system, is that it can, as demonstrated in this chapter, improve the quality of care for patients without increased costs and investment. Reducing infections by changing existing processes and practices can be accomplished without adding additional costs to patient care; in fact, the shorter hospital stays and reduced readmission rates for patients that result can decrease costs and provide an incentive to expand the use of collaboration and partnership. Similar cost savings can result from other improvements in patient safety, including the reduction in falls and faster responses to emergency codes.

While most of the cost savings cited are almost serendipitous (and secondary to) the primary goal, which is improved quality of care, the potential for collaboration and partnership to directly address the issue of cost reduction is great. RNs and other health care workers are very much aware that the continued increase in health care costs threatens their ability to provide care, which ultimately affects their own job security. This awareness provides significant incentives for those health care workers to use collaboration and partnership mechanisms that have proven successful in addressing the problem of health care costs.

Unfortunately, at the moment, successful collaboration and partnership programs involving nurses and other health care workers are the exception and not the rule. As long as there is willingness to do so, there is little reason that health care workers, the unions that represent them, and hospital administrations cannot expand this promising approach to health care workplaces across the United States. And the fact that many hospitals remain non-union does not mean that this approach is unavailable to those workplaces. The desire for, and the efficacy resulting from, increased voice are ubiquitous. While there is a need for greater experience with collaboration and partnership programs in the non-union sector, this approach, in theory, could bring many of the same across-the-board benefits it has created in the unionized health care sector.

The first step in moving in this direction is greater awareness—on the part of all parties—about the improvements that collaboration and partnership approaches can have in health care settings. Until then, nurses unions can continue to use collective bargaining and political/legislative work to try to improve patient care in American hospitals.

REFERENCES

Aiken, L. H., D. M. Sloane, J. P. Cimiotti, S. P. Clarke, L. Flynn, J. Seago, J. Spetz, and H. L. Smith. 2010. "Implications of the California Nurse Staffing Mandate for Other States." *Health Services Research* 45, no. 4: 904–21. doi:10.1111/j.1475-6773.2010.01114.x.

American Association of Critical-Care Nurses. 2016. "Mandatory Overtime." http://bit.ly/29rxm9S.

American Nurses Association. 2016a. "About ANA." http://bit.ly/29Qqmyd.

American Nurses Association. 2016b. "Nurse Staffing." http://bit.ly/29rxdmG.

American Nurses Association. 2016c. "ANA State Government Affairs on Mandatory Overtime." http://bit.ly/29Qqdek.

American Nurses Association. 2016d. "Mandatory Overtime: Summary of State Approaches." http://bit.ly/29rxpCG.

Association for Union Democracy. 2010 (Jan./Feb.). "New National Union Aims to Unite Nurses." *Union Democracy Review* 183.

Business Wire. 2002 (Sep. 6). "California Nurses Association Wins Mandatory Overtime Ban, Record Gains at Kaiser Permanente in Nation's Largest RN Contract." *Business Wire.* http://bit.ly/29ry8Ui.

California Healthcare Association. 2003 (Apr.). "Nurse to Patient Ratios." CHA Special Report, p. 4.

California Nurses Association. 2008 (Jun. 23). "The Kaiser AFL-CIO Partnership: Silencing Patient, Union, and Caregiver Voice." California Nurses Association.

California Nurses Association. 2015 (Oct.). "Conversations with Kay." *National Nurse: The Voice of National Nurses United,* p. 9.

California Nurses Association. 2016a. "CNA/NNU 101: Your Guide to Joining the RN Movement." http://bit.ly/29sPSdY.

California Nurses Association. 2016b. "Professional Standards for RNs." http://bit.ly/29sPXOU and http://bit.ly/29sPHPJ.

Clark, P. F., and D. A. Clark. 2006. "Union Strategies for Improving Patient Care: The Key to Nurse Unionism." *Labor Studies Journal* 31, no. 1: 51–70. doi:10.1353/lab.2006.0003.

Clark, P. F., and D. A. Clark. 2008 (Jun.). Interviews with CNA officials, including executive director, co-presidents, director of research, and director of Kaiser Permanente Division, Oakland, CA.

Clarke, S. P., J. L. Rockett, D. M. Sloane, and L. H. Aiken. 2002. "Organizational Climate, Staffing, and Safety Equipment as Predictors of Needlestick Injuries and Near-Misses in Hospital Nurses." *American Journal of Infection Control* 30, no. 4: 207–16. doi:10.1067/mic.2002.123392.

Cotterman, D. 2015 (Sep. 28). "ValleyCare Calls Arbitrator's Overtime Decision Disappointing." *WFMJ.com.* http://bit.ly/29sRTqi.

de Castro, A. B., K. Fujishiro, T. Rue, E. A. Tagalog, L. P. Samaco-Paquiz, and G. C. Gee. 2010. "Associations Between Work Schedule Characteristics and Occupational Injury and Illness." *International Nursing Review* 57, no. 2: 188–94. doi:10.1111/j.1466-7657.2009.00793.x.

Dziuba-Ellis, J. 2006. "Float Pools and Resource Teams: A Review of the Literature." *Journal of Nursing Care Quality* 21, no. 4: 352–59. doi:10.1097/00001786-200610000-00013.

Eakin, P. 2016. "Welcome to PASNAP's Newest Members!" *Pennsylvania Association of Staff Nurses and Allied Professionals*. http://bit.ly/29sRdl3.

GovTrack.US. 2016. "S. 1842 (110th): Safe Nursing and Patient Care Act of 2007." http://bit.ly/29sRnZB.

Hirsch, B., and D. Macpherson. 2016. "Union Membership and Coverage Database." Unionstats.com. http://bit.ly/29sRqol.

Indest, G. 2012 (May 20). "Registered Nurses in Florida Finalize Union Agreement with HCA." *The Health Law Firm Newsletter*. http://bit.ly/29sRDYE.

Kaiser Permanente. 2010 (Oct. 1). "National Agreement." http://bit.ly/29sRxQv.

Kane R. L., T. Shamliyan, C. Mueller, S. Duval, and T. Wilt. 2007 (Mar.). "Nursing Staffing and Quality of Patient Care." Evidence Report/Technology Assessment No. 151. AHRQ Publication No. 07-E005. Agency for Healthcare Research and Quality.

Labrador, R. 2014 (Jun. 11). "Labor Secretary Praises Allegheny General Hospital During Visit." *Pittsburgh Post-Gazette*. http://bit.ly/29sSgkU.

Lafer, G. 2005. "Hospital Speedups and the Fiction of a Nursing Shortage." *Labor Studies Journal* 30 (1): 27–46. doi:10.1353/lab.2005.0029.

Larson, N., S. Sendelbach, B. Missal, J. Fliss, and P. Gaillard. 2012. "Staffing Patterns of Scheduled Unit Staff Nurses vs. Float Pool Nurses: A Pilot Study." *Research in Practice* 21, no. 1: 27–39.

Lazes, P. M., M. Figueroa, and L. Katz. 2012. "How Labor–Management Partnerships Improve Patient Care, Cost Control, and Labor Relations: Case Studies of Fletcher Allen Health Care, Kaiser Permanente, and Montefiore Medical Center's Care Management Corporation." Cornell University, ILR School. http://bit.ly/29sSvws.

Massachusetts Nurses Association 2011. "Tufts, St. Vincent RNs Win Staffing Language, Ratify Contracts and Avoid Strikes." *Labor Action News*, Massachusetts Nurses Association. http://bit.ly/29sSEjq.

Massachusetts Nurses Association. 2014. "News Bulletin: This Is a Historic Step in Our Ongoing Campaign for Safe Limits in All Units." http://bit.ly/29sSCIe.

McDonagh, M. 2014. "Nurse Unions Continue to Push for Nurse-Patient Ratio Legislation." Littler. http://bit.ly/29rCFGo.

Michigan Nurses Association. 2001. "Michigan Nurses Association Health Care Survey Results."

Minnesota Nurses Association. 2004. "Contract Agreement Between MNA and Methodist Hospital."

Molyneux, G. 2001. "Professional Employees: The Next Frontier for Organized Labor." *Public Perspective*, March/April: 29–32.

National Nurses Union. 2016. "About NNU." http://bit.ly/29rDeju.

New York State Nurses Association. 2015 (Aug. 6). "NY State's Largest Nurses Union Celebrate Historic Contract Settlement Across New York City." Press release. http://bit.ly/29rDbUO.

Pruitt, J. 2016 (Jun. 22). Interview with James Pruitt, Vice President, LMP and Labor Relations, Kaiser Permanente

Rogers A. E., W. T. Hwang, L. D. Scott, L. H. Aiken, and D. F. Dinges. 2004. "The Working Hours of Hospital Staff Nurses and Patient Safety." *Health Affairs* 23, no. 4: 202–12.

Rogowski, J. A., D. Staiger, T. Patrick, J. Horbar, M. Kenny, and E T. Lake. 2013. "Nurse Staffing and NICU Infection Rates." *JAMA Pediatrics*, no. 5: 444–50. doi:10.1001/jamapediatrics.2013.18.

Sachs, A. 2014 (Dec. 18). "Public Ranks Nurses as Most Honest, Ethical Profession for 13th Straight Year." Press release, American Nurses Association. http://bit.ly/29rEPFU.

Service Employees International Union. 2015 (Apr.). "Improving Care, Lowering Costs: How Front-Line Hospital Workers Are Transforming Healthcare." http://bit.ly/29rFE1F.

Service Employees International Union. 2016a. "Nurses United for Quality Care." http://bit.ly/29TOSlN.

Service Employees International Union. 2016b. "SEIU Agreement: July 1, 2015–June 30, 2017. A Collective Bargaining Agreement Between Board of Regents, State of Iowa and Service Employees International Union Local 199." http://bit.ly/29rGifc.

Service Employees International Union. 2016c. "Agreement Between SEIU Healthcare 1199 NW and Sweden Medical Center (Registered Nurse Unit)." http://bit.ly/29rFHKG.

Sochalski, J., and L. H. Aiken. 1999. "Accounting for Variation in Hospital Outcomes: A Cross-National Study." *Health Affairs* 18 (3): 256–59. doi:10.1377/hlthaff.18.3.256.

Strategic Alliance. 2007. "Strategic Alliance Report 2007: Creating Competitive Advantage in a Changing Health Care Environment Through Worker Participation." Cornell University, ILR School. http://bit.ly/29rGH1B.

Tate, S. 2005. "Patient Advocacy: The Nurse's Responsibility." *Topics in Advanced Practice Nursing eJournal* 5, no. 2. http://wb.md/29rHfVc.

Trinkoff, A. M., M. Johantgen, C. L. Storr, A. P. Gurses, Y. Liang, and K. Han. 2011. "Nurses' Work Schedule Characteristics, Nurse Staffing, and Patient Mortality." *Nursing Research* 60, no. 1: 1–8. doi:10.1097/nnr.0b013e3181fff15d.

Trinkoff, A. M., R. Le, J. Geiger-Brown, and J. Lipscomb. 2007. "Work Schedule, Needle Use, and Needlestick Injuries Among Registered Nurses." *Infection Control and Hospital Epidemiology* 28, no. 2: 156–64. doi:10.1086/510785.

Wood, D. 2012 (Aug. 17). "Massachusetts Latest State to Outlaw Mandatory Nurse Overtime." *NurseZone Newsletter*.

Zobrist, Z. 2016 (Jan. 11). Interview with Zack Zobrist, SEIU Pennsylvania Healthcare Staff Representative.

Chapter 6

Labor–Management Partnerships in Health Care: Responding to the Evolving Landscape

Adrienne E. Eaton
Rebecca Kolins Givan
School of Management and Labor Relations
Rutgers University

Peter Lazes
Joseph S. Murphy Institute for Worker Education and Labor Studies
City University of New York

INTRODUCTION

Over the past 20 years or so, unions and management have developed several significant joint projects in health care organizations to improve labor–management relations, increase efficiency, improve patient care and satisfaction, and create more meaningful work (Kochan, Eaton, McKersie, and Adler 2009). These partnerships have also helped the parties respond to changes in the health crare landscape. In the U.S., labor–management partnerships have been an important and powerful process to improve the quality of services/products, control costs, and improve the quality of work life of employees as a result of front-line staff and union involvement (Eaton, Rubinstein, and Kochan 2008; Kochan et al. 2008; Rubinstein and Kochan 2001). Partnerships are both a business and a labor relations approach and are typically customized to address the issues of a particular organization, its workforce, and workforce representatives.

Partnerships feature increased union and worker involvement in managerial decision making and work reform. These processes have helped organizations remain competitive, create high-quality products and services, and provide meaningful work for employees (Lazes, Figueroa, and Katz, 2012; Maimonides Medical Center 2007). While overall there has likely been a decline in the number of labor–management partnerships in the United States, health care is one of the few sectors where they have continued to grow and develop (Eaton, Cutcher-Gershenfeld, and Rubinstein 2016).

Although there is also a record of partnerships and other forms of union–management collaboration in long-term care, in this chapter, we focus on hospitals and health systems. We ask how labor–management collaboration in health care comes about, and when and how collaboration is successful.[1] We are guided in this by the general literature on labor–management partnership. Kochan and colleagues (2008), for instance, argue that partnerships are precarious and that to survive and flourish they need to put in place structures or practices that solve three specific strategic challenges: initiation, governance, and sustainability.

Eaton, Rubinstein, and McKersie (2004) identify, on the basis of data collected from more than 50 partnerships, specific factors that deal with a very similar list of challenges. Specifically, they argue that partnerships are usually formed in the context of a crisis, but they also require talented leadership and facilitation, "enabling language," and "union capacity to engage in managerial decision making while maintaining [its representational role]" (Eaton, Rubinstein, and McKersie 2004: 9). Eaton, Rubinstein, and McKersie (2004) also identify factors associated with sustainability including, among others, achieving improvements in productivity or quality and ongoing management of the tension between collaborative and adversarial relations. This last factor has particular implications for how collective bargaining is conducted (Kochan, Eaton, McKersie, and Adler 2009: 87; Rubinstein 2001: 426). We attempt to explore these issues using six in-depth cases.

The health care industry has been rapidly changing in recent years. The high cost of care coupled with poor quality is pressuring health systems to change how they provide services. In addition, more patients, as a result of the Affordable Care Act (ACA), now have access to health insurance, which has resulted in increased demand at the same time that many hospital systems are merging and consolidating. More specifically, health systems are undergoing major changes that shift the focus from hospital-based care to integrated and more community-based care.

As the health care landscape continues to transform as a result of new quality requirements and changes in reimbursement, labor–management partnerships increasingly play a role in identifying and developing new systems of care. These changes require staff to work together in different ways. The jobs themselves are also significantly changing as a result of reimbursement shifting from a fee-for-service reimbursement process (getting paid for what is done during a particular hospital or physician visit) to an outcome-based process (Porter and Lee 2013).

SIX KEY CASES

We selected six critical cases in order to understand the nature of collaboration between labor and management in health care.[2] Four of these cases are defined by the parties themselves as, and meet our definition of, "partnership," while two involve more-limited forms of collaboration—

although they may evolve into partnerships. Space limitations did not allow for inclusion of additional cases, but we believe the cases we discuss are among—if not *the*—most extensive and interesting examples of labor–management collaboration currently ongoing in health care organizations in the United States.[3] We also wanted our cases to involve different unions to the extent possible.

The case studies were based on interviews, observation (sometimes participant observation), and documentary research. We examined meeting minutes, reports, collective bargaining agreements, and secondary literature. In most of the cases, at least one of us has had a consulting relationship to the partnership at some point. We interviewed key actors in each case, which generally included representatives of both union and management.

Labor–management projects in health care vary in origin—some emerge from crises in relationships, where conflicts arising from the bargaining and implementation of contracts were clearly detrimental to the functioning of the hospital organization. In other cases, parties saw an opportunity to make improvements to their organizations before crisis struck. The cases vary from broad partnership, in the case of Kaiser Permanente, to fairly narrow joint work, as in the case of the Committee on Interns and Residents' quality improvement program. In each case, we try to draw out the origins of the partnership, the key areas for collaboration, the major stumbling blocks and successes, and the results of the collaboration.

We detail the collaborative processes, the resources that were allocated by labor and management, and some of the outcomes for the relevant stakeholders. We show that, while each case retains unique attributes, there are some common factors that demonstrate that collaborative relationships can be particularly productive in the health care workplace. We argue that health care is special, or exceptional, because it does not produce cars or steel rods, but rather it involves the care of human beings—with individual well-being and even lives at stake. Health care employees tend to identify with the mission of the organizations they work for, and it is likely easier for them to find common cause with management toward the goal of better patient care.

University of Massachusetts Memorial Hospital and SHARE

SHARE, an AFSCME affiliate, represents 2,800 clerical, technical, and health care employees at the UMass Memorial Medical Center and another 500 at the UMass Medical School, both in Worcester, Massachusetts. UMass Memorial is a three-campus hospital system with almost 800 beds and more than 9,500 employees; it is also the clinical partner of the UMass Medical School (UMass Memorial Medical Center 2016).

SHARE was organized in 1997 and is part of a network of unions called the New England Organizing Project (NEOP), at the core of which is the

Harvard Union of Clerical and Technical Workers (HUCTW). HUCTW organized under the banner, "It's not anti-Harvard to be pro-union" and has from its beginning taken a collaborative approach to labor relations. This has involved using interest-based, problem-solving tools to deal with grievances, as well as formal departmental level labor–management committees to work on various problems.[4] The NEOP model emphasizes one-on-one relationships between union staff and members and "participation by members in decisions at work, and partnership and collaboration with the employer" (New England Organizing Project, no date). As such, SHARE has taken the initiative to push for greater voice for members in patient care and quality improvement.

Recently, SHARE's interest has been met with an open reception from the new CEO, Eric Dickson, and Dickson's newly hired chief human resource officer, Bart Metzger, at UMass Memorial Healthcare. Dickson and Metzger are interested in improving what have been fractious relations with the system's various unions and in involving workers in quality improvement efforts. Metzger has experience in the New York City health care system, where he was able to observe the important joint work done at Maimonides Medical Center (another case discussed in this chapter) and other hospitals, and more recently from Allegheny General Hospital, which has an ongoing joint labor–management partnership with the union SEIU Healthcare PA.[5]

More recently, SHARE has become heavily involved, working closely with the hospital's internal process improvement office, the Center for Innovation and Transformational Change (CITC), in efforts to strengthen the hospital's quality improvement efforts. The union has had a full-time union staff person assigned to this work since late 2014 and added a second person on a part-time basis in fall 2015. The full-time union staffer provides training for the workforce in "lean management" under the auspices of the CITC and coaches individual union members on their process improvement work. He also supports the two central, institution-wide elements of the process improvement work: Idea Boards and huddles.

Each department is supposed to have a bulletin board for identifying and posting work problems and new ideas for work processes and is supposed to huddle—that is, regularly meet in a fairly fluid and informal way—to discuss ideas posted on the board and move them through an implementation process. There is, in practice however, wide variation in how often departmental huddles are held and in who runs them—varying from management, doctors, SHARE members, or a rotation—and in the quantity and quality of ideas generated. Depending on the nature of the problem, it may be addressed internally by department staff or passed along to a department manager or supervisor or to CITC staff. Idea Boards and huddles are available (but not mandatory) for all hospital units, not just those providing clinical care. For example, in Central Scheduling—not a direct care unit—there is a project focused on improving patient satisfaction by improving the quality of interactions with this call center.

It is interesting to note that, as of yet, there are no written agreements between labor and management about this process improvement work. Nor have the parties engaged in interest-based bargaining. There is, however, an innovation fund of $1 million available to pay for improvements (generated from Idea Boards) that departments could not otherwise pay for.

There is also a history—again in some units—of Joint Working Groups that bring together managers, providers, union members, and union staff to discuss issues more generally. SHARE is talking with management about a more structured partnership with management, but at the time of this writing had decided to engage in this more bottom-up effort. The union believes strongly that members want to have a more direct role in process improvement activities as well as in improving quality of work-life issues. The main challenge thus far is the unevenness of implementation: some departments are quite invested and committed to the process, while others have not adopted any of the new practices, as evidenced by blank Idea Boards dotted around some units.

University of Vermont Medical Center[6] and AFT Nurses and Healthcare Professionals 5221

The University of Vermont Medical Center (formerly Fletcher Allen Medical Center) serves as the main university teaching hospital in Vermont, comprising the Medical Center Hospital, University Health Center, and UVM College of Medicine. There are also 30 outpatient and community clinics serving approximately 51,000 patients annually. More than 1,650 registered nurses work in the University of Vermont Medical Center alongside 450 physicians and 147 advanced-practice registered nurses and physician assistants. The Vermont chapter of the AFT Nurses and Healthcare Professionals (VTNHP) division represents nurses and ancillary staff at the Medical Center Hospital only.

The joint labor–management partnership was forged in 2006 as a response to insufficient nursing staff ratios in the hospital, building on a previous 2003 agreement to set up a "safe staffing" joint committee. By 2006, it had become clear that management had not followed the recommendations of the joint committee. Initially, the union filed a grievance, which it was pursuing to arbitration. While preparing for the hearing, Jennifer Henry, then-president of the VTNHP local, traveled to Sunnyside Medical Center in Clackamas, Oregon (a Kaiser Permanente facility), to learn about partnership work there. She returned to Vermont committed to creating a similar process and became convinced that to achieve an effective "staffing composition," the union and management needed to develop a less adversarial and more problem-solving relationship with each other.

Henry convinced both the administration and her executive committee to drop the arbitration and design a joint process to implement strategies to improve staffing and restructure responsibilities in each unit of the hospital. This became known as the Model Unit Process (MUP), and it was eventually written into future agreements.

The MUP provides staff nurses, their managers, and nurse educators time to analyze patient and staff needs and determine the appropriate staffing of the unit to improve care delivery and work processes. Non-nurses, such as social workers, nursing assistants, ward clerks, physicians, and pharmacists, are included in these activities when appropriate. The MUP was written into the 2009–2011 collective bargaining agreement, "with the intent of creating a collaborative culture, reducing financial impact and building a systemwide approach to quality improvement."[7]

In 2008, after careful review, labor and management leaders, along with their consultant, decided to take steps to improve their MUP program. Management and labor agreed that future MUP teams would work on two systemwide and two unit-based projects instead of working on as many projects as staff identified. This change helped future MUPs to focus so that they could develop concrete solutions by the time their education and analysis work was completed, usually taking six months. The unit-based projects were identified by a survey compiled by each unit before it started its MUP. Teams were encouraged to start with easy projects—ones considered "low-hanging fruit"—to be able to achieve results quickly so that staff nurses could see that the MUP would result in real decision making. Two of the common systemwide projects were infection prevention and improving communications.

A second goal was to expand opportunities for MUP teams to learn from each other as they went through their six-month cycle of education, analysis, and solution development. To facilitate that, MUP teams from several departments held their educational workshops together and shared their progress during the analysis phase of their work. At the end of the six-month process, they shared their results at an "Outcomes Congress" with the director of nursing and the president of the local union.

In addition to resolving significant staffing issues, staff nurses gained access to departmental budgets, enabling them to make informed decisions about resource use and understand what it takes to run a department from the perspective of a manager. Managers and nurse educators learned more details about the needs and issues of front-line staff. All units of the hospital have now been through a MUP, and the process has begun in outpatient and community health centers.

Along with hiring a consultant (jointly funded by the union and management) to conduct the seven educational/learning sessions, the hospital agreed to free up a union leader to work part-time to support MUP activities. As well as attending the educational sessions, this union leader is available to assist MUP teams by suggesting ways to gather data on specific problems and help team leaders address both systemwide and unit-based problems. This MUP advisor also works with Professional Practice Committees (PPCs)[8] to prepare them for their role in implementing agreements established by their MUP.

Once each MUP team finalizes its recommendations, as a result of feedback from other staff on their unit, they obtain approval for any changes and modified staffing levels from the president of the union and the director of nursing. It is the responsibility of the PPC for a particular unit to implement and sustain these activities.

The tangible results achieved included a reduction in patient falls (from three to two falls per 1,000 patient days) and a reduction in nurse position vacancies—resulting in $8 million in cost savings and improved morale. Union membership has increased by 12% since the inception of the MUP, and the local's members now include 300 tech workers. There are now about 2,100 members in the local union. As a result of improving PPCs and creating better communications among MUP teams, floor nurses are now more aware of the role of the union in creating a voice for them in the decision making in their unit.

Importantly, the labor–management effort at UVM has been able to weather turnover in labor and management leadership. There have now been three changes in the leadership of the local union and management since the inception of the MUP program in 2006. There remains a strong commitment to providing members with the opportunity to improve working conditions and patient care through the program.

There remain some significant challenges. One has been strengthening the work of the PPCs so that they are better able to implement and sustain MUP recommendations. As stated in the labor contract, physicians and other front-line staff members are not members of an MUP or a PPC, but they do attend specific education and training sessions on an as-needed basis. Their absence as active MUP team members reduces the ability of the teams to have access to their insights and knowledge and their involvement to make sure changes are implemented. There also continue to be difficulties documenting and communicating specific changes and outcomes. To some extent this is a result of the nurses not having time (other than during MUP training) to spend on documenting results. Finally, there doesn't seem to be labor involvement in quality improvement and delivery system changes beyond the MUP program. Given the progressive nature of Vermont health care, it would seem UVM might be an appropriate system in which to go beyond unit-based work to explore joint ways to provide more coordinated and integrated care for patients.

Los Angeles Department of Health Services and SEIU Local 721[9]

The Los Angeles Department of Health Services (LA-DHS) is the second largest public safety-net health system in the United States. It includes four hospitals, two former hospitals that are now multiservice ambulatory care centers, 17 community health centers, and 161 community partner clinics (primarily Federally Qualified Health Centers) that provide primary care. It treats 750,000 patients annually, most of whom receive Medicaid or are uninsured, and employs 18,460 staff. The unions that represent workers at LA-DHS are SEIU Local 721, which represents most workers, including nurses; the Committee for Interns and Residents (CIR); and the Union for American Physicians and Dentists (UAPD), which represents attending physicians and dentists.

Since the appointment of LA-DHS director Mitch Katz and his team in 2011, labor and management have begun a comprehensive process of developing opportunities to work together. Both the SEIU international and SEIU Local 721 agreed that it was necessary to create a more integrated delivery system as a result of the ACA as well as to focus on improving access to care and the patient experience. An integrated delivery system focused on treating patients in a coordinated and proactive way could help meet the goal of keeping patients healthier and reducing unneeded hospitalizations.

In late 2011, the leadership of SEIU Local 721 began discussions with the new leadership of LA-DHS. The initial focus was on culture change, the re-enrollment of county residents so that they were eligible to receive LA-DHS services, and the expansion of unit-based teams known as care improvement teams (CITs). The interest in CITs was based on the awareness among union and management leaders of the success of similar activities at other health care institutions, such as Kaiser Permanente, and a recent labor–management partnership process with the Environmental Services Department at the Los Angeles County–USC Medical Center.

By 2013, both union and management leaders decided to deepen their joint process. A one-day retreat was conducted for senior union and management leaders to establish strategic areas of work as well as develop clear principles of engagement (a charter) for joint efforts. The four strategic areas were improving the patient experience, developing a systemwide quality and safety improvement process, expanding the development of CITs, and improving current labor–management committees. In addition, a Labor–Management Transformation Council (LMTC)[10] was created to set strategic priorities, monitor key areas of work, and take corrective actions to ensure that needed changes were implemented. This group was also responsible for making sure that resources were available to support the development and implementation of changes and to develop appropriate tracking and monitoring systems for all joint work.

A social contract was created (i.e., principles of engagement) to make sure joint labor–management work was encouraged within all departments of LA-DHS. The composition of the LMTC includes senior management responsible for operations and medical staff in all four hospitals; Quality Improvement, CIT, and labor relations staff; and senior union leaders and the health care division staff of SEIU Local 721. When CIR and UAPD joined the labor–management partnership process, they were included on the council as well.[11]

At the LMTC retreat, specific groups were created to work on the strategic goals for the labor–management partnership process. Each labor–management work group had a labor and management co-chair and chose members from the LMTC or elsewhere within LA-DHS. In addition to the LMTC, the LA-DHS created the position of director of CITs to oversee the expansion of unit-based teams. Another four staff members (most of them rank-and-file employees) were released from their current jobs to serve as coaches/mentors to CITs. The union agreed to release one full-time staff person to work on the partnership with LA-DHS management.

In addition, the LMTC developed a comprehensive educational program known as CRMs (conference room meetings) to inform all front-line staff (from environmental service employees to attending physicians) why changes were needed to improve access, quality, and coordination of patient care. These educational activities were quite important because a large number of front-line staff were not aware of changes in reimbursement and the need to become a "provider of choice" as a result of the ACA (i.e., patients could now go elsewhere for care) and changes in state funding for uninsured and underinsured patients.

As the labor–management partnership process has deepened in terms of specific activities to improve the patient experience (such as reducing wait times) and patient care (access to a primary care provider), being an effective partner with management has been a challenge for the union and its staff. The union staff has had to develop new skills for this role. The union leadership also realized they needed to develop an extensive member communications strategy so that the union doesn't come across as "management sellouts," given that the union had not previously been involved in quality and system improvement activities.

So far, the LA-DHS/SEIU partnership has produced some significant positive outcomes. For instance, a systemwide set of emergency codes for all four hospitals and 17 ambulatory care settings has been implemented, replacing multiple codes that were confusing and dangerous for both patients and staff. Patient satisfaction scores have improved for outpatient services in key locations as a result of greater access to care and reduced wait time to be seen by a primary care provider. A comprehensive training program has been developed for coders to ensure that LA-DHS receives appropriate reimbursement for services rendered.

Another positive outcome is that the local union has discovered a huge cadre of members who want to work with the union to give front-line staff a voice in decision making. Partnership activities "have mobilized significant numbers of members who see their union as providing them with opportunities to develop a voice and dignity at work while improving patient care," said Gilda Valdez, chief of staff for SEIU Local 721.

Although the joint effort has resulted in major progress, the partnership still faces significant challenges. One is moving beyond unit-based activities to more outcome- or value-based work that is cross-functional or cross-unit (Porter 2010). A further challenge is moving from just treating a patient's current condition to improving a patient's overall health. Such an approach would build on the current quality improvement processes. An additional challenge for labor and management at LA-DHS is how to internally integrate current quality improvement and partnership activities, a common challenge in labor–management efforts (Eaton 1995; Litwin and Eaton, forthcoming). It will also be important to accelerate the coordination and integration of services between primary care, behavioral health, community organizations, and public health because many LA-DHS patients have complicated and co-morbidity conditions. Improving the coordination and integration of primary care and behavioral health services will help ensure that patients have greater access to mental health services as well.

Maimonides Medical Center and CIR, NYSNA, and 1199SEIU[12]

Almost 100 years old, Maimonides Medical Center is the pre-eminent treatment facility in Brooklyn, New York. Maimonides has approximately 600 beds, a staff of renowned physicians, and more than 70 primary care and subspecialty programs. In 2015, the hospital delivered over 8,500 babies and had more than 110,000 adult and pediatric ER visits. It is one of the largest independent teaching hospitals in the nation and trains more than 400 medical and surgical residents annually.

Maimonides started its labor–management partnership process (referred to as its Strategic Alliance process) in 1997—about the same time as Kaiser Permanente started its partnership. The joint vision of executive vice president Pam Brier (later CEO and president) and John Reid, vice president of 1199SEIU (later an executive vice president of the union), was to create ways for labor and management to work together to meet the challenges of the rapidly changing health care environment. The innovative 1994 collective bargaining agreement between 1199SEIU and the League of Voluntary Hospitals and Nursing Homes (Maimonides is a member of the League) created language to encourage labor and management to work together to improve patient care in League hospitals and nursing homes. This innovative contract expanded the joint job security fund and the training and upgrading fund of the League to include additional money for education and consulting services for hospital and nursing homes, such as the 1199/League's Labor–Management Project (Kochan, Eaton, McKersie, and Adler 2009; Maimonides Medical Center 2007).

From the beginning, 1199SEIU was an active partner[13] in the Strategic Alliance work at Maimonides. The New York State Nurses Association (NYSNA) was an original member of the Strategic Alliance but withdrew from 2002 to 2004 as a result of a jurisdictional conflict with 1199SEIU. The Committee of Interns and Residents (CIR) became recognized as a bargaining unit in 2004 and joined Strategic Alliance activities at that time.

The full involvement of physicians as well as all other front-line staff has been a key aspect of the partnership at Maimonides. Attending physicians sit on the Labor–Management Strategic Alliance Council (LMC), which oversees all of the partnership activities. All unions are members of departmental labor–management committees that have been established throughout the hospital.

From the inception of the Strategic Alliance, there have been three key structures. The LMC oversees and supports all joint work; it meets on a monthly basis to share information about changes in the hospital and community as well other issues that impact the hospital (i.e., funding issues, political action, joint lobbying, and innovation grants from the Centers for Medicare and Medicaid Services). This group establishes yearly goals for the Strategic Alliance process and priorities for joint work.

The council operates in a manner similar to that of the LMTC in Los Angeles. It assigns staff to support various work groups and departments. The council consists of senior management of the hospital (including the CFO), as well as several supervisors, leaders from the three unions, human resource/labor relations (HR/LR) staff, quality improvement and performance improvement staff, and front-line staff from specific departments where alliance work is taking place. In addition to this structure, the leaders from each of the three unions and senior management meet regularly (via the Joint Oversight Committee). At the department level are departmental labor–management committees (DLMCs) that oversee training, education and joint problem solving, and redesign activities. DLMCs are composed of union and management representatives and front-line staff. The Strategic Alliance process at Maimonides has been focused on improving patient care and the patient experienc and on creating meaningful jobs for staff. It is seen as a business strategy and therefore has the support of top management. It is driven by operations managers, not by labor relations.

Sizeable resources have been freed up to help establish and sustain the joint work. Three full-time front-line staff (called "developers"—one from each participating union) are assigned to support alliance activities, along with a manager in charge of organizational effectiveness. The developers, paid for by the hospital, are trained in process improvement and system innovation techniques by Cornell University advisors, quality improvement staff, and 1199/League Labor–Management Project staff. The developers are assigned to work with departments or work groups by the LMC. When work groups are established, front-line staff are released from their patient care responsibilities to work on problem-solving and work redesign activities (other staff on those units are scheduled to backfill the positions while staff work on Strategic Alliance activities). There is a hospital-wide budget for backfill for staff, the three developer positions, and for training of union and management about how to support the alliance process.

The Strategic Alliance process has developed over time, starting in its early phase with educational workshops for all employees about the importance of joint work to improve patient care and the quality of work life of employees, moving to establishment of DLMCs to work on a broad range of quality of care, workforce, and labor relations issues. The Strategic Alliance process deepened in the mid-2000s by creating several interdepartmental and systemwide areas of work. This process consisted of the following:

- Creating a joint hiring process for screening and hiring of managers and supervisors
- Establishing a "community of workers" process to improve respect and dignity among Environmental Service workers
- Establishing an environmental services study action team— an intensive employee-driven process to improve the cleanliness of the hospital
- Instituting a cardiology project to improve patient care that resulted in reducing call-bell response time and improving nurse-to-patient ratios
- Setting up a dispute resolution process for handling workforce and management issues appropriately and quickly

Driven by the commitment of the CEO, the Maimonides strategic alliance process has been proactively supported by HR/LR staff (something that is not always true in partnerships). These staff members have developed workshops for managers and supervisors to help them see the value in and master the skills necessary for front-line staff engagement in activities to improve the quality of patient care. In addition, HR staff have helped to revise the employee orientation program in conjunction with the unions to highlight the importance of front-line engagement. HR staff have incorporated into the annual performance review of managers the extent to which their workers are involved in departmental changes. Finally, HR/LR staff have been members of the work group developing an alternative dispute resolution process to help resolve work-related problems, reducing the need for grievances and write-ups.

One strong indicator of the degree of the level of cooperation present in this partnership is the joint hiring process for all supervisors in which workers participate from the start of the process to the final recommendation. Top management assigned the HR department to support the joint process when they found it was being unevenly implemented, and the department produced a guide to the process.

In addition to internal funding by Maimonides Medical Center, the Labor–Management Project of the League of Voluntary Hospitals and Nursing Homes and 1199SEIU has funded some of the consulting and education services of the Cornell University Healthcare Transformation Project, as well as provided mentoring and coaching by their own staff.

Among the significant outcomes from the Strategic Alliance process at Maimonides are the following:

- A redesign of the preparation and delivery of special dietary meals by Food and Nutrition Department staff so that meals are delivered on time more than 90% of the time
- A reduction in wait time from Patient Transport for ER Radiology by 40%
- Increases in Hospital Consumer Assessment of Healthcare Providers and Systems scores (HCAHPS scores of patient experience) by 50% for cleanliness of patient rooms and public areas
- A reduction in response times to cardiac patient alarms of less than one minute
- Joint development of a contact/call center to provide appointment for patients and referral for physicians and to enable physician-to-physician communications
- A reduction in the number of patients returning to the intensive care unit after transferring to a step-down unit
- Improved psychiatric care for seniors
- A 36% reduction in labor-related grievances

Challenges ahead for the Strategic Alliance include forthcoming leadership changes (both the CEO of the hospital and the vice president of the union will be leaving the hospital) and a greater emphasis on ambulatory coordinated care.

Committee of Interns and Residents

The Committee of Interns and Residents (CIR), has 14,000 members nationally, with concentrations in New York, California, and a handful of other states. In recent years, the union has placed considerable emphasis on quality improvement initiatives and patient safety. This focus has been for a number of reasons, including member physicians' emphasis on improving patient care, and strategically reaching members who may be less engaged by more traditional bread-and-butter union issues. The union first attempted to implement programs at the hospitals that seemed most amenable to joint quality improvement work, but those early efforts were sometimes a struggle, given the parties' lack of experience and the challenge of coordination. However, CIR did achieve some positive results and helped to build a better roadmap for future efforts.

With more experience and better language in collective bargaining agreements, including clear structures and processes, the next round of projects achieved better results. Those programs included creating house staff safety councils as a forum for residents to lead improvements in patient safety; instituting a blame-free culture for reporting errors and near misses; improving the process of medication reconciliation; and making follow-up calls to primary care physicians following patient discharge from the hospital. CIR's work has been aided by the new American Council for Graduate Medical Education requirement that quality improvement be part of medical training (Institute of Medicine 2010).

As CIR took on more—and more diverse—quality improvement projects, the union bargained for additional resources to build support structures for this work. This included funding for a Joint Quality Improvement Association (a separate nonprofit organization focused on quality improvement activities) and joint funds to pay for and incentivize quality improvement. CIR was able to negotiate funding for quality improvement projects as a result of surpluses in the health benefit fund for these employees; medical residents tend to be young and healthy, and thus are relatively inexpensive to insure. CIR was able to divert some of the savings from the benefit fund surpluses into quality improvement initiatives that would directly benefit patients. As one chief resident stated, "As residents we felt it was very important we tie in the benefits we were getting in our contract with the care we were providing to our patients; we wanted to connect those two in some way" (Jaltenor 2013).

The union is now working at numerous hospitals to implement quality improvement programs, although the status and progress of the programs are mixed. Current quality improvement activities by CIR (as of this writing) are initiated by residents and supported by a director who is a black belt in Lean Six Sigma (a certificate program to help develop process and quality improvement activities). She was hired in 2011 and promoted to direct the initiative in 2014.

The most successful quality improvement programs have active member-leaders and receptive hospital managers and medical directors. In some cases, committees have been formed, and communication between residents and attending physicians has improved. At times, however, it has been difficult to quantify outcomes. In some cases, the residents have developed a commitment to quality improvement and have begun to see it not only as a strategy to improve patient care but also a useful avenue for their own research and publications. The example of quality improvement at Maimonides Medical Center demonstrates a successful collaborative case where the union was instrumental in achieving a positive outcome with a direct impact on patient care.

There are about 450 residents working at Maimonides Medical Center (Maimonides Medical Center 2015). The residency program at Maimonides is one of the largest free-standing programs in the country (Cohen and Kantrowitz 2012). In addition to the involvement in the Strategic Alliance activities with Maimonides Medical Center as previously described, CIR has engaged in specific quality improvement work at the medical center. The parties established a Joint Quality Improvement Committee in their 2011 collective bargaining agreement. The 2011 contract also included incentive bonuses for residents, to be paid out if the quality improvement initiatives were successful. In the most recent contract (2013–2016), the hospital contributed $180,000 to the incentive pool to reward quality improvement work. The contract also provides funding for a quality fellowship, to be filled by a post-graduate resident.

One of the significant quality improvement activities at Maimonides was the medication reconciliation project. Medication reconciliation is a fundamental aspect of the safe provision of health care. It involves "collecting and maintaining a complete and correct list of patient medications" when the patient is discharged and at all transition points within the hospital (such as a transfer from the emergency room to an inpatient unit) to make sure the medications are safe and appropriate (Sedgh et al. 2013: 357; see also Institute for Healthcare Improvement, no date). This activity is essential in avoiding dangerous medication interactions and providing appropriate care; incomplete medication reconciliation is a massive problem in most health care settings, causing numerous avoidable errors (for more, see Duguid 2012).

The CIR intervention allowed resident leaders to educate their peers on reconciliation and why it matters; they implemented a smartphone-based tool that provided the reference material necessary for medical reconciliation. Some residents (members of the Joint Quality Improvement Committee) also became "super users." That status allowed them to serve as a resource on the wards for other residents to observe and support the reconciliation process. These activities were extremely critical as Maimonides transitioned from a paper-based medication reconciliation process to one that used electronic medical records. After one year, residents received an incentive bonus in several departments where compliance had improved by 20% or more (Sedgh et al. 2013). In some departments, medication reconciliation improved by more than 40% (Jaltenor 2013).

While it is clear that there are numerous routes to improved medication reconciliation, the successful path here depended on the partnership among the union, front-line staff, and management. The seed for the work emerged from bargaining, with the decision to create a joint committee and make incentive funds available (provided by the hospital) to achieve needed outcomes. The development and implementation of this comprehensive medication reconciliation process was overseen by a joint labor–management committee. CIR leaders, staff, and members were directly involved in the success of the project. As a medical director and executive vice president Dr. David Cohen stated, "The idea was that this had to be a project that materially improved patient care, materially changed the hospital operations in a positive way and that there would be a bonus attached if quantitative measures were achieved by the house staff" (Cohen and Kantrowitz 2012).

The outcomes of this labor–management partnership were clear improvements. Accurate medication reconciliation dramatically improved, and residents and management (who are also the faculty) were extremely positive about the experience of working together on this project. The improved accuracy of the medical reconciliation translates directly into improved patient care and patient safety. Residents were able to take ownership of their work and develop expertise that they passed on to new classes of residents. As one resident put it, "The residents own this process. We didn't have the higher-ups in the hospital telling us what to do; we told them what we need to fix and how we were going to fix it and they gave us the institutional support to do it" (Cohen and Kantrowitz 2012).

Challenges to quality improvement initiatives for CIR have come when management was not interested in union involvement or when the members themselves did not show the interest or initiative to take on these projects.

Kaiser Permanente and the Coalition of Kaiser Permanente Unions[14]

Kaiser Permanente is a complex organization. It brings together separate entities: the Kaiser Foundation Hospitals, the Kaiser Foundation Health Plans, and the Permanente Medical Groups operating in multiple regions of the country. Together, these organizations serve more than 10 million members (the vast majority in California) and employ almost 18,000 physicians and more than 200,000 other workers. The majority of these employees are represented by several national unions and 27 local unions and are covered, in addition to the national agreement negotiated by the

Coalition of Kaiser Permanente Unions, by around 40 local contracts. SEIU has the largest membership of all the unions. There are also unions representing workers at Kaiser that by choice do not participate in the partnership, the most significant of which, the California Nurses Association (CNA), represents thousands of nurses in Kaiser's Northern California region.[15]

Kaiser is sometimes known as the HMO that labor built, an acknowledgment of the important role that union health plans played in the earliest days in bolstering and expanding the organization. It is a history that, at least arguably, helped pull the parties together. Despite this foundation, competitive pressures arising from the entry of new HMOs into Kaiser's markets and Kaiser's entry into new geographic areas put downward pressures on labor costs and led to labor strife beginning in the 1980s. The first step toward partnership took place in 1995 and involved the Kaiser unions forming a coalition to strategize how to confront Kaiser's labor relations practices.

As Kochan, Eaton, McKersie, and Adler describe it, "Almost from the beginning … the union coalition pursued two tracks: an adversarial approach focused on a corporate campaign and an approach to Kaiser around a partnership" (2009: 37). In large part, the push for partnership among some union leaders came from a desire to avoid, if possible, fundamental and lasting damage to what was a heavily unionized employer.[16] But partnership also gained enormous legitimacy through being supported by union leaders willing to use an adversarial approach if necessary (Eaton, Rubinstein, and Kochan 2008).

Kaiser leadership had also been thinking about a partnership approach for a long time, and eventually the leadership on both sides of the table came together in 1997 to hash out a partnership agreement that spelled out six initial goals:
- Improve quality health care for Kaiser Permanente members and the communities we serve.
- Assist Kaiser Permanente in achieving and maintaining market-leading competitive performance.
- Make Kaiser Permanente a better place to work.
- Expand Kaiser Permanente's membership in current and new markets, including designation as a provider of choice for all labor organizations in the areas we serve.
- Provide Kaiser Permanente employees with the maximum possible employment and income security within Kaiser Permanente and/or the health care field.
- Involve employees and their unions in decisions.[17]

In 2002, the parties added a seventh goal: consult on public policy issues and jointly advocate when possible and appropriate.

Early on, the parties negotiated a union security/organizing agreement calling, among other things, for employer neutrality in regard to new union organizing, and an employment security agreement protecting individual employees. The parties also created a structure (called the Senior Partnership Council) to enable top leaders from management and unions to meet regularly to oversee all labor–management partnership work within Kaiser. A staff structure was developed at the national level, eventually to be known as the Office of Labor Management Partnership (OLMP). The OLMP was funded by the collectively bargained Labor Management Partnership trust, which by 2005 had an annual budget of $16 million.

In its early stages, the partnership resulted in some intense, localized, and very successful projects. Two of those projects have received the most attention: one keeping open an optical lab that had been slated for closure and another involving the rapid opening of a new hospital through a joint process (Baldwin Hospital).

As is often the case, the partnership also changed how the parties approached collective bargaining. In the year 2000, for the first time, labor and management leaders engaged in a complex, interest-based process involving almost 400 representatives from the two sides. Perhaps even more importantly, and running counter to the dominant trend in labor relations, they also conducted centralized national bargaining. Since 2000, the parties have continued with both national and interest-based bargaining, adjusting the details of the process over the years (for details see Kochan, Eaton, McKersie, and Adler 2009, Chapter 6).

The partnership in its first decade generally did a good job repairing the labor relationship and at focused projects aimed at improving quality or cutting costs while preserving employment security. Employees indicated in both employer and union surveys that they were more satisfied with their work, and many organizational metrics had improved (see Kochan, Eaton, McKersie, and Adler 2009, Chapter 11, for a thorough discussion of outcomes). At the same time, given Kaiser Permanente's size and complexity, the partnership took different forms and levels of intensity from facility to facility. Overall, it struggled to involve wide swathes of members in workplace decisions or in transforming care delivery.

In 2005, the parties negotiated ambitious language to create unit-based teams (UBTs) throughout the organization; the language included specific targeted percentages of the workforce for each year. In the course of implementing the UBT language and the 2005 agreement generally, the parties concluded that UBTs would also be the vehicle to work on other organizational improvements, one of which was service quality, throughout the organization. Each region set goals for UBTs, including region-specific issues such as reduced absenteeism (southern California) and improved collection of patient/member co-payments (also known as revenue capture, which was a northern California issue).

The parties claimed to have reached the goal of 100% coverage of the partnership workforce with UBTs by 2010. In the new agreement reached in that year, the goals focused on steadily increasing the portion of teams that were "high performing" as measured on an internal five-point scale. According to Kochan (2016: 256), "By January 2012, 3,458 teams were operating [within the organization]. … [B]y December 2012, 40 percent of teams had reached the 'high performance' level." The latest collective agreement, reached in 2015, calls on UBTs, for the first time, to include member and patient voices.[18]

Despite a serious effort by the parties to track both the functioning and outcomes of UBTs, because teams work on a huge array of specific projects with very different goals, systematic research on outcomes has been difficult. Internal Kaiser research has found, however, that higher-performing UBTs are associated with significantly higher HCAHPS (patient experience survey) scores on four specific measures, the overall hospital rating, and with much lower injury rates (Kochan, 2016, Figures 11.1 and 11.3: 257–258).

Overall, the partnership at Kaiser has been reasonably successful at accomplishing the parties' mutual goals. If nothing else—and there is in fact a lot else—simply surviving almost 20 years through leadership changes on both sides of the table, intense environmental pressures, and equally intense inter- and even intra-union conflict is remarkable. Interestingly, President Obama recently credited the LMP with helping to make Kaiser one of the leading providers of health care in the United States.[19] The deep institutionalization of the partnership would appear to increase the likelihood that the parties will be able to take on the challenge of providing lower-cost health care needed to compete in the new ACA-created individual markets and to weather the shift of health care to more community settings.

COMMON THEMES FROM CASE STUDIES

As hospitals, health systems, and unions representing health care workers adjust to extensive changes in the health care landscape, the record so far on labor–management partnerships indicates that they can play a major role in achieving sustainable outcomes of improved patient care and control of inappropriate costs while creating meaningful work for employees through front-line staff involvement. On the basis of the case studies presented and lessons from other significant labor–management partnership processes in health care, we now summarize common themes. We begin with points that are common to these cases but that are not particularly new to those familiar with labor–management partnerships. We then turn to themes that are new and particular to health care.

Applying the Labor–Management Partnership Literature to Health Care

One of the challenges identified in the partnership literature is the handling of modes of interaction across the different areas of the labor–management relationship, including collaborative work, collective bargaining, and grievance handling. The parties often find it contradictory to engage in joint problem-solving approaches to improve patient care while conducting daily labor relations and bargaining in more traditional ways (Kochan, Eaton, McKersie, and Adler 2009: 87; Rubinstein 2001: 426). Most of the organizations discussed in this chapter make use of a combination of interest-based bargaining and alternative dispute resolution to achieve some degree of alignment in the relationship. That is, they engage in a problem-solving approach for all interactions.

The literature also references the importance of enabling contract language (Eaton, Rubinstein, and McKersie 2004). Specific contract language has been quite helpful in sustaining and spreading partnership activities, particularly when there is a leadership change for either party. For at least two decades, the labor movement has pushed for partnership language to be included in contracts (AFL-CIO 1994; Lazes, Figueroa, and Katz 2012) to clarify the methods and principles of engagement as well as to create needed structures and resources that will help sustain this new way of working together and can't be eliminated at the whim of new management.[20] Most of the cases presented in this chapter have developed specific contract language that denotes the focus, structure, goals, and resources.

As was the case in prior labor–management partnerships, governance structures and principles of engagement (which include agreements to free up staff to support and assist the partnership), budgets to allow frontline staff time to work on designated problems, and employment security clauses have been critical for the success and sustainability of joint problem solving and system redesign (Kochan, Eaton, McKersie, and Adler 2009; Lazes, Figueroa, and Katz 2012). Eaton, Rubinstein, and McKersie (2004) point to the need for both strong, proactive labor and management leaders and the restructuring of union locals to build capacity and to convince staff and employees to work together in new ways (see also Lazes and Savage 2000; Rubinstein 2001).

In many of the cases cited in this chapter, additional resources and release time were bargained, sometimes supplemented with resources from joint labor–management funds. Proactive union and management leadership continues to be a critical factor in creating and sustaining a significant labor–management partnership process. Eaton, Rubinstein, and McKersie (2004) also point to the achievement of important outcomes such as productivity or quality gains as a foundation for sustainability of partnership, and we clearly see those kinds of gains in the cases we examined, although sometimes limited to particular organizational niches.

We know from the literature on partnership that, historically, some learning took place among and across partnerships. Many labor–management partners interested in developing a partnership, for instance, visited GM's Saturn plant during its heyday (Rubinstein and Kochan 2001: 112–15). Indeed, leaders of one of the earliest joint projects under the Kaiser partnership visited Saturn as well as other joint models during the development phase of their partnership process (Kochan, Eaton, McKersie, and Adler 2009: 56). Union and management representatives at Kaiser also visited and learned from the multi-employer health care partnership in the Twin Cities of Minnesota (see endnote 3).

We think it is important to note that the cases described here have influenced one another because the key stakeholders have directly learned from each other. Representatives from SHARE are learning from the UVM case and from Allegheny Health Network. Union and management stakeholders in the Los Angeles case as well as union leaders from UVM have also looked to Kaiser for lessons. Union representatives from many locals cited in this chapter attended workshops at Cornell University in 2008, 2009, and 2010 specifically to share their different experiences. Consultants for all of our case studies have helped connect clients with others doing similar work and shared lessons learned from previous partnerships. In short, there has been much cross-learning taking place that influences the approaches of the organizations discussed in this chapter.

Lessons for the Health Care Sector

There are also several aspects of these cases that we see as new and challenging, either because of the point at which they've developed in the trajectory of labor–management partnerships in the United States (i.e., they have learned from earlier cases and been able, therefore, to take things to another level) or because of the unique aspects of health care as a sector.

What is particularly striking across these cases is the extent to which unions have been proactive in driving these efforts. Each of the partnerships were developed either mutually (Kaiser Permanente, Maimonides) or as a result of long-term, determined pushes from the union(s) involved (AFT at UVM, CIR at Maimonides, and SHARE at UMass). In some cases, these efforts are a result of strategic approaches by the unions—either at the national or local level—to get out in front of the constantly changing health care landscape. AFT, CIR, and SEIU internationals have taken the initiative to learn about best practices for improving health care outcomes (e.g., a sector strategy moving to an integrated care delivery system, improving the quality of each aspect of patient care, creating patient-centered medical homes, integrating psychiatric and primary care services, workforce development) and have encouraged their locals to incorporate these new areas of work within the goals and practices of their local. This being said, it has been a challenge for union locals to free up and prepare their staff to partner with management to develop new services and new jobs.

Another aspect of health care labor–management partnerships that is different from most previous partnerships is the presence of multiple unions[21] and the need to include all front-line staff involved in departmental and system changes. These health care organizations, to a large extent, have multiple bargaining units. At the most extreme end, we see the Kaiser partnership with ten different national unions participating, but other unions representing significant numbers of workers that are, for ideological reasons, choosing not to be part of the partnership.

Fundamentally, given the nature of health care delivery as a cross-functional, interdisciplinary enterprise, team work and collaboration are critical: it is a major barrier when important stakeholders are not at the table (whether in a union or not) in efforts to alter work practices and policies. At Kaiser, this issue has arisen with nurses in the northern California region and, at times, with physicians throughout the organization. At UVM and Allegheny General Hospital, only the nurses are involved in labor–management partnership activities. To some extent, this situation has been an issue of design. At UVM, management and the AFT local have structured their partnership process to focus on AFT members, whereas at LA-DHS and Maimonides all stakeholders are included in partnership work—even employees who are not members of a union. Layered on top of the problem of multiple occupations and multiple unions is the strong nature of hierarchy in health care. While it's important for all occupational groups to participate, it is also challenging for less-educated or -skilled workers to use their voices and to have them heard.

Also essential to understanding partnerships in health care is the 24/7 nature of operations and the tight staffing in most acute care facilities. Partnership activities necessitate front-line worker involvement in gathering data, problem solving, and testing solutions. This means time away from direct patient care. At Kaiser this issue was defined largely as one of "backfill"—how to fund workers to free up other workers for partnership training and work sessions (Kochan, Eaton, McKersie, and Adler 2009: 83). With the arrival of UBTs at Kaiser, the organization solved the problem, at least in part, with quick huddles (see Eaton, Konitsney, Litwin, and Vanderhorst 2011 for a discussion of huddles and other innovative solutions to the problem of meetings for UBTs).

UMass Memorial is also using huddles and has assigned executives to huddles; SHARE also has a union staff member assigned to work solely on process improvement activities. CIR and Maimonides, LA-DHS, and UVM have established agreements so that front-line staff have the time to meet in work groups and serve on governance committees. This has sometimes meant having other staff come in early or stay over their shift. Even with these agreements, it can remain difficult to free up staff to join a partnership activity if there is a need for direct patient care.

Several partnerships have also decided to address both bottom-up problems (e.g., departmental and unit quality problems identified by front-line staff) as well as to focus on strategic needs (e.g., integrating primary care and behavioral health; establishing patient-centered medical homes) to transform their systems to be more integrated and patient centered. This joint focus on delivery system transformation goes well beyond what was typically seen in prior non–health care partnerships. These efforts also demonstrate the differences between hospital workers and those working in manufacturing settings. Rather than just being employed, health care workers have chosen to work in occupations that have a direct impact on others. They therefore seem to be more open to opportunities that give them voice in improving patient outcomes. We speculate that in manufacturing, workers may be less likely to offer suggestions that might simply increase profits for the owners of the business.[22] It is interesting to note in this regard that two of our cases—Kaiser Permanente and UMass Memorial—seek to involve patients directly in the problem identification and solving process. This suggests both the centrality of the patient in health care and possibly a new direction in labor–management collaboration whereby an additional stakeholder is not just discussed but actually is present in quality improvement processes.

Another development in health care partnerships has been a significant deepening of the role of labor relations staff in operational matters and extensive involvement of operations staff. Under a partnership, LR staff focus more on understanding and supporting operational changes (the creation of patient-centered medical homes, the implementation of electronic health records, etc.). They typically have primary responsibility to develop and deepen the use of interest-based tools and alternative dispute resolution that we discussed in this chapter. HR and LR staff have also been important in helping labor and management leaders anticipate and develop training of employees for new roles and responsibilities as the health care industry changes (community health workers, mental health advisors, etc.). Although some of those areas cited in this chapter were the responsibility of LR staff in prior partnerships—there is a deeper involvement in all of these areas.

Health care partnerships have also required intensive work to increase the knowledge and skills of the union staff about changes in the industry and methods that are needed to achieve them. This has been a priority for AFT, CIR, and SEIU at the national as well as local levels. These unions have decided that helping their members have a voice in improving care will result in more meaningful work and greater connection/engagement of members to the union. The unions in these cases see partnership as a mode of union building as well as a path to improving both patient care and relationships with management.

CONCLUSION

Although labor–management partnerships have existed in other sectors of the economy, the pace of change in health care organizations creates an environment where collaborative work may have a high chance of success. Unlike manufacturing organizations where many jobs have the potential of being outsourced and moved outside of the United States (giving employers a strong exit option), health care is still largely delivered in person. Health care's rootedness creates incentives for unionized employers to engage collaboratively with their unions. Collaborative projects and broader labor–management partnerships can ensure there are processes in place to allow continuous improvement, develop new systems to improve access and coordination of care, and maintain the financial health of the facility to avoid cuts and layoffs. The organizations we've described in this chapter have also had the advantage of learning from roughly three decades of labor–management partnership practice in other sectors.

The literature on labor–management partnership has identified many challenges and barriers to successful partnerships and union–management collaboration more broadly. Our review of six key cases suggests that those same challenges exist in health care along with several unique to the industry. At the same time, these challenge can be met and barriers overcome. For practitioners on either side of the table thinking about pursuing a collaborative path, it is important to recognize the problems that will be encountered along the way.

Proactive labor and management leaders have been a critical prerequisite for a robust partnership process. In an environment where change is rapid and continuous, union and management health care leaders will need the dexterity and readiness to adapt their approach to partnership and collaboration in order to respond to ever-changing patient and organizational needs.

ENDNOTES

[1] We use the terms "partnership" and "collaboration" somewhat interchangeably here. In our view, partnerships are more extensive and involve deep and wide forms of both union and worker participation in decisions formerly reserved for management. By "deep," we mean the extent to which they provide opportunities for decision making for front-line staff. By "wide," we mean the scope of decisions being made or range of topics discussed. While all partnerships feature union–management collaboration, some forms of collaboration are more focused or narrow and do not rise to the level of partnership.

[2] Critical cases are those that are most likely to "yield the most information and have the greatest impact on the development of knowledge" (see Patton 2002: 236).

[3] There are other important health care cases worth noting here. One is the on-again, off-again (but currently off) multi-employer, multi-union partnership in the Twin Cities (Minnesota), along with the spin-off partnership based in the Allina system (see Preuss 1998 and Preuss and Frost 2003). The second is the 1199SEIU–League of Voluntary Hospital and Nursing Home process. The third is the relatively recent labor–management partnership, again involving SEIU, at Allegheny Health Network in western Pennsylvania. The authors of this chapter have reviewed material on and are familiar with these three cases and have taken them into account in the analysis at the end of the chapter. In addition to these cases, there was a significant level of labor–management partnership in the Veterans Health Administration during the Clinton administration (Masters, Albright, and Eplion 2006).

[4] For a discussion of their problem-solving approach, see http://bit.ly/29JZOSK.

[5] Allegheny General Hospital has developed an important labor–management partnership with their SEIU local that is focused primarily on quality improvement and nursing issues.

[6] Peter Lazes, one of the authors of this chapter, provided limited consulting assistance to the leadership of AFT Local 5221 several years ago.

[7] Article 20B, 2009–2011 collective bargaining agreement.

[8] A professional practice committee is a work group composed of staff nurses, their nurse educator, and nurse manager on each unit of the hospital. This group is responsible for identifying and working on important nurse practice issues. The agreement to have PPCs is written into the union contract.

[9] Peter Lazes, one of the authors of this chapter, has been a consultant to the leadership of LA-DHS and SEIU Local 721 for several years.

[10] At the time that the LMTC was developed, there were about 20 unit-based CITs at one of the ambulatory care facilities. These teams were not connected at that time to an overall partnership process.

[11] Eventually, operations staff from the Los Angeles Department of Mental Health and the Los Angeles Department of Public Health joined the LMTC.

[12] Peter Lazes, one of the authors of this chapter, was a consultant to Maimonides Medical Center, CIR, NYSNA, and 1199SEIU from 1997 to 2013.

[13] There was a brief period when 1199SEIU withdrew from the Strategic Alliance during negotiations in 2009.

[14] Adrienne Eaton, one of the authors of this chapter, served as a consultant to the Coalition of Kaiser Permanente Unions for many years and received grants from both the coalition and Kaiser Permanente to conduct research on the partnership.

[15] For a discussion of CNA's objections in the early stages of the labor–management partnership with Kaiser Permanente, see Kochan, Eaton, McKersie, and Adler 2009: 43–45.

[16] This was also a moment in time when there was a lot of discussion about partnership floating around the labor movement following publication of *The New American Workplace* in 1994 by the AFL-CIO. Further, Peter diCicco, at the time the head of the AFL-CIO's Industrial Union Department but eventually the first executive director of the Coalition of Kaiser Permanente Unions, drew on his personal experience with job enrichment as an officer of the International Union of Electrical Workers at a General Electric plant in Massachusetts.

[17] See Kochan, Eaton, McKersie, and Adler 2009: 46 for excerpts or http://bit.ly/29K15cy for the full original partnership agreement.

[18] See http://bit.ly/29EiHDd.

[19] See http://bit.ly/29K1xYj.

[20] But see also "Partnerships of Steel" (Rubinstein 2003) for a discussion of the costs as well as benefits of a top-down contractual approach.

[21] The AT&T Workplace of the Future partnership did include two different unions. Eaton (1995) reports that the relations between the two unions were often as fraught as the relationship between the unions and management. For a full discussion of inter-union relationships at Kaiser, see Kochan, Eaton, McKersie, and Adler 2009, Chapter 7; and Eaton, Rubinstein, and Kochan 2008.

[22] While this is truly speculative on our part, we do know that Kaiser Permanente conducted internal research in 2004 (the Looking Glass project) that showed very strong identification with the mission of the organization and desire to provide or contribute to providing high-quality care throughout its workforce.

REFERENCES

AFL-CIO. 1994. "The New American Workplace: A Labor Perspective." Washington, DC: Committee on the Evolution of Work.

Cohen, D., and M. Kantrowitz. 2012. "Resident Physician Engagement in Medication Safety Through a Labor–Management Partnership." Video. http://bit.ly/29KthMv.

Duguid, Margaret. 2012. "The Importance of Medication Reconciliation for Patients and Practitioners." *Australian Prescriber* 35, no. 1: 15–19.

Eaton, A. E. 1995. "Educating for AT&T, CWA and IBEW's Workplace of the Future." In *Proceedings of the Forty-Seventh Annual Meeting of the Industrial Relations Research Association*, Washington, DC, January, pp. 383–90.

Eaton, A. E., J. Cutcher-Gershenfeld, and S. A. Rubinstein. 2016. "Labor–Management Partnership in the United States: Islands of Success in a Hostile Context." In *Developing Positive Employment Relations: International Experiences of Labour Management Partnership*, edited by A. Wilkinson and S. Johnstone. New York, NY: Palgrave Macmillan.

Eaton, A. E., D. Konitsney, A. S. Litwin, and N. Vanderhorst. 2011. "The Path to Performance: A Study of High-Performing Unit-Based Teams at Kaiser Permanente." Kaiser Permanent Labor Management Partnership, February. http://www.lmpartnership.org/rutgers.

Eaton, A. E., S. A. Rubinstein, and T. A. Kochan. 2008. "Balancing Acts: Dynamics of a Union Coalition in a Labor Management Partnership." *Industrial Relations: A Journal of Economy and Society* 47, no. 1: 10–35. doi:10.1111/j.1468-232x.2008.00502.x.

Eaton, S. C., S. A. Rubinstein, and R. B. McKersie. 2004. "Building and Sustaining Labor Management Partnerships: Recent Experiences in the U.S." *Advances in Industrial and Labor Relations* 13: 137–56. doi: 10.1016/s0742-6186(04)13005-9.

Institute for Healthcare Improvement. No date. "Reconcile Medications at All Transition Points." http://bit.ly/2aolnsT.

Institute of Medicine. 2010. "ACGME Board of Directors Approved New Requirement for Residency Programs." Washington, DC: National Academies of Sciences. http://bit.ly/29GD2aX.

Jaltenor. 2013. "Maimonides Residents Gain Notice for Medication Reconciliation." *CIR Vitals*, February 25. http://bit.ly/29GD3LL.

Kochan, T. A. 2016. "The Kaiser Permanente Labour Management Partnership: 1997–2013." In *Developing Positive Employment Relations: International Experiences of Labour Management Partnership*, edited by A. Wilkinson and S. Johnstone. New York, NY: Palgrave Macmillan.

Kochan, T. A., P. S. Adler, R. B. McKersie, A. E. Eaton, P. Segal, and P. Gerhart. 2008. "The Potential and Precariousness of Partnership: The Case of the Kaiser Permanente Labor Management Partnership." *Industrial Relations: A Journal of Economy and Society* 47, no. 1: 36–65. doi:10.1111/j.1468-232x.2008.00503.x.

Kochan, T. A., A. Eaton, R. McKersie, and P. Adler. 2009. *Healing Together: The Labor Management Partnership at Kaiser Permanente*. Ithaca, NY: ILR Press/Cornell University Press.

Lazes, P., M. Figueroa, and L. Katz. 2012. "How Labor–Management Partnerships Improve Patient Care, Cost Control, and Labor Relations." Washington, DC: American Rights at Work.

Lazes, P., and J. Savage. 2000. "Embracing the Future: Union Strategies for the 21st Century." *Journal for Quality and Participation* 23, no. 4: 18–23.

Litwin, A. S., and A. E. Eaton. Forthcoming. "Complementary or Conflictual? Formal Participation, Informal Participation, and Organizational Performance." *Human Resource Management*.

Maimonides Medical Center. 2007. "Creating Competitive Advantage in a Changing Health Care Environment through Worker Participation: Strategic Alliance Report 2007." Brooklyn, NY: Maimonides Medical Center.

Maimonides Medical Center. 2015. "Medical Education: Fellowship, Residency and More." Brooklyn, NY: Maimonides Medical Center. http://bit.ly/29GNvmv.

Masters, M. F., R. R. Albright, and D. Eplion. 2006. "What Did Partnerships Do? Evidence from the Federal Sector." *Industrial and Labor Relations Review* 59, no. 3: 367–85.

New England Organizing Project, no date. "About New England Organizing Project." http://bit.ly/2aLjinA.

Patton, M. Q. 2002. *Qualitative Research and Evaluation Methods* (3rd edition). Thousand Oaks, CA: Sage.

Porter, M. 2010 (Dec. 23). "What Is Value in Health Care?" *New England Journal of Medicine*, pp. 2447–81.

Porter, M., and T. E. Lee. 2013 (Oct.). "The Strategy That Will Fix Health Care." *Harvard Business Review*, pp. 1–19.

Preuss, G. A. 1998. "Committed to Care: Labor–Management Cooperation and Hospital Restructuring." Washington, DC: Economic Policy Institute. http://bit.ly/29GOuDw.

Preuss, G. A., and A. Frost. 2003. "The Rise and Decline of Labor–Management Cooperation: Lessons from Health Care in the Twin Cities." *California Management Review* 45, no. 2: 85–106.

Rubinstein, S. A. 2001. "The Local Union Revisited: New Voices from the Front Lines." *Industrial Relations: A Journal of Economy and Society* 40, no. 3: 405–35.

Rubinstein, S. A. 2003. "Partnerships of Steel—Forging High Involvement Work Systems in the US Steel Industry: A View from the Local Unions." *Advances in Industrial and Labor Relations* 12: 117–46.

Rubinstein, S. A., and T. A. Kochan. 2001. *Learning from Saturn*. Ithaca, NY: ILR Press/ Cornell University Press.

Sedgh, S., M. Kantrowitz, S. Shamah, A. Agarwal, V. Fernandez, and D. Cohen. 2013. "Q-Tip: Resident-Driven Quality Improvement to Inpatient Medication Reconciliation in an Academic Setting." *American Journal of Medical Quality* 28, no. 4: 357. http:// bit.ly/29GQZ8P.

UMass Memorial Medical Center. 2016. "About Us: Statistics." http://bit.ly/29GRlfE.

CHAPTER 7

Leading Change Together: Kaiser Permanente's Partnership Strategy for Innovation

JIM PRUITT
The Permanente Federation

PAUL M. COHEN
Kaiser Permanente

INTRODUCTION

In 2008, Joann Horton, a medical clerk at a Kaiser Permanente medical center in Northern California, learned her job might be eliminated when an electronic medical record system came online. At the time, she said, "I was terrified."

A year later, Joyce Lee, an imaging transcriptionist at a Kaiser Permanente medical center in Southern California, found herself in the same boat. With the organization shifting to a new voice-to-text technology for transcribing radiology results, her future was uncertain.

But unlike many other American workers whose jobs in recent years have been eliminated, Horton, Lee, and thousands of other Kaiser Permanente workers—75% of whom are union represented—landed safely. Today, Lee is working as a Kaiser Permanente phlebotomist, a job she says she always wanted. Horton retired in 2014, after retraining as a secretary in her facility's Home Health Department.

Along the way, Kaiser Permanente's electronic medical record system—the largest civilian system in the world—changed the way workers, managers, and physicians do their jobs. Many, like Horton and Lee, saw their old jobs go away. But all were protected by an employment and income security agreement, and they received career counseling and retraining. As a result, workers and their unions not only accepted the new system but helped design it, test it, and train co-workers to use it. Everyone who wanted to stay at Kaiser Permanente ended up with a comparable or better position. (For more information, see the appendix, Preparing for the Work of the Future.)

The positive outcomes were possible thanks to Kaiser Permanente's Labor Management Partnership, the largest, longest running, and most comprehensive labor partnership in the country. It is a forward-looking, joint strategy to answer questions that have bedeviled the entire health care industry. This strategy focuses on how to

- Innovate in a time of change
- Reduce the cost of care while improving quality
- Spread successful practices across the organization
- Engage a diverse workforce in continuous improvement
- Resolve labor relations and operational issues without destroying work relationships

By bringing together diverse points of view and providing a framework for joint problem solving, the Labor Management Partnership has helped Kaiser Permanente tackle these and other difficult issues. We believe such partnerships can be a model for other health care organizations and workers as the industry prepares for a new wave of disruptive change, including telemedicine, storefront drop-in clinics, growing consumer choice, and health care reform.

In this chapter, we examine how and why the partnership formed, what it has achieved, and how it has sustained success. We begin with the historical context for formation of the Labor Management Partnership. We then summarize the performance outcomes achieved in partnership. That's followed by a discussion of four key success factors that have enabled Kaiser Permanente—and its partnership unions—to adapt and grow. We conclude with the perspective of an outside observer and an overview of a joint initiative to prepare today's workforce for a new wave of change.

WHY PARTNERSHIP?

Kaiser Permanente's Labor Management Partnership achieved its vast scope and scale in part as a result of both parties' history. To know what makes the partnership tick, it's useful to start with the organization's social and economic roots, the rise of a diverse union coalition, and a shared willingness to negotiate sweeping labor agreements.

Social and Economic Roots

Kaiser Permanente's model of care and coverage grew from the efforts of industrialist Henry J. Kaiser and public health innovator Dr. Sidney Garfield during the Great Depression and World War II to provide medical care to Kaiser's industrial workers and their families. After the war, Kaiser Permanente opened to the public, offering comprehensive, prepaid care at its own facilities. With the support of organized labor, it grew to be the largest nonprofit health plan in the United States—staffed by more than 186,000 employees (139,000 represented by unions) and 18,000 physicians serving more than 10.6 million health plan members in eight states and the District of Columbia. Annual revenue exceeds $63 billion.

The organization's early labor history laid a foundation for a partnership that has helped it maintain leadership in multiple measures of quality, service, and labor standards. The Labor Management Partnership started in 1997 as a handshake agreement between then-CEO David Lawrence and then-president of the AFL-CIO, John Sweeney. It was a gamble for both parties. At the time, Kaiser Permanente faced serious financial and competitive pressures. The unions' early support for the organization had given way to acrimony and a series of bitter strikes. More than two dozen local unions formed a coalition to strengthen their hand in bargaining and mount a corporate campaign against Kaiser Permanente. But hoping to avoid a mutually destructive war, the parties chose another path.

They created a way to engage workers, managers, and physicians in issues affecting the quality and affordability of care, the patient experience, and the workplace experience. To implement change, the Labor Management Partnership provides, among other things:

- Jointly established criteria and targets for team performance
- A database to track team innovations and results
- Peer advisors who help teams improve work processes and solve problems

A Diverse Union Coalition

The partnership is jointly led and funded by Kaiser Permanente and the Coalition of Kaiser Permanente Unions, now comprising 28 local unions (Table 1, next page).

Six unions representing about 27,000 employees have chosen not to join the union coalition or participate in the partnership. The largest of these is the California Nurses Association, representing more than 18,000 registered nurses at Kaiser Permanente, mostly in Northern California. And Kaiser Permanente's experience with both partnership and nonpartnership unions provides a vivid picture of what is possible in traditional versus nontraditional labor relations.

Thomas Kochan, professor of management at the MIT Sloan School of Management, has studied the Labor Management Partnership from its early days. His 2013 report on the accomplishments and challenges of the partnership included this conclusion:

> Kaiser Permanente is now one of the nation's leaders in the use of frontline teams to improve health care delivery.… The Kaiser Permanente Labor Management Partnership continues to serve as the nation's largest and most successful labor management partnership. As such it demonstrates the potential value of this approach for … labor relations in the 21st century and as a model for health care delivery and improvement. (Kochan 2013: 32)

TABLE 1
Members of the Coalition of Kaiser Permanente Unions (as of April 2016)

International Union	Participating Locals	Members Represented
American Federation of State, County and Municipal Employees	1	18,531
American Federation of Teachers	2	3,726
International Brotherhood of Teamsters	1	525
International Federation of Professional and Technical Engineers	1	1,379
International Longshoremen's and Warehousemen's Union	1	61
International Union of Operating Engineers	1	24
Kaiser Permanente Nurse Anesthetists Association	1	355
Office of Professional Employees International Union	4	12,247
Service Employees International Union	4	58,493
United Food and Commercial Workers	11	10,003
United Steel Workers	1	6,733
Total	**28**	**112,077**

Sweeping Labor Agreements

Through the partnership, Kaiser Permanente and the Coalition of Kaiser Permanente Unions have negotiated five national labor agreements. All of them have gone far beyond the scope of traditional union contracts. While providing industry-leading wages and benefits, the agreements also address service and quality improvement; workforce planning, training, and development; workforce health, safety, and wellness; joint efforts to grow the business and union membership; and enhancements to partnership practices.

Each agreement also has included at least one achievement that has had lasting impact on the organization, the workforce, and our health plan members and patients. Innovations coming out of past agreements include the following:

- 2005: Jointly led work teams established to drive front-line performance improvement
- 2008 (reopener): Shared strategy to grow health plan and union membership

- 2010: Uniform performance goals and metrics for teams across the organization
- 2012: Total Health Incentive Plan, a voluntary program that rewards employees for collective participation in confidential health screenings and improvements
- 2015: Joint assessment of future workforce needs and increased investment in workforce training and technology deployment

PERFORMANCE BENEFITS OF PARTNERSHIP

While the parties' shared history and ambitious agreements allowed the partnership to take root, the partnership's success is due to the performance benefits delivered to all involved—including Kaiser Permanente members and patients.

The Labor Management Partnership has contributed to industry-leading performance. For example, in J.D. Power's 2015 Member Health Plan Study, Kaiser Permanente was ranked highest in member satisfaction among commercial health plans in five regions of the United States. In addition, leading public and private agencies have given Kaiser Permanente top marks on a wide range of quality indicators.

Leaders inside and outside Kaiser Permanente have recognized our partnership strategy as a driver of organizational performance. In a White House Summit on Worker Voice in October 2015, President Obama said:

> There are businesses out there who are taking the high road and enlist their employees as partners in their shared future, and understand that if they're investing in their employees and making them partners, that they'll actually do better, not worse.... Kaiser Permanente works with 28 different unions to provide good pay and benefits, but also educational programs, and avenues for employees to help improve quality and care throughout the company—which is why they're considered one of the premier health organizations in the country.

Link to Performance

Kaiser Permanente and the Coalition of Kaiser Permanente Unions track organizational as well as clinical outcomes, down to the front-line team level. Kaiser Permanente researchers have found important linkages between teams that report having an effective work environment and performance outcomes such as good attendance, lower injuries, and better service scores. For instance, in the 2015 survey of more than 144,000 Kaiser Permanente employees, departments that scored high on an index of 18 measures of workforce effectiveness and engagement also reported the following:

- 4% higher patient satisfaction scores
- 21% fewer lost workdays
- 38% fewer workplace injuries
- 60% fewer patient falls with injuries

In addition, employees who report feeling highly involved in their partnership teams are far more likely to say they have influence in decisions affecting work and that their input is used. They are more comfortable voicing opinions and more likely to speak out when there are problems. They're also more likely to understand the mission of the organization and the goals of their department, and, in general, they have more favorable opinions about their work and the workplace.

Better Outcomes for Patients, Workers, and the Organization

By engaging rank-and-file workers, managers, and physicians, the partnership is slowly transforming the culture of the organization. It is doing so both through a top-down and a bottom-up, team-based approach. We're seeing results in improved cost structure, patient care, and service. Here are just a few examples:

- A neonatal intensive care unit in Downey, California, gave voice to parents who were concerned that they couldn't visit during shift changes, when nurses exchange information about the babies they are caring for. The team devised a system that allows parents to listen in on these exchanges, then discuss their child's care with the incoming nurse.
- An ambulatory surgery team in Gaithersburg, Maryland, ran a drill to test their response time to malignant hyperthermia—a rare but dangerous side effect of anesthesia. Not satisfied with their results, they expedited lab processes, redesigned supply carts, and devised checklists. The team cut its response time by two minutes, doubled its self-assessed level of expertise, and shared its new practices with other teams across the organization.
- A San Jose, California, in-patient pharmacy team worked with physicians to analyze prescription patterns and saved more than $600,000 by increasing the use of cost-effective equivalents and reducing waste.
- Colorado-based couriers averted the outsourcing of their jobs by assessing their internal clients' needs and improving their own routes, workflows, and information systems. Their new processes also are saving $375,000 a year.

- Redwood City, California, hospital discharge assistants developed a new protocol for scheduling follow-up appointments, dramatically increasing the number of post-discharge appointments kept by patients and reducing costly readmissions.

More broadly, both parties have grown stronger since forming the partnership. Kaiser Permanente's membership has grown to more than 10.6 million people, from about 7.4 million in 1997. At the same time, while unions nationally have lost members and clout, union coalition membership has nearly doubled, from 57,000 to more than 112,000, with steady annual wage growth of 2% to 3% and preservation of health and retirement benefits.

KEY SUCCESS FACTORS

The Labor Management Partnership formed because conditions demanded change. It has endured because it has achieved measurable results. And it continues to flex and grow because we follow a few key principles and practices. These include self-directed work teams, interest-based problem solving and honest conversations, a shared guidepost for action, and a willingness to respond to challenges and skeptics.

Self-Directed Work Teams

Many large organizations seek to tap the ingenuity of front-line workers and managers, enable continuous improvement, and build a culture of learning and accountability. Increasingly, and especially in health care, this happens through high-performing teams, not individual performers.

Amy Edmondson, professor of leadership and management at Harvard Business School, has studied team learning and innovation at many organizations, including Kaiser Permanente. She has observed that in knowledge organizations such as hospitals, employees have to feel safe "to give tough feedback and have difficult conversations—which demand trust and respect—without the need to tiptoe around the truth." In such settings, she has noted:

> Performance is increasingly determined by factors that can't be overseen: intelligent experimentation, ingenuity, interpersonal skills, resilience in the face of adversity. … People rely on their own and their colleagues' judgment and expertise, rather than on management direction, to decide what to do. (Edmondson 2008: 62–63)

The Labor Management Partnership has provided a home for this way of working. The concept of self-directed work teams as a means to accomplish organizational goals was put forward in 2000, in our first national negotiations; the emergence of what we call unit-based teams under the 2005 National Agreement established them as the formal operating strategy for the organization and unions. Today there are about 3,500 such teams in place across the organization, in virtually every work setting.

Interest-Based Solutions and Honest Conversations

Kaiser Permanente and the union coalition are leading practitioners of interest-based bargaining. The interest-based approach—which we also use for day-to-day problem solving—has guided the successful negotiation of all our national agreements. The interest-based process consists of

- Defining the issue that needs to be resolved
- Having each party identify its underlying interests and concerns
- Jointly developing issues that address each party's interests
- Selecting solutions, through consensus, that address all parties' interests

Our bargaining involves people from all levels, specialties, and regions of the organization. In 2015, there were 150 workers, managers, and physicians on bargaining teams. In addition, about 300 workers and 50 managers served as observers in all bargaining sessions and caucuses. They bargained in a compressed time frame that encouraged quicker resolution of issues than is typical in bargaining large-scale agreements. In 2015, we agreed on a complex, far-reaching contract over the course of four 3-day sessions.

The process brings broader perspective, more novel ideas to the table, and more support for the agreement afterward. Interest-based bargaining also is a powerful learning experience for emerging leaders—some of whom have had little previous exposure to contract bargaining and most of whom gain insights and relationships that last for years.

"We have frontline workers with management, and the presidents of [Kaiser Permanente] regions all sitting at the table together talking," said Maureen Meehan-Golonka, president of the Hawaii Nurses Association. "It's not something that happens every day."

"What stands out for me is the honest conversations we have," said Jerry Vincent, director of labor relations, Northern California, about interest-based bargaining. "Everyone is comfortable expressing themselves and offering their own point of view. It's very different from traditional labor negotiations."

A Shared Guidepost

Unit-based teams are guided in their work by the Kaiser Permanente Value Compass—a tool adopted jointly by our partner unions and Kaiser Permanente and included in the 2010 national agreement.

Teams use the Value Compass (Figure 1) to identify and develop performance improvement projects that address one or more points of the compass. They are supported in their work by peer advisors as well as more senior union and management sponsors. Because teams are an important part of operations, we closely monitor their progress and rate the performance of every team, quarterly, on a five-point scale. The measurements typically have to do with such standards as whether teams meet regularly; have a sponsor; and are trained in problem-solving techniques, data analysis, business literacy, and other skills.

This tracking includes the types of improvement projects launched by each of our 3,500 front-line teams, their alignment with the organization's clinical and business goals, and their use of advanced tools in specific areas, such as waste and cost reduction.

Answering Challenges and Skeptics

As noted previously, honestly addressing difficult issues is essential to sustaining a successful partnership. And the partnership does face challenges. Leaders from both sides have deep experience in traditional labor–management settings and can attest that partnership is more demanding—personally and institutionally. For example, collective bargaining and decision-making processes can be slower and more taxing because more people are involved and more interests may need to be considered.

FIGURE 1
Kaiser Permanente Value Compass

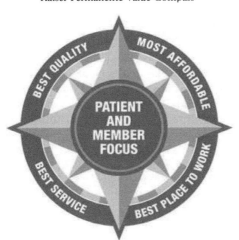

In addition, the union coalition faces opposition from those in the labor movement who reject partnership per se as a union strategy. Moreover, adherence to and accountability for partnership practices vary. For instance, some physicians are more visibly involved in partnership activities than others. And even in our most successful units, there are skeptics on both sides who remain uninvolved.

However, research suggests that managers, especially front-line supervisors and middle managers, have good reason to work in partnership. Studies by Kaiser Permanente Organizational Research have connected levels of team engagement with quality, service, safety, and attendance results, as discussed previously. Simply put, where the work environment is perceived to be better, patients give higher overall ratings to their hospital, and workers have a safer, more productive work experience.

Additional research has identified four building blocks of performance at Kaiser Permanente (Figure 2). They are largely behavioral—and highly dependent on the environment established by the manager within the team or work unit.

Beyond the workplace dynamics at the unit level, performance is determined by interdependent relationships with other departments and physicians, organizational systems and support, and foundational principles such as trust and accountability.

All four performance drivers are influenced by communication across and within departments—and all can be strengthened by applying partnership practices, says Deborah Konitsney, director of Organizational Research, Kaiser Permanente.

CONCLUSION

In 2004, Jeffrey Pfeffer, author and professor of organizational behavior at Stanford Graduate School of Business, offered this assessment of the Labor Management Partnership:

> Kaiser and its unions are attempting to build an innovative model of management—a relationship of mutual respect. What makes this even more unusual, and more difficult, is that they're attempting to institutionalize this model, rather than relying on a single, charismatic leader. (Pfeffer 2004: 6)

At the time, the partnership was still in its formative years. But Pfeffer's insight has passed the test of time. Since the partnership's founding, three CEOs and three executive directors have led Kaiser Permanente and the Coalition of Kaiser Permanente Unions, respectively. Each was different but remained committed to the partnership and built support for it among constituents.

FIGURE 2

Performance Drivers at Kaiser Permanente: Model Based on Kaiser
Permanente Linkage Research of What Drives Performance Outcomes

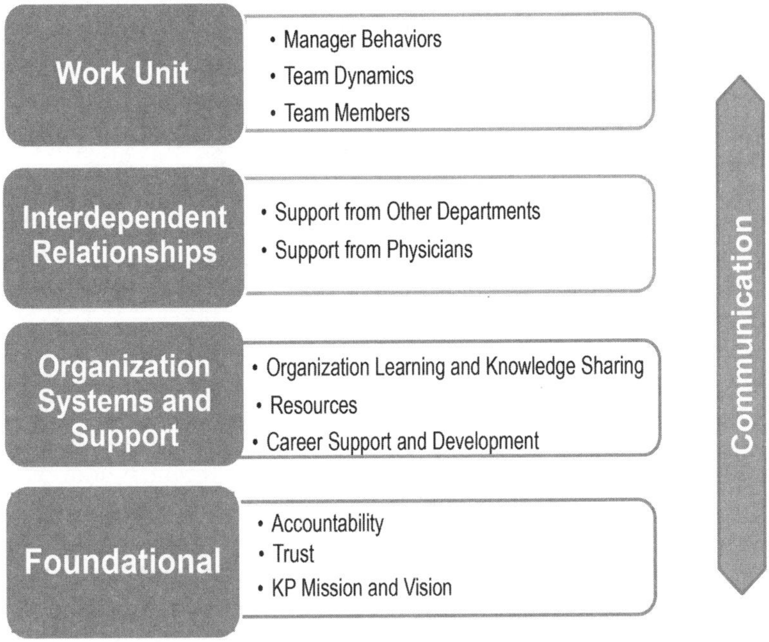

Work Unit	• Manager Behaviors • Team Dynamics • Team Members	
Interdependent Relationships	• Support from Other Departments • Support from Physicians	Communication
Organization Systems and Support	• Organization Learning and Knowledge Sharing • Resources • Career Support and Development	
Foundational	• Accountability • Trust • KP Mission and Vision	

Source: Kaiser Permanente

As health care becomes ever more complex, team based—and expensive—the partnership provides a model for managing change. It is expanding the possibilities for labor–management relations in health care. It has measurably improved care delivery, helped reduce costs and waste, and given patients and caregivers a voice. And it is helping a leading health care organization and its unionized workforce adapt to the deep changes reshaping the industry.

The Labor Management Partnership is far from perfect. It has not eliminated disagreements. After 18 years, we are still learning as we go. But it is a powerful alternative to traditional models of care delivery and labor relations. We have lived through traditional workplace approaches and partnership approaches, and we know from experience: partnership works better.

APPENDIX: PREPARING FOR THE WORK OF THE FUTURE

Workforce planning and development has been a long-term commitment—and a multimillion dollar investment—of Kaiser Permanente's Labor Management. Programs to enhance worker skills, certification, and continuing education have benefited the organization, its members and patients, and thousands of Kaiser Permanente workers. Programs include the following:

- Two education trusts that funded more than 32,000 course enrollments for more than 100,000 eligible workers in 2015
- Tuition reimbursements of $3,000 or more per enrolled worker
- Time off with stipends to replace lost wages for workers taking approved training
- One-on-one career counseling to help workers take charge of their professional advancement
- In-house mentorships and preceptorships to help newly trained workers meet experience requirements

Kaiser Permanente's 2015 national agreement with the Coalition of Kaiser Permanente Unions makes the "work of the future" a priority for both parties. The agreement establishes a collaborative, transparent process for managing job redeployments. In addition, union–management jobs committees in every operating region will assess training opportunities, identify emerging and hard-to-fill positions in the organization, help employees meet minimum experience requirements, and work to eliminate barriers to job placement and training.

A member of the union bargaining team in our 2015 negotiations noted that preparing the workforce for change is a personal issue and a shared interest. "When I was younger, I was given opportunities and I ran with it," said Julie Markiewicz, an officer of SEIU Local 49 in Oregon. "We want to give the younger generation the same kind of opportunities so they stay with Kaiser Permanente and build a future here."

REFERENCES

Edmondson, A. C. 2008 (Jul.–Aug.). "The Competitive Imperative of Learning." *Harvard Business Review*, 60–67.

Kochan, T. A. 2013. "The Kaiser Permanente Labor Management Partnership, 2009–2013." Report. Cambridge, MA: MIT Sloan Management Institute for Work and Employment Research.

Pfeffer, J. 2004 (Dec). "The Key to a High-Performing Workplace: People." *Hank: Frontline News for KP Workers, Managers and Physicians*, 6.

CHAPTER 8

Caring Health Care Work Environments and Patient-Centered Care

CHERYL RATHERT
JESSICA N. MITTLER
LAURA E. MCCLELLAND
Virginia Commonwealth University

INTRODUCTION

The idea that health care delivery should be "patient centered" (PC) has been around for several decades (Gerteis, Edgman-Levitan, Daley, and Delbanco 2002). Dozens of studies have attempted to understand what PC care is (see Rathert, Vogus, and McClelland 2016 for a review) and the extent to which it influences patient outcomes (Rathert, Wywrich, and Boren 2013). Yet there is no consensus on how PC care should be defined or operationalized (Rathert, Vogus, and McClelland 2016). For this chapter, we conceptualize PC care as "the experience (to the extent the individual patient desires it) of transparency, individualization, recognition, respect, dignity, and choice in all matters, without exception, related to one's person, circumstances, and relationships in health care" (Berwick 2009: w560).

In addition, we assume that to provide true PC care, providers must take the lead in establishing a therapeutic alliance with patients (Epstein, Fiscella, Lesser, and Stange 2010; Mead and Bower 2000)—one of compassion, caring, and reducing patient vulnerabilities (Epstein, Fiscella, Lesser, and Stange 2010; Hobbs 2009; McClelland and Vogus 2014). Care providers must be able to get to know "the patient as a person" (Epstein, Fiscella, Lesser, and Stange 2010: 1490). Providers also should be equipped with leadership skills in order to engage the patient as an active participant.

Too often, however, organizations believe PC care means individualizing systems that are disease or provider focused rather than creating work environments that sustain compassion and patient-centeredness (Epstein and Street 2011). We assert that true patient-centeredness can be achieved only when organizations provide work environments that facilitate caring and therapeutic relationships for their workers as well as their patients.

Although some health systems have focused on providing PC care since the 1980s, the 2010 Affordable Care Act's Value-Based Purchasing (VBP) program (Centers for Medicare and Medicaid Services 2013) created a sense of urgency for PC care. VBP ties a portion of participating hospitals' Medicare reimbursement to its performance on patient experience scores and other outcomes. In addition to influencing Medicare reimbursement dollars, patient experience data are now publicly reported using a standardized survey, the Hospital Consumer Assessment of Healthcare Providers and Systems (HCAHPS) (www.medicare.gov/hospitalcompare). Medicare calculates VBP scores using the HCAHPS patient experience metrics (Centers for Medicare and Medicaid Services 2013) (constructs measured appear in Table 1).

There are also standardized CAHPS surveys for many additional care settings, and the federal government continues to evaluate VBP implementation in other delivery settings. For example, the Centers for Medicare and Medicaid Services (CMS) implemented a nine-state mandatory pilot program for home-health organizations in 2016 (Centers for Medicare and Medicaid Services 2015). Although CAHPS administration in most delivery settings is not required, many nonhospital health care organizations (HCOs) increasingly use CAHPS surveys in response to the evolving federal mandates to improve the quality of health care. As a result, many HCOs now focus on systems and processes that influence care

TABLE 1
HCAHPS Patient Experience Survey Domains

Domain	Number of Items
Communication with nurses	3
Communication with doctors	3
Responsiveness of hospital staff	2
Pain management	2
Communication about medicines	2
Cleanliness of hospital	1
Quietness of hospital	1
Discharge information	2
Care transition	3
Overall care rating	1
Recommend the hospital	1

Source: www.medicare.gov/hospitalcompare

quality, and many have moved away from a sole emphasis on efficiency and added the aim of providing "customer satisfaction" (Mikesell and Bromley 2012).

WORK ENVIRONMENTS

The health care work environment became of interest to scholars and policy makers after several reports by the Institute of Medicine (IOM) (2000, 2001, 2004) found that quality and patient safety were more likely to be influenced by the work environment and its systems and processes than by individual behaviors or competencies (Berwick 2002; Institute of Medicine 2004). Nursing scholars had focused on work environment research prior to these reports (Kramer and Schmalenberg 2005a); however, the IOM reports triggered a flurry of research into health care work environments. The IOM (2004) proposed that threats to quality and patient safety are found in four basic features of the work environment: (1) management practices, (2) workforce deployment practices, (3) work design, and (4) organizational culture.

In this chapter, we review some of this research. First, we discuss fruitful scholarship that linked customer service climates and customer outcomes (Subramony and Pugh 2014; Vogus and McClelland 2016). Next we discuss the extensive work environment research on Magnet® hospitals. We then discuss some studies that investigated how organization-level characteristics (e.g., collaboration, cultural competence) influence HCAHPS patient experience ratings, and conclude with some recent research that examined specific work environment characteristics (e.g., compassion practices) that influence worker and patient outcomes.

We conclude that when organizations take care of their workers, there are better outcomes for patients as well. We argue that "care" is a defining characteristic of health care, and care should encompass workers as well as patients. Given that patients are usually suffering to some extent and are vulnerable (Hobbs 2009), compassion is required for true caring. When care workers experience supportive and compassionate work environments, they are better able to meet patient needs (McClelland and Vogus 2014). Such work environments should lead to better employee outcomes as well, and hence contribute to better overall organizational performance.

CULTURE/CLIMATE RESEARCH

A service is a unique product based on three attributes: (1) it is intangible and does not exist until it is provided to the customer, (2) it is nonstandardized, and (3) it is produced and consumed simultaneously with the customer observing and participating in the production process (Morrison

1996: 494). This co-production of service means that the customer is inseparable from the person delivering the service (Lengnick-Hall 1996). Health care is a very complex service, which unfolds over time and potentially has life and death implications for the customer, as well as implications for care workers and organizations (Vogus and McClelland 2016). Not surprisingly, much of what facilitates high-quality PC care depends on the nature of the health care work environment.

Some of the most fruitful work environment research, mostly outside of health care, links organizational climates for customer service with customer perceptions and satisfaction (Subramony and Pugh 2014). Although organizational culture and climate are not the same, and although the terms are often used interchangeably, here we focus on climates; see Denison 1996 for discussion of the differences. Climates are the shared perceptions among employees about what types of activities, behaviors, and attitudes their organization or unit values. Organizational structures and processes, hierarchies, policies, and unspoken rules that define appropriate behavior shape these perceptions (Wiley and Brooks 2000). Specific types of climate have been shown to predict specific outcomes (Carr, Schmidt, Ford, and DeShon 2003). For example, research on service climates in banking and retail organizations found strong linkages to customer satisfaction (Subramony and Pugh 2014). That research was the foundation for the nascent climate–patient outcome research in health care.

Strong customer service climates develop when organizations identify what customers expect and need in terms of the services they are seeking and deliberately manage the work environment to achieve those needs (Subramony and Pugh 2014). In health care, customer service climates should be designed for PC care (Avgar, Givan, and Liu 2011; Rathert, Ishqaidef, and May 2009; Rathert and May 2007). Rathert and May (2007) studied health care worker perceptions of the climate for PC care in their work units. Their study found that nurses who perceived that their units' climates were more patient centered reported fewer medication errors on their units.

Likewise, Rathert and colleagues (2009) found that participants who rated their work units as more oriented toward continuous quality improvement felt more psychologically safe and rated their units higher on patient safety. While these studies found support for climate–customer relations in health care, they were limited in that their data came only from workers. More rigorous service-climate research should include data from customers and other sources such as clinical outcomes (Subramony and Pugh 2014).

Recent studies that use two or more data sources and/or are longitudinal support those findings. Avgar, Givan, and Liu (2011) used hospital performance data, staff surveys, and patient surveys to examine relationships at the organization-level of analysis. They found that climates for PC care had positive effects on patient perceptions and negative effects on medical errors. Moreover, PC care climates had lower employee turnover intentions, which is desirable because turnover intentions were negatively related to quality. These findings were stronger for organizations that used high involvement work practices (e.g., employee voice, teamwork, autonomy).

Similarly, Weinberg, Avgar, Sugrue, and Cooney-Miner (2013) examined high-performance work environments (HPWE) at the unit-level of analysis. Employees in units that had more HPWEs (e.g., promotion of employee discretion) had higher patient experience ratings and lower odds that patients would experience adverse outcomes. Patient safety climate interventions also have been shown to reduce nosociomial infection rates (Larson et al. 2000).

More recently, a study in the outpatient primary care setting examined the relationship between voice climate (workers feeling safe to speak up) and patient experiences of receiving timely care (Nembhard, Yuan, Shabanova, and Cleary 2015). Patients who visited clinics where front-line workers reported stronger voice climates reported receiving more timely care in terms of getting an appointment, seeing their doctors within 15 minutes of arrival, and timely receipt of test results.

Nembhard and colleagues (2015) suggested that when workers have more voice, they feel more comfortable speaking up about problems or ideas that can improve the efficiency of care as well as quality. Although HPWEs and voice climate include front-line care providers and may influence PC care, it is important to note that they are not necessarily instances of PC care. When workers feel empowered to speak up and are supported in discretionary behaviors, PC care may be one of several positive outcomes that may result. Nevertheless, focusing on aspects of climates that improve worker outcomes may ultimately lead to better PC care.

MAGNET® HOSPITALS

Another fruitful research stream has focused on the quality of the nursing work environment as a means to improve patient care quality and employee outcomes. The term "Magnet® hospital" is an official designation ascribed by the American Nurses Credentialing Center (ANCC) for hospitals that meet specific criteria indicating they have a "magnetic work environment" for nurses and provide top-quality care for patients. The development of this program began in the early 1980s, mostly in response to projected nursing shortages. The ANCC wanted to understand what types of working conditions were necessary to attract and retain top-quality nurses to acute care hospital and nursing home settings (Kramer and Schmalenberg 2005a). Forty-one top-performing hospitals were selected as benchmarks for nursing work environments on the basis of criteria such as low nursing vacancy and turnover rates, and nominations by members of the American Academy of Nursing (Kramer and Schmalenberg 2005a). The term "Magnet hospital" emerged because the top hospitals had characteristics that served to attract and retain quality nursing staffs (Buchan 1999). In 1994, the ANCC began its Magnet Recognition Award program.

Magnet research identified valued outcomes for nurses and the hospital characteristics that were successful for attaining them. It identified three criteria associated with the best hospitals for nurses: (1) nurses perceived that the hospital was a good place to work, (2) the hospital had lower than average turnover during nursing shortages, and (3) the hospital was located in an area where it was competing with other hospitals for nursing staff (Institute of Medicine 2004). The research examined the structural characteristics in the top facilities (see Kramer and Schmalenberg 2005a for review), identifying 14 "forces of magnetism," of which eight are considered essential (Table 2).

Magnet hospitals emphasize nursing leadership as the key for obtaining the magnetic work environment. Importantly, the hospital's chief nursing officer (CNO) must sit at the highest level of executive decision making and strategic planning and must have at least a master's degree in nursing. The hospital must also implement the American Nurses Association's Scope and Standards for Nurse Administrators—it must have policies and procedures in place so that nurses can express concerns without fear of reprisals (voice), and the applicant organization cannot have been involved in any unfair labor practices as determined by the National Labor Relations Board or a state agency during the three years prior to the application. Magnet hospitals must undergo criteria verification, a site visit, and a public comment period. As of late 2015, there were 424 Magnet hospitals in the United States, three in Australia, two in Saudi Arabia, and one each in Canada and Lebanon (American Nurses Credentialing Center 2016).

A notable finding from the Magnet work is the necessity to establish an organizational "culture where concern for the patient is paramount" (Kramer, Schmalenberg, and Maguire 2004: 45). Kramer and colleagues (2004) surveyed 4,320 staff nurses in 26 hospitals to explore cultural values that differed between Magnet and non-Magnet hospitals. Ninety percent of respondents employed in Magnet hospitals said that "concern for the patient is paramount" compared with 78% of those employed in hospitals that were preparing to apply for Magnet status and only 58% in non-Magnet hospitals. Respondents also judged organizational concern for patients as a key cultural value, with higher priority than for other values such as controlling costs and addressing physician needs. Further, Magnet hospital respondents were more likely to say that PC cultural

TABLE 2
The Eight Essentials of Magnetism

Characteristic	Attributes
Nurse–physician relationships	Collegial, collaborative relationships in which each has power. Nurses decide what to communicate to physicians.
Autonomous nursing practice	Freedom to make independent decisions that exceed standard nursing practice but are in the best interest of the patient. Nurses perceive they have sufficient knowledge and support to be autonomous.
Control over nursing practice	Nurses have input plus decision-making power; collective accountability.
Clinically competent co-workers	Includes specialty certifications, degree education, formal and informal peer review, and organizational reinforcement.
Perceived adequacy of staffing	Care delivery models, mix of staff at each shift, patient acuity, and "enough for what?" can all affect perceptions of staffing adequacy, but perceptions must be rated as adequate.
Nurse manager support	Counseling staff, orienting physicians, providing opportunities for growth, procuring and allocating resources, facilitating a highly professional staff.
Support for education	Financial assistance, availability of opportunities, others' valuing education, rewards for education.
Culture in which concern for the patient is paramount	Nurses say the culture expects "concern for the patient" more than other values (i.e., cost of care, pleasing physicians). Nursing leadership primarily responsible for initiating and maintaining culture.

Source: Kramer and Schmalenberg 2004.

values were regularly updated, promoted, and communicated to new employees. Although the Magnet research has not been framed as "PC climate," Magnet strategies mirror approaches put forth in service climate–customer satisfaction research.

NURSE WELL-BEING AND PATIENT OUTCOMES

The empirical research on characteristics of magnetic work environments and their effects on the well-being of nurses is extensive. Nurses are more satisfied with their jobs and have lower levels of burnout in Magnet hospitals (Brady-Schwartz 2005; Kelly, McHugh, and Aiken 2011; Kramer and Schmalenberg 2005b; Kutney-Lee et al. 2009; Lake 2002; Laschinger, Shamian, and Thompson 2001; Laschinger, Almost, and Tuer-Hodes

2003; Upenieks 2002). Research also shows that Magnet hospitals have better patient outcomes. Lower mortality rates were found in Magnet than in non-Magnet hospitals (Aiken, Smith, and Lake 1994) and HIV–AIDS patients were less likely to die in Magnet hospitals than in non-Magnet hospitals—even in non-Magnet hospitals that had dedicated AIDS patient beds (Aiken, Sloane, and Lake 1997).

Chen, Koren, Munroe, and Yao (2014) found that Magnet hospitals in Illinois were rated by patients significantly higher on six of seven HCAHPS composites (nurse communication, explanation about medicines, pain well controlled, discharge information, overall rating of care, and willingness to recommend) than non-Magnet hospitals. Similarly, Smith (2014) examined HCAHPS scores for all U.S. hospitals and found that Magnet hospitals performed significantly better than Magnet-in-process and non-Magnet hospitals. Magnet-in-process hospitals also performed better than non-Magnet hospitals. One study of trauma centers in Pennsylvania found 20% lower mortality rates for trauma patients who were treated at Magnet hospitals than those who were treated at similar non-Magnet hospitals (Evans et al. 2014). Taken together, these studies provide compelling evidence that hospital work environments that support nurse well-being also produce better patient outcomes.

HOSPITAL WORK ENVIRONMENTS AND HCAHPS

Other recent non-Magnet hospital research has used publicly available HCAHPS data to examine hospital work environments and how they relate to patient experiences of care. Some studies have identified common features among hospitals where patients report better experiences. For example, hospitals with higher nurse-to-patient-days ratios exhibited significantly higher HCAHPS scores, and patients rated not-for-profit hospitals significantly better than for-profit hospitals on the HCAHPS overall care measure (Jha, Orav, Zheng, and Epstein 2008).

Another study found that hospitals with more collaborative cultures had higher HCAHPS scores (Manary et al. 2014). Hospitals that focused on improving their cultural competence found that minority patient disparities were reduced, and they had higher HCAHPS scores as well (Weech-Maldonado et al. 2012). As will be discussed in more detail in this chapter, one study found that hospitals with practices that supported and incentivized workplace compassion had significantly higher HCAHPS scores (McClelland and Vogus 2014). HCAHPS scores also have been linked to patient safety. Specifically, significantly fewer hospital-acquired infections were found among patients discharged from hospitals with higher HCAHPS ratings (Stein et al. 2014).

Overall, these studies found that organizational factors such as collaborative culture, decentralization, nurse-to-patient-days ratios, and compassion practices influence an important indicator of patient experience (i.e., HCAHPS ratings) and potentially provide guidance to practitioners regarding practices they might implement to improve patient care experiences.

COMPASSION PRACTICES AND WORKER–PATIENT OUTCOMES

While progress has been made in improving health care work environments, particularly for nurses, we posit that further improvements can be made when organizations value compassionate work environments (McClelland and Vogus 2014). Despite an increasing emphasis in health care education on collaboration and compassion, the way people actually treat each other often undermines compassion (Lown and Manning 2010).

Policy makers and patient advocates argue that PC care should be central to all health care delivery (Berwick 2009; Epstein, Fiscella, Lesser, and Stange 2010; Institute of Medicine 2001), but care currently is predominantly "organized around care rather than caring" (Chochinov 2013: 757). Caring and compassion are keys to the therapeutic relationships central to PC care (Hobbs 2009). Research increasingly suggests that creating work environments in which providers can thrive—that focus on caring and compassion rather than trying to standardize PC care through scripts, checklists, and amenities—may be the best way to improve patient experiences (McClelland and Vogus 2014; Rathert, Vogus, and McClelland 2016).

Caring in the context of PC care includes understanding that people respond to illness differently, honoring every patient's dignity and personal autonomy, and helping all patients to reach their healing potential (Grilo, Santos, Rita, and Gomes 2014). Health care workers who exhibit caring and compassion generally aim to be competent and authentic: they listen, provide emotional support and encouragement, and they sense patient needs (Beck 1993).

Workplace compassion is defined as "noticing another person's suffering, empathically feeling that person's pain, and acting in a manner intended to ease the suffering" (Lilius et al. 2008: 194–95). Workplace compassion is particularly relevant for health care, given that patient "customers" are there to have their vulnerabilities and suffering alleviated. Compassion from care provider to patient is a defining characteristic of a therapeutic relationship and is central to patient-centeredness. Compassion is a component of caring and includes action or behavior that is the "intersection between empathy ... and sympathy" (Lown, Rosen, and Marttila 2011: 1772). A compassionate health care worker takes action based on hearing a patient's unique concerns (empathy) and feeling the patient's emotions (sympathy) (Lown, Rosen, and Marttila 2011). Despite two

decades of focus on PC care and improving care provider work environments, only about half of patients report that they experienced
"compassion" in their recent health care experiences (Lown, Rosen, and
Marttila 2011).

COMPASSIONATE WORKPLACE EXAMPLES

Health care organizations with compassionate work environments provide
compassionate support for their care providers, and in turn, facilitate caring
and better interpersonal relationships with patients (McClelland and Vogus
2014). Indeed, McClelland and Vogus (2014) found that hospitals with
organizational practices that supported and rewarded compassion had significantly better overall HCAHPS ratings. One example of such practices
is Schwartz Rounds (Lown and Manning 2010). Schwartz Rounds are
regular meetings of interdisciplinary clinicians in which participants focus
on improving support and communication with one another and with patients and family. Each meeting focuses on a specific case, and participants
discuss its psycho-social elements as opposed to only clinical issues (Lown
and Manning 2010). One evaluation found that clinicians who had attended five or more Schwartz Rounds in the previous year were more likely
to report that they have more compassion for patients and their families,
were better able to focus on patients' nonverbal and emotional cues, felt
better able to discuss sensitive situations with patients and families, and felt
more energized about their work (Lown and Manning 2010).

Another example of a compassionate practice, developed by the Cleveland
Clinic, is the use of "Code Lavender" teams (McClelland and Vogus 2014).
These teams consist of employees who respond immediately when employees have a work-related trauma, often involving a patient (e.g., harmful
medical error, ethical dilemma). Code Lavender teams offer spiritual and
emotional support to help employees recover and reduce their stress. These
organizational practices legitimate workplace compassion, and compassion
becomes an integral part of the work environment. When health care leaders support compassionate acts among workers, patients and families are
then treated more compassionately (McClelland and Vogus 2014) and
worker well-being is improved (Lown and Manning 2010; Rathert, Vogus,
and McClelland 2016).

SUMMARY AND CONCLUSION

In this chapter, we have brought together several distinct but related
streams of research to highlight the importance of health care work
environments in improving health care worker and patient outcomes. In

light of the health care industry's pursuit of PC care, we have illustrated how caring, compassionate work environments that facilitate therapeutic alliances among workplaces, care providers, and patients should lead to better outcomes for all.

Going forward, we recommend research that further drills down into organizational work environments. The research on Magnet hospitals and their attributes has been particularly insightful at the broader organizational level, but additional focus on specific climate attributes of the work environment may provide valuable evidence for designing activities to improve work environments and PC care (McClelland and Vogus 2014; Nembhard, Yuan, Shabanova, and Cleary 2015).

While HCOs will continue to focus on their organizations' overall HCAHPS scores, future research also should look more closely at unit-level climates to identify actions that influence patient ratings of specific experience domains (nurse–doctor communication, discharge information, etc.). Through continued emphasis on understanding and building healthy work environments, health can be improved for workers and patients alike.

REFERENCES

Aiken, L. H., D. M. Sloane, and E. T. Lake. 1997. "Satisfaction with Inpatient Acquired Immunodeficiency Syndrome Care: A National Comparison of Dedicated and Scattered-Bed Units." *Medical Care* 35, no. 9: 948–62. doi:10.1097/00005650-199709000-00007.

Aiken, L. H., H. L. Smith, and E. T. Lake. 1994. "Lower Medicare Mortality Among a Set of Hospitals Known for Good Nursing Care." *Medical Care* 32, no. 8: 771–87. doi:10.1097/00005650-199408000-00002.

American Nurses Credentialing Center (ANCC). 2016. "American Nurses Credentialing Center Magnet Recognition Program." American Nurses Credentialing Center. http://bit.ly/2cOibJH.

Avgar, A. C., R. K. Givan, and M. Liu. 2011. "Patient-Centered But Employee Delivered: Patient Care Innovation, Turnover Intentions, and Organizational Outcomes in Hospitals." *Industrial and Labor Relations Review* 64, no. 3: 423–40. doi: 10.1177/001979391106400301.

Beck, C. T. 1993. "Caring Relationships Between Nursing Students and Their Patients." *Nurse Educator* 18, no. 5: 28–32. doi:10.1097/00006223-199309000-00015.

Berwick, D. M. 2002. "A User's Manual for the IOM's 'Quality Chasm' Report." *Health Affairs* 21, no. 3: 80–90. doi:10.1377/hlthaff.21.3.80.

Berwick, D. M. 2009. "What 'Patient-Centered' Should Mean: Confessions of an Extremist." *Health Affairs* 28, no. 4. doi:10.1377/hlthaff.28.4.w555.

Brady-Schwartz, D. C. 2005. "Further Evidence on the Magnet Recognition Program." *JONA: The Journal of Nursing Administration* 35, no. 9: 397–403. doi:10.1097/00005110-200509000-00009.

Buchan, J. 1999. "Still Attractive After All These Years? Magnet Hospitals in a Changing Health Care Environment." *Journal of Advanced Nursing* 30, no. 1: 100–108. doi:10.1046/j.1365-2648.1999.01054.x.

Carr, J. Z., A M. Schmidt, J. K. Ford, and R. P. Deshon. 2003. "Climate Perceptions Matter: A Meta-Analytic Path Analysis Relating Molar Climate, Cognitive and Affective States, and Individual-Level Work Outcomes." *Journal of Applied Psychology* 88, no. 4: 605–19. doi:10.1037/0021-9010.88.4.605.

Centers for Medicare and Medicaid Services. 2013. "Hospital Value-Based Purchasing Program." Rep. ICN 907664. Centers for Medicare and Medicaid Services. http://go.cms.gov/1Yv0GMr.

Centers for Medicare and Medicaid Services. 2015 (Oct. 29). "Final Rule for Home Health Pilot Mandate." Centers for Medicare and Medicaid Services. http://go.cms.gov/23ez4fa.

Chen, J., M. E. Koren, D. J. Munroe, and P. Yao. 2014. "Is the Hospital's Magnet Status Linked to HCAHPS Scores?" *Journal of Nursing Care Quality* 29, no. 4: 327–35. doi:10.1097/ncq.0000000000000062.

Chochinov, H. M. 2013. "Dignity in Care: Time to Take Action." *Journal of Pain and Symptom Management* 46, no. 5: 756–59. doi:10.1016/j.jpainsymman.2013.08.004.

Denison, D. R. 1996. "What Is the Difference Between Organizational Culture and Organizational Climate? A Native's Point of View on a Decade of Paradigm Wars." *Academy of Management Review* 21, no. 3: 756–59.

Epstein, R. M., K. Fiscella, C. S. Lesser, and K. C. Stange. 2010. "Why the Nation Needs a Policy Push on Patient-Centered Health Care." *Health Affairs* 29, no. 8: 1489–95. doi:10.1377/hlthaff.2009.0888.

Epstein, R. M., and R. L. Street. 2011. "The Values and Value of Patient-Centered Care." *Annals of Family Medicine* 9, no. 2: 100–103. doi:10.1370/afm.1239.

Evans, T., K. Rittenhouse, M. Horst, T. Osler, A. Rogers, J. A. Miller, C. Martin, C. Mooney, and F. B. Rogers. 2014. "Magnet Hospitals Are a Magnet for Higher Survival Rates at Adult Trauma Centers." *Journal of Trauma and Acute Care Surgery* 77, no. 1: 89–94. doi:10.1097/ta.0000000000000262.

Gerteis, M., S. Edgman-Levitan, J. Daley, and T. L. Delbanco. 2002. *Through the Patients' Eyes: Understanding and Promoting Patient-Centered Care* (2nd edition). San Francisco, CA: Jossey-Bass.

Grilo, A. M., M. C. Santos, J. S. Rita, and A. I. Gomes. 2014. "Assessment of Nursing Students and Nurses' Orientation Towards Patient-Centeredness." *Nurse Education Today* 34, no. 1: 35–39. doi:10.1016/j.nedt.2013.02.022.

Hobbs, J. L. 2009. "A Dimensional Analysis of Patient-Centered Care." *Nursing Research* 58, no. 1: 52–62. doi:10.1097/nnr.0b013e31818c3e79.

Institute of Medicine, Committee on Quality of Health Care in America. 2000. *To Err Is Human: Building a Safer Health System*, edited by L. T. Kohn, J. M. Corrigan, and M. S. Donaldson. Washington, DC: National Academies Press.

Institute of Medicine, Committee on Quality of Health Care in America. 2001. *Crossing the Quality Chasm: A New Health System for the 21st Century*. Washington, DC: National Academies Press.

Institute of Medicine, Committee on the Work Environment for Nurses and Patient Safety. 2004. *Keeping Patients Safe: Transforming the Work Environment of Nurses*, edited by A. Page. Washington, DC: The National Academies Press.

Jha, A. K., E. J. Orav, J. Zheng, and A. M. Epstein. 2008. "Patients' Perception of Hospital Care in the United States." *New England Journal of Medicine* 359, no. 18: 1921–31. doi:10.1056/nejmsa0804116.

Kelly, L. A., M. D. McHugh, and L. H. Aiken. 2011. "Nurse Outcomes in Magnet® and Non-Magnet Hospitals." *JONA: The Journal of Nursing Administration* 41, no. 10: 428–33. doi:10.1097/nna.0b013e31822eddbc.

Kramer, M., and C. Schmalenberg. 2004. "Development and Evaluation of Essentials of Magnetism Tool." *JONA: The Journal of Nursing Administration* 34, no. 7: 365–78. doi:10.1097/00005110-200407000-00010.

Kramer, M., and C. E. Schmalenberg. 2005a. "Best Quality Patient Care: A Historical Perspective on Magnet® Hospitals." *Nursing Administration Quarterly* 29, no. 3: 275–87. doi:10.1097/00006216-200507000-00013.

Kramer, M., and C. Schmalenberg. 2005b. "Revising the Essentials of Magnetism Tool: There Is More to Adequate Staffing Than Numbers" *JONA: The Journal of Nursing Administration* 35, no. 4: 188–98. doi:10.1097/00005110-200504000-00008.

Kramer, M., C. Schmalenberg, and P. Maguire. 2004. "Essentials of a Magnetic Work Environment, Part 4." *Nursing* 34, no. 9: 44–48. doi:10.1097/00152193-200409000-00039.

Kutney-Lee, A., M. D. McHugh, D. M. Sloane, J. P. Cimiotti, L. Flynn, D. F. Neff, and L. H. Aiken. 2009. "Nursing: A Key to Patient Satisfaction." *Health Affairs* 28, no. 4. doi:10.1377/hlthaff.28.4.w669.

Lake, E. T. 2002. "Development of the Practice Environment Scale of the Nursing Work Index." *Research in Nursing and Health* 25, no. 3: 176–88. doi:10.1002/nur.10032.

Larson, E. L., E. Early, P. Cloonan, S. Sugrue, and M. Parides. 2000. "An Organizational Climate Intervention Associated with Increased Handwashing and Decreased Nosocomial Infections." *Behavioral Medicine* 26, no. 1: 14–22. doi:10.1080/089 64280009595749.

Laschinger, H. K. S., J. Almost, and F. Tuer-Hodes. 2003. "Workplace Empowerment and Magnet® Hospital Characteristics: Making the Link." *JONA: The Journal of Nursing Administration* 33, no. 7/8: 410–22. doi:10.1097/00005110-200307000-00011.

Laschinger, H. K. S., J. Shamian, and D. Thompson. 2001. "Impact of Magnet® Hospital Characteristics on Nurses' Perceptions of Trust, Burnout, Quality of Care and Work Satisfaction." *Nursing Economics* 15, no. 5: 209–19.

Lengnick-Hall, C. A. 1996. "Customer Contributions to Quality: A Different View of the Customer-Oriented Firm." *Academy of Management Review* 21, no. 3: 791–824. doi:10.2307/259002.

Lilius, J. M., M. C. Worline, S. Maitlis, J. Kanov, J. E. Dutton, and P. Frost. 2008. "The Contours and Consequences of Compassion at Work." *Journal of Organizational Behavior* 29, no. 2: 193–218. doi:10.1002/job.508.

Lown, B. A., and C. F. Manning. 2010. "The Schwartz Center Rounds: Evaluation of an Interdisciplinary Approach to Enhancing Patient-Centered Communication, Teamwork, and Provider Support." *Academic Medicine* 85, no. 6: 1073–81. doi:10.1097/acm.0b013e3181dbf741.

Lown, B. A., J. Rosen, and J. Marttila. 2011. "An Agenda for Improving Compassionate Care: A Survey Shows About Half of Patients Say Such Care Is Missing." *Health Affairs* 30, no. 9: 1772–78. doi:10.1377/hlthaff.2011.0539.

Manary, M., R. Staelin, K. Kosel, K. A. Schulman, and S. W. Glickman. 2014. "Organizational Characteristics and Patient Experiences with Hospital Care: A Survey Study of Hospital

Chief Patient Experience Officers." *American Journal of Medical Quality* 30, no. 5: 432–40. doi:10.1177/1062860614539994.

McClelland, L. E., and T. J. Vogus. 2014. "Compassion Practices and HCAHPS: Does Rewarding and Supporting Workplace Compassion Influence Patient Perceptions?" *Health Services Research* 49, no. 5: 1670–83. doi:10.1111/1475-6773.12186.

Mead, N., and P. Bower. 2000. "Patient-Centredness: A Conceptual Framework and Review of the Empirical Literature." *Social Science and Medicine* 51, no. 7: 1087–1110. doi:10.1016/s0277-9536(00)00098-8.

Mikesell, L., and E. Bromley. 2012. "Patient Centered, Nurse Averse? Nurses' Care Experiences in a 21st-Century Hospital." *Qualitative Health Research* 22, no. 12: 1659–71. doi:10.1177/1049732312458180.

Morrison, E. W. 1996. "Organizational Citizenship Behavior as a Critical Link Between HRM Practices and Service Quality." *Human Resource Management* 35, no. 4: 493–512. doi:10.1002/(sici)1099-050x(199624)35:4<493::aid-hrm4>3.3.co;2-n.

Nembhard, I. M., C. T. Yuan, V. Shabanova, and P. D. Cleary. 2015. "The Relationship Between Voice Climate and Patients' Experience of Timely Care in Primary Care Clinics." *Health Care Management Review* 40, no. 2: 104–15. doi:10.1097/hmr.0000000000000017.

Rathert, C., G. Ishqaidef, and D. R. May. 2009. "Improving Work Environments in Health Care: Test of a Theoretical Framework." *Health Care Management Review* 34, no. 4: 334–43. doi:10.1097/hmr.0b013e3181abce2b.

Rathert, C., and D. R. May. 2007. "Health Care Work Environments, Employee Satisfaction, and Patient Safety: Care Provider Perspectives." *Health Care Management Review* 32, no. 1: 2–11. doi:10.1097/00004010-200701000-00002.

Rathert, C., T. J. Vogus, and L. E. McClelland. 2016. "Re-Humanizing Health Care: Facilitating 'Caring' for Patient-Centered Care." In *Oxford Handbook of Health Care Management*, edited by E. Ferlie, K. Montgomery, and A. R. Pedersen. Oxford, UK: Oxford University Press.

Rathert, C., M. D. Wyrwich, and S. A. Boren. 2013. "Patient-Centered Care and Outcomes: A Systematic Review of the Literature." *Medical Care Research and Review* 70, no. 4: 351–79. doi:10.1177/1077558712465774.

Smith, S. A. 2014. "Magnet Hospitals: Higher Rates of Patient Satisfaction." *Policy, Politics, and Nursing Practice* 15, no. 1–2: 30–41. doi:10.1177/1527154414538102.

Stein, S. M., M. Day, R. Karia, L. Hutzler, and J. A. Bosco. 2014. "Patients' Perceptions of Care Are Associated with Quality of Hospital Care: A Survey of 4605 Hospitals." *American Journal of Medical Quality* 30, no. 4: 382–88. doi:10.1177/1062860614530773.

Subramony, M., and S. D. Pugh. 2014. "Services Management Research: Review, Integration, and Future Directions." *Journal of Management* 41, no. 1: 349–73. doi:10.1177/0149206314557158.

Upenieks, V. V. 2002. "Assessing Differences in Job Satisfaction of Nurses in Magnet and Nonmagnet Hospitals." *JONA: The Journal of Nursing Administration* 32, no. 11: 564–76. doi:10.1097/00005110-200211000-00004.

Vogus, T. J., and L. E. McClelland. 2016. "When the Customer Is the Patient: Lessons from Healthcare Research on Patient Satisfaction and Service Quality Ratings." *Human Resource Management Review* 26, no. 1: 37–49. doi:10.1016/j.hrmr.2015.09.005.

Weech-Maldonado, R., M. Elliott, R. Pradhan, C. Schiller, A. Hall, and R. D. Hays. 2012. "Can Hospital Cultural Competency Reduce Disparities in Patient Experiences with Care?" *Medical Care* 50: S48. doi:10.1097/mlr.0b013e3182610ad1.

Weinberg, D. B., A. C. Avgar, N. M. Sugrue, and D. Cooney-Miner. 2013. "The Importance of a High-Performance Work Environment in Hospitals." *Health Services Research* 48 (1): 319–32. doi:10.1111/j.1475-6773.2012.01438.x.

Wiley, J. W., and S. M. Brooks. 2000. "The High-Performance Organizational Climate." In *Handbook of Organizational Culture & Climate*, edited by N. M. Ashkanasy, C. P. M. Wilderom, and M. F. Peterson, 177–91. Thousand Oaks, CA: Sage.

CHAPTER 9

Changing Forms of Organization and Implications for Managing Across Boundaries

SIMON BISHOP
JUSTIN WARING
Nottingham University Business School

PUBLIC POLICY AND THE CHANGING ORGANIZATIONAL LANDSCAPE OF THE ENGLISH NHS

From a distance, the English National Health Service (NHS) can appear to be a single entity, or at least an integrated system of defined organizational types and relationships. Up close, a much more complex picture emerges, and a common view is that we are now seeing rapid increases in the variety of organizations supplying health care across the United Kingdom (Peel and Harding 2013; Sheaff 2013). This fragmentation can be considered in relation to successive periods of NHS reform and reorganization; beginning with a vision of an integrated and centralized bureaucracy at its inception in 1948 (Greener 2009; Rivetts 1998), the NHS has been through periods in which organizational management, market mechanisms, and professional networks have been promoted as primary organizing ideals (Exworthy, Powell, and Mohan 1999; Klein 2010).

Sediments of successive periods of reform can be seen as shaping the landscape of today's organizational arrangements. This can be observed in the current Conservative-led government reforms, which have brought a renewed focus on market mechanisms while maintaining and, in some places, strengthening central regulations, performance standards, and national bodies. To consider the current organizational environment of the NHS, here we very briefly introduce the NHS, focusing on the policy reforms taking place since 2010—most notably the 2012 Health and Social Care (HaSC) Act.

To provide a thumbnail sketch: the NHS is the oldest single-payer health system in the world and provides a comprehensive range of health services to the people of England, employing some 1.7 million people and treating nearly 1 million people every day (Binleys 2016). Certain distinctive features of the NHS have endured through periods of reform, including its founding principles of funding through general taxation, services free at the point of use, and treatment decisions based on clinical need rather than ability to pay. Although the structure has changed a number of times through the decades, the NHS has remained a comparatively hierarchical and centralized health system, with power extending down from the central government Department of Health to regional bodies that oversee the care provided by hospitals, ambulance services, and community care organizations (which today are known as NHS trusts) for a given population.

Crucial to the functioning of the NHS has been the distinctive role of general practitioners (GPs). These are family physicians who are also funded by general taxation but operate as independent contractors and act as the gatekeepers to specialist services by making referrals based on the clinical need of their patients. For most patients, GPs are the "front door" to NHS services and are their most frequent point of contact with the health system.

By international criteria for judging health care quality, the NHS often rates as highly cost efficient in terms of outcomes for spending, with the percentage of GDP spent on health care in England comparatively low at 9% compared with 11% in France and 16% in the United States (Organisation for Economic Co-operation and Development 2013), although it falls slightly behind the leading OECD countries for performance on certain health conditions as well as personalization measures (Organisation for Economic Co-operation and Development 2013; World Health Organization 2014).

As the latest set of government reforms to "modernize" the NHS, the 2012 HaSC Act was introduced by the coalition Conservative–Liberal Democrat government. This followed on from the 2010 white paper *Equity and Excellence: Liberating the NHS* (Department of Heath 2010), published soon after the coalition government came to power. Although not detailed in the Conservative manifesto before the 2010 general election, the plans for reform were led by the Conservative Secretary of State for Health, Andrew Lansley. Promoted against a backdrop of funding shortfalls—as well as perennial calls to improve efficiency, effectiveness, and innovation—the reforms were extended as the Conservatives' vision for the future of the health service in England.

The three ambitions for reform promulgated by Conservative ministers were (1) reducing the bureaucracy of purchasing and governing health services by moving decisions "closer to the patient," (2) increasing diversity and choice, and (3) improving the efficiency of providers through competition. When announced, the reforms were hugely controversial and became the topic of intense political debate, with several commentators claiming the 2012 reforms to be the most dramatic in the history of the NHS (Timmins 2012), in particular because the reforms were seen to open health care to much greater levels of competition, including from new entrants in the private sector (Peedell 2011), as well as shifting the power—and responsibility—for health service provision away from the central government.

The central plank of reforms involved a reinvention of the way health care services are commissioned across England. This mandated the closure of existing commissioning bodies, 151 primary care trusts (PCTs) and 10 strategic health authorities (SHAs). Although PCTs and SHAs had only themselves been established in the late 1990s, they represented a continuation of the long-standing NHS structural arrangement in which regional bodies (of changing shape and scale) attached to particular geographic regions held responsibility for the health care of a defined population of citizens. Following the 2012 reforms, PCTs and SHAs were replaced by a system in which new clinical commissioning groups (CCGs) of primary care physicians (GPs) are to commission care services on behalf of their patient groups.

In many ways, these changes echoed the first wave of marketization led by the Conservative government in the early 1990s, in which certain willing GPs (who became known as fundholders) were given a budget to purchase services for their patients on the "internal" market (Rosen and Mays 1998). However, while in earlier reforms it had been expected that the care-providers commissioned would themselves largely be from NHS organizations, the 2012 act greatly extended the invitation to enter the contracting processes, ostensibly opening the market to new for-profit and nonprofit providers. Further, the extent of GPs' involvement in purchasing services had previously been open to local interpretation, with many GPs resisting fundholding while others were keen to take up the expanded role (Timmins 2012). In contrast, current reforms mandated a comprehensive set of commissioning responsibilities for GPs and tight deadlines for new CCGs to be established. Commissioning responsibilities entail contracting services for patients, alongside additional requirements for governance of quality and improvement.

Although the government promised to maintain the principle that health care services would remain free at the point of delivery and funded by general taxation, the 2012 act was widely considered a radical break from NHS traditions and continues to stimulate significant political debate and professional and public unrest and protest (Campbell 2012; Edwards 2013; Pollock, MacFarlane, and Godden 2012).

Under the new commissioning arrangements, the 212 CCGs control approximately 60% of the £108 billion overall NHS budget for England—approximately 7.5% of GDP (Department of Health 2014)—with the remainder spent on national coordinating bodies, most notably NHS England, specialist centrally commissioned services, and public health initiatives under local government control. The CCGs use their budget to commission community, primary, and acute health services for patient groups under their coverage.

An important part of the new commissioning arrangements was the demand that all service contracts be made available for competitive tender (Krachler and Greer 2015), with an enforced separation between the commissioning and provision of services. These elements were intended to provide more open forms of competition than had been seen in previous eras and were upheld by a new regulatory body, Monitor, which was tasked with overseeing the contracting arrangements as well as preventing conflicts of interests and other market distortions. An additional important aspect of reforms was the transfer of public health responsibilities from the NHS to local authorities, distancing CCGs from the requirement to consider issues of universal geographic coverage and equitable access (Wenzl, McCuskee, and Mossialos 2015).

The direction of reforms also further emphasized the divergent paths taken by the NHS in England, Wales, and Scotland that mirror the political devolution a decade earlier. Reflecting differences in the political landscape across the United Kingdom, the governments of Wales and Scotland have sought to distance themselves from the push toward marketization taking place in England.

Before moving on to outline some of the implications of reforms for provider organizational forms, it is important to note that despite the ongoing controversy surrounding the reforms, there are also considerable areas of continuity from past political periods. Since its inception, the NHS has been composed of multiple types of organizations, with considerable variations in care specialties and across regions (Klein 2010). In addition, although widely viewed as a comprehensively public system, NHS care has always mixed public and private sectors. General practitioners have never been employed directly by the NHS, but rather provide services under independent contracts.

In the past 30 years, there have been numerous policy initiatives to allow for-profit organizations to participate in the provision and management of publicly funded health services. Central government attempts to bring in additional (non-NHS) providers go back at least to the 1990s, and a proportion of ancillary services, long-term care, elderly care, and mental health and dentistry services funded by the NHS have been contracted out to nonprofit and for-profit providers since this period (Pollock and Leys 2005). As some commentators have suggested, rather than a radical break from the past, the 2012 HaSC Act can alternatively be read as continuing the long-running neoliberal reforms begun by Thatcher's government in the 1980s and maintained and, in some respects, extended under the 1997–2010 New Labour government (Speed and Gabe 2013).

Therefore, while it is clear that the latest reforms are having an impact on the organizational structures, processes, and activities of delivering services operating under the NHS banner, these changes should be seen in light of long-term shifts in health policy and management. There are signs that the pace of change is increasing, with a growing proportion of new contracts now being won by non-NHS organizations (NHS Support Federation 2013), as discussed in the following section.

In this chapter, we suggest that instances in which we do see new organizational forms taking hold have been particularly telling in regard to the current challenges for management across the NHS as a whole. In the next section, we introduce an illustrative range of new organizational forms, before moving on to discuss the management challenges stemming from these changes in the final part of this chapter.

CHANGING ORGANIZATIONAL FORMS IN THE NEW NHS

For-Profit Involvement

The organizational change that has gained the widest public attention is the increasing involvement of private sector organizations in the provision of NHS services. During the early 1990s, high-profile efforts to build bridges between the NHS and the private sector generally focused on securing new lines of investment in health infrastructure projects in order to avoid large up-front public costs funded through additional taxation or public borrowing. The Private Finance Initiative (PFI) allowed consortia of private contractors to fund, design, construct, and in some cases, maintain and run new buildings and facilities (Hodge, Greve, and Boardman 2010). Between 1997 and 2010, 80% of hospital building projects were financed this way (Pollock and Price 2010). Despite widespread public concern about the threat to core service principles and evidence of the poor value of many of these deals (Pollock and Kirkwood 2009), experience in the health sector has led the United Kingdom to help export the PFI model across the world (Hodge, Greve, and Boardman 2010).

In the 2000s, the role of the private sector was further extended to allow for new forms of partnership working in the management of infrastructure as well as the co-delivery of front-line services including pre-existing NHS care pathways and clinical teams. This was initially outlined in the comprehensive *NHS Plan* (Department of Health 2001), which set out a long-term strategy to tackle the endemic problems of undercapacity, lack of choice, and lack of competition within the NHS by allowing private providers to work within the NHS system. A prominent example was the introduction between 2003 and 2009 of independent sector treatment centers (ISTCs) that deliver high-demand, low-risk elective diagnostic and treatments services, such as day surgery (Bishop and Waring 2011; Pollock and Kirkwood 2009). ISTCs could be wholly or partly owned and managed by a private provider, who was also under contract to provide clinical services in coordination with the wider public health care system. Approximately 50 such centers were set up in the 2000s during two distinct waves of contracting, with most contracts set to run for an initial period of five years.

Since the 2012 HaSC Act, a much greater range of acute, primary, and community health care services has been made available to private contractors. Between 2013 and 2015, approximately one third of available contracts were won by national and international private sector organizations (Iacobucci 2014). For the first time in the history of the NHS, private sector organizations have won a small number of contracts to manage and run existing NHS acute general hospitals, with those cases gaining significant public attention (Levitt 2015). More commonly, private health companies have won contracts to provide specialist support services or activities seen as on the periphery of mainstream care, such as after-hour services.

Adding nuance to this picture, Krachler and Greer (2015) argue that there are enduring boundaries to market entrants from the private sector. Embedded professional relationships, public distrust, and institutional norms, as well as the ongoing requirement for universal coverage and tight budgets, result in difficulties for new entrants trying to compete with existing NHS organizations. Public NHS organizations continue to directly deliver an estimated 80% of services, and private sector contracting often takes place only in response to a particular central government policy initiative such as additional financial incentives. Indeed, there have been a number of occasions in which private companies have pulled away from the provision of NHS services, suggesting that conditions for an "open" market do not exist (British Broadcasting Corporation 2015; Plimmer 2015a, 2015b). Although the proportion of NHS expenditures going to the private sector has doubled in the past ten years, as of 2014 this amount was estimated to be approximately 6% of NHS spending (Iacobucci 2014).

One difficulty in delineating the current extent of private sector involvement in the NHS is that relationships between public and private sectors come in many forms. In some instances of private involvement, we see relatively "loose" or "arm's-length" financial arrangements whereby private companies provide care infrastructure or support services away from front-line care, such as in Local Improvement Financial Trust (LIFT) schemes that established partnership arrangements for private investment in primary care facilities. In other cases, we see "tight" joint ventures in which there is a full partnership working across service financing, planning, and delivery, such as in ISTCs (Waring, Currie, and Bishop 2013).

Further, the gradual rise in openly for-profit organizations supplying NHS services has taken place at the same time as changes in the regulation, governance, and management of NHS organizations—which means that they have taken on several elements of for-profit business themselves. Since the early 2000s, many NHS organizations became NHS foundation trusts, granting them independent legal status and partial—and often contested (Brettingham 2005)—autonomy from central government. Since passage of the HaSC Act, this independent legal status has become universal, and the cap on the amount of revenue NHS trusts could themselves make from treating privately insured patients has been raised to 49%.

There has been a widespread increase in NHS trusts engaging in private revenue-generating activities, particularly the trusts in more affluent areas of the country (Watt 2014). This suggests that aside from new private entrants, the distinction between sectoral backgrounds of organizations working within the NHS is becoming increasingly vague. This development is significant because the involvement of private interests in health care provision has remained central to political and public debate about the NHS since it was founded (Tallis and Davis 2013). While the public remains firmly against privatization, the gradual mixing of public, for-profit, and nonprofit organizational elements is a less tangible topic for public debate (Bishop and Waring 2016). Further, the increasingly intersectoral "hybrid" character of the NHS is reflected in contemporary issues of management and employment, as discussed in more detail in the next section of this chapter.

Nonprofit Involvement and New Relationships

Aside from the introduction of profit elements into NHS organizations, the NHS has also recently witnessed an increase in social enterprises and in mutual and charitable organizational forms. Again, these models have been strongly encouraged by central government over the past 20 years, with New Labour identifying social enterprises and nonprofit organizations as illustrative of their advocated "third way" of public governance. However, the adoption of these forms was quite limited until the current era, when the managerial "right to request" transition to social enterprise forms was written into policy (Department of Health 2011).

Additional funding streams have been made available for those willing to make the leap to charitable status, and a growing number of organizations have been keen to take the opportunity to push for increased autonomy from NHS regulations and bureaucracy and adopt more flexible business models of funding and care (Cabinet Office 2011; Millar, Lyon, and Gabriel 2010). For others more reluctant to make the change, the HaSC Act also included a stick to force certain organizations to adopt charitable status in the form of new competition regulations (Hall, Miller, and Millar 2012). Specifically, prior to the HaSC Act, community care services such as district nursing, physiotherapy, and other home services had often been supplied directly by the PCT commissioners. To separate the provision of such services from the new CCGs, those PCT services were required to break off as social enterprises or charities, with some including a degree of employee ownership and others involving systems of wider cooperative membership. While there is yet no clear evidence on the outcomes for these organizations, the move plays into a scene of increasing organizational fragmentation and poses challenges of governance and integration across the health system, as discussed later in this chapter.

Additional movement in the organizational landscape comes from changes to the interorganizational relationships among and between providers, commissioners, and regulatory authorities, with new forms of hierarchy and networks coming into effect. Aside from the stronger split between commissioning and providing community care services, additional changes have been brought about by the establishment of CCGs.

One key area is the relationships among GP practices, and between GPs and other aspects of primary and community care. While GPs have historically operated in independent surgeries or in small partnerships, we now see examples of larger practice groups or federations of GPs developing new models of primary care—for example, with salaried GPs under a common corporate management structure, adopting shared operational processes, systems, and care pathways (Williams 2015). Although such groups were not completely unheard of in eras under previous policies, the commissioning environment is now in place for successful or entrepreneurial GPs to expand the scope and/or scale of their activities, such as by operating in multiple locations with the potential to share back-office functions, staffing, and other resources.

This uptick in organizational innovation has been strongly encouraged by the Department of Health and NHS England, who have sought to develop a new mindset among willing GPs by offering the possibility of efficiency savings and providing direct financial incentives for adopting new organizational forms. For example, as one of the largest examples in the country, Our Health Partnership in the West Midlands is rapidly adding practices to its group of more than 150 GPs, aiming to allow smaller practices to remain cost effective as part of a "super partnership" model (Matthews-King 2015). This model seeks to share costs such as information systems development and other back-office functions. It also offers the chance for new approaches to care—for example, with patients registered to a practice group rather than to an individual GP and directed toward a range of health services and professionals based on need instead of booking appointments directly with GPs.

Similar activities can be seen in other spheres of care, with multiple forms of partnerships and mergers between providers, such as new horizontal relationships (e.g., between acute providers to share services across localities or with organizations such as major trauma hubs playing an enlarged role by becoming regional specialist centers). Also included are new vertical relationships, with a handful of examples of public and for-profit providers commissioned to supply integrated services for conditions across primary and acute care pathways, either directly themselves or through "prime contractor" models (Addicott 2014).

Also notable are ongoing efforts to reshape the relationship between physical health, mental health, and social care providers, who have been subject to long-standing divisions. A significant example includes the devolution of health spending in Greater Manchester through the creation of a new superordinate authority to oversee spending for both health (NHS) and social care (historically controlled by local government) across the region, with the aim of increasing coordination or potentially reorganizing these previously separate functions. Although those changes are not yet complete, the effort appears to counter the market focus on national reforms, and it illustrates the growing diversity across the country. More generally, it highlights the dynamic tension between market and government forces in the control of health care in England, with each presented as a solution to the excesses of the other—resulting in cyclical change.

KEY ISSUES FOR MANAGEMENT: GOVERNANCE, EMPLOYMENT, AND STAFF COMMITMENT

In considering the implications of the latest "re-disorganization" of the NHS (Hunter et al. 2015), there is certainly some difficulty in distinguishing issues caused by changes to organizational forms from broader trends in the contemporary public service environment. As has been seen in many developed countries, public spending since 2008 has been constrained in the United Kingdom, and although direct health care funding has been protected from cuts, reductions in local authority budgets for social care more broadly have varying implications for health budgets (Kings Fund 2015a).

Nevertheless, evidence from case studies, as well as industry and organizational reports, has suggested ways in which ongoing fragmentation of the health system has resulted in challenges for health care management. Here we focus on two of the issues gaining most attention since the reforms: governance and employment, particularly changes in the ethos and commitment of staff.

First, there have been widespread debates over the impact of reforms on governance structures and processes. Part of the rationale promulgated by the government for closer involvement of GPs in commissioning was the failure of existing governance mechanisms to identify and intervene in instances of failing care. High-profile cases, such as the poor care that led to the Mid Staffordshire NHS Trust scandal [explored at length in the Francis report (2013)], highlighted ambiguity in the accountability of over-lapping government bodies. General practitioners were given control of spending and responsibility for quality in an effort to reduce ambiguity and move decisions closer to patients. However, fragmentation in health provision continues to bring challenges, particularly about the balancing of risks, rewards, and responsibilities between the new commissioners and competing providers (Grimsey and Lewis 2007). In a number of health care public–private health care partnerships, asymmetries in information led the public sector to overpay for services provided by the private sector (Shaoul 2005) or locked the state into paying large sums for services for which there was insufficient demand or were no longer required (Pollock and Kirkwood 2009).

With commissioning having been transferred to CCGs from PCTs, an early concern was the loss of expertise to cope with the complexity of the commissioning environment and ensure appropriate contracts were in place (Checkland et al. 2012). Indeed, there were instances of large (>£1 billion) contract failures in the early years of the new arrangements because multifaceted service contracts proved impossible to deliver in practice (Plimmer 2015b).

An additional widely noted issue with the current reforms is the split role of GPs as both commissioners and providers of services, with a good deal of uncertainty about how GP-led primary care services should be commissioned by CCGs without conflicts of interests arising (Iacobucci 2013). Aside from their own practices, many GPs have financial interests in private companies that are bidding for contracts from the CCGs of which they are themselves members (Iacobucci 2013).

To cope with such issues and bolster the governance of market arrange-ments, new and altered regulatory bodies were added to the commission-ing system. At the regional level, there were two mechanisms. First, health and well-being boards, hosted in local authorities, provide oversight of access to care and health outcomes. Second, Healthwatch, a charitable watchdog organization, represents patient interests and provides informa-tion to facilitate patient choice. At the national level, Monitor and the Care Quality Commission regulate care standards and commercial ac-tivities, respectively.

NHS England has taken an increasingly active role in setting standards and measuring performance, and it has exercised its power to take over the management of NHS trusts deemed to be failing. These regulatory bodies have become necessary additions that aid in the transition to locally led commissioning arrangements and strengthen the governance and accountability of providers, but they also increase the complexity of the new system—specifically, they create significant overlaps between the governance responsibilities of the various authorities (Checkland et al. 2013). In contrast to the market rhetoric associated with the 2012 HaSC Act, the expanding authority of these bodies raises large questions about the sovereignty of commissioners and providers and further alters the mix of market, state, and network controls in the delivery of health care. The reforms since 2012 were, at the very least, intended to offer a clear direction for the health system in England; however, there is evidence that for leaders, managers, and clinicians, confusion about the intended organization of services continues to reign (Peckham et al. 2015).

A second area of significant concern during the course of reforms is maintaining a high-quality health workforce. Prior to the 1990s and 2000s, the NHS was traditionally seen as a highly integrated employer. This picture has changed in recent years to one characterized by increasingly local flexibility for management to shape employment within national frameworks. Allowing greater organizational control over employment systems and work roles has been one of the driving forces behind market reforms. However, attempting to move away from central control of employment has also changed the balance of power between health care staff, professional groups, and employing organizations, creating new problems for management and employees.

Opportunities for new winners and losers have been created, which are based on the relative power of the actors in this more open and competitive labor market. In earlier bouts of private contracting, it was mainly the lower-status workgroups and support staff who were transferred out of public employment, and concerns were raised about the creation of a two-tiered public service workforce because those workers were separated from public sector employment protection, favorable terms and conditions, and public pensions (Grimshaw, Vincent, and Willmott 2002).

In more recent reforms, professional clinical staff are increasingly more directly involved in organizational change, and they retain greater power to resist or challenge aspects that threaten their work conditions and employment. Given the shortages of many professional specialties, more autonomous and less powerful employers have been losing out and struggle to maintain minimum safe staffing levels (Lintern 2013). In several instances, higher-status professionals have been able to disrupt changes at the local level by refusing to cooperate with management and campaigning against reforms (Campbell and Syal 2015). Alternatively, clinicians have used the arrival of for-profit and nonprofit organizations to their own benefit by increasingly contracting out their own work to other suppliers or locum (temporary) employment agencies (Cooper 2014).

Leading on from this, tight networks of commissioners, providers, and subcontractors can also create ambiguity about the lines of accountability and control over employment, underpinned by the employment regulations surrounding public professional and clinical work (Forrer, Kee, Newcomer, and Boyer 2010). Previous research has spelled out the complexities of employment across close, interorganizational networks (Cooke, Earnshaw, Marchington, and Rubery 2004; Marchington, Grimshaw, Rubery, and Willmott 2005); these issues are exemplified when NHS staff are transferred to private or nonprofit organizations. For example, in a number of public–private partnership arrangements, clinical professionals previously in the public sector have seen their work either fully or partially moved to private service providers (Bishop and Waring 2011). However, in certain circumstances, transferred staff have public sector employment conditions protected—meaning the new employers are limited in their ability to manage employees and alter how they carry out their work, thus undermining the objectives of reform. Similarly, under current reforms, primary and community care providers reopened as independent organizations face significant constraints in their ability to make changes to employment as a result of existing service agreements and integrated working arrangements.

Within these struggles for more autonomous organizations to make efficiency changes while maintaining a competent workforce, there are indications that pursuing efficiency introduces significant difficulties in the levels of the commitment of health care staff. Throughout the public service literature is widespread evidence of the commitment and ethos of public sector employees waning during recent market reforms (Hebson, Grimshaw, and Marchington 2003; Hoque, Kirkpatrick, Lonsdale, and De Ruyter 2011; Smith 2012). Since 2012, there has been substantial unrest among staff groups and professional associations, with repeated strike action by midwives, led by the Royal College of Midwives, and junior doctors, led by the British Medical Association. These actions, while certainly related to wider reforms, have been in direct response to attempted changes and restrictions to national agreements regarding pay and working conditions.

There is also widespread anecdotal evidence of clinical staff leaving their professions or emigrating in increasing numbers overseas (Doward 2015), with regular reports of staffing crises within individual trusts (Royal College of Nursing 2016). However, given the size of the NHS workforce, this picture is inevitably complex, and, overall, the number of staff within the NHS continues to steadily rise (Kings Fund 2015b).

Without up-to-date studies examining this issue, it is not clear how the latest round of organizational and commissioning reforms relate to wider changes in the political and public service landscape in shaping the work, commitment, and ethos of contemporary health professionals (Evetts 2016; Noordegraaf 2013).

CONCLUSION

This chapter was written in early 2016, making it difficult to provide a thorough review of the latest set of political health reforms in England and the implications for the organization of care. The HaSC Act has certainly prompted an upturn in the degree of marketization, with increasing variation in provider types and important changes to the relationships among providers and between providers and commissioners.

At the same time, there remain significant barriers to private providers expanding their position within the health market, and for-profit services remain the exception rather than the rule (Krachler and Greer 2015). Further, the supposed local autonomy of commissioners and providers is heavily constrained by an expanded set of regulatory and performance structures and processes. The need for open competition, emphasized during the early part of the Conservative government's time in power, has become less a focus in more recent NHS strategy documents (Stevens 2014).

There are also important political battles currently being fought, most notably between the British Medical Association over a new employment contract for junior doctors, which appear important in shaping the distribution of power among the medical profession, organizational management, and central government. The balance of power among managers, government, and professionals has shaped the organization of health activities over the long run (Klein 2010), with the 2012 reforms being the latest chapter in the history of the NHS—an institution perpetually declared to be "at a breaking point" but which nevertheless is celebrated as a central part of British public life, with enduring public support.

This is not to say cyclical reform is inconsequential because continual change has had a dramatic impact on front-line staff and managers in terms of their professional identities, well-being, and commitment to the service (Robinson, Jones, Fevre, and Lewis 2012; Waring and Bishop 2011), with benefits and risks shifting over time. This contested terrain helps to explain why organizational researchers are drawn to the NHS, which remains a lively domain for studying the intersection of policy and professionals—and which holds important outcomes for organizations, their workforce, and society.

REFERENCES

Addicott, R. 2014. "Commissioning and Contracting for Integrated Care." London, UK: The Kings Fund.

Binleys. 2016. *Binley's NHS Guide*, Winter/Spring 2016 edition. Basildon, UK: Beechwood House.

Bishop, S., and J. Waring. 2011. "Inconsistency in Health Care Professional Work: Employment in Independent Sector Treatment Centres." *Journal of Health Organization and Management* 25, no. 3: 315–31.

Bishop, S., and J. Waring. 2016 (May 20). "Becoming Hybrid: The Negotiated Order on the Front Line of Public-Private Partnerships." *Human Relations.* doi:10.1177/0018726716630389.

Brettingham, M. 2005. "Local Control Over Foundation Trusts Is 'Rhetoric.'" *British Medical Journal* 330, no. 7505: 1408. doi:10.1136/bmj.330.7505.1408-d.

British Broadcasting Corporation. 2015 (Jan. 9). "Hinchingbrooke Hospital: Circle to Withdraw from Contract." BBC News.

Cabinet Office. 2011. "Business Support for Social Enterprises." London, UK: Her Majesty's Stationary Office.

Campbell, D. 2012 (Mar. 7). "Save Our NHS: Thousands March in Health Bill Protest.'" *The Guardian.* http://bit.ly/29igsVi.

Campbell, D., and R. Syal. 2015 (Feb. 2). "NHS Paying Locum Doctors £1,760 a Day to Cover Chronic Staff Shortages." *The Guardian.* http://bit.ly/2c8CPng.

Checkland, K., P. Allen, A. Coleman, J. Segar, I. McDermott, S. Harrison, C. Petsoulas, and S. Peckham. 2013. "Accountable to Whom, for What? An Exploration of the Early Development of Clinical Commissioning Groups in the English NHS." *BMJ Open* 3, no. 12. doi:10.1136/bmjopen-2013-003769.

Checkland, K., A. Coleman, J. Segar, I. McDermott, R. Miller, A. Wallace, C. Petsoulas, S. Peckham, and S. Harrison. 2012. "Exploring the Early Workings of Emerging Clinical Commissioning Groups: Final Report." London, UK: Policy Research Unit in Commissioning and the Healthcare System (PRUComm).

Cooke, F. L., J. Earnshaw, M. Marchington, and J. Rubery. 2004. "For Better and for Worse: Transfer of Undertakings and the Reshaping of Employment Relations." *The International Journal of Human Resource Management* 15, no. 2: 276–94. doi:10.1080/0958519032000158518.

Cooper, C. 2014 (Dec. 17). "NHS Services Cut in Nottingham after Doctors Quit Rather than Work for Private Firm." *The Independent.*

Department of Health. 2001. "The NHS Plan." London, UK: Her Majesty's Stationery Office.

Department of Health. 2010. "Equity and Excellence: Liberating the NHS." London, UK: Her Majesty's Stationery Office.

Department of Health. 2011. "Making Quality Your Business: The Right to Provide." London, UK: Her Majesty's Stationery Office.

Department of Health. 2014. "Annual Report and Accounts 2013–14." London, UK: Her Majesty's Stationery Office.

Doward, J. 2015 (Aug. 22). "Thousands of New Doctors Opt for a Better Life Abroad." *The Guardian.* http://bit.ly/2c8DMMk.

Edwards, N. 2013 (Apr. 3). "Implementation of the Health and Social Care Act." *The BMJ* 346. doi:10.1136/bmj.f2090.

Evetts, J. 2016. "Hybrid Organizations and Hybrid Professionalism: Changes, Continuities and Challenges." In *Perspectives on Contemporary Professional Work: Challenges and Experiences,* edited by A. Wilkinson, D. Hislop, and C. Coupland. Cheltenham, UK: Edward Elgar.

Exworthy, M., M. Powell, and J. Mohan. 1999. "The NHS: Quasi-Market, Quasi-Hierarchy and Quasi-Network?" *Public Money and Management* 19, no. 4: 15–22. doi: 10.1111/1467-9302.00184.

Forrer, J., J. E. Kee, K. E. Newcomer, and E. Boyer. 2010. "Public–Private Partnerships and the Public Accountability Question." *Public Administration Review* 70, no. 3: 475–84. doi:10.1111/j.1540-6210.2010.02161.x.

Francis, R. 2013. "Report of the Mid Staffordshire NHS Foundation Trust Public Inquiry." London, UK: Her Majesty's Stationery Office.

Greener, I. 2009. "Towards a History of Choice in UK Health Policy." *Sociology of Health and Illness* 31, no. 4: 309–24.

Grimsey, D., and M. Lewis. 2007. *Public–Private Partnerships: The Worldwide Revolution in Infrastructure Provision and Project Finance*. Cheltenham, UK: Edward Elgar.

Grimshaw, D., S. Vincent, and H. Willmott. 2002. "Going Privately: Partnership and Outsourcing in UK Public Services." *Public Administration* 80, no. 3: 475–502. doi:10.1111/1467-9299.00314.

Hall, K., R. Miller, and R. Millar. 2012. "Jumped or Pushed: What Motivates NHS Staff to Set up a Social Enterprise?" *Social Enterprise Journal* 8, no. 1: 49–62. doi: 10.1108/17508611211226584.

Hebson, G., D. Grimshaw, and M. Marchington. 2003. "PPPs and the Changing Public Sector Ethos: Case-Study Evidence from the Health and Local Authority Sectors." *Work, Employment and Society* 17, no. 3: 481–501. doi:10.1177/09500170030173005.

Hodge, G. A., C. Greve, and A. E. Boardman. 2010. *International Handbook on Public–Private Partnerships*. Cheltenham, UK: Edward Elgar.

Hoque, K., I. Kirkpatrick, C. Lonsdale, and A. De Ruyter. 2011. "Outsourcing the Procurement of Agency Workers: The Impact of Vendor-Managed Services in English Social Care." *Work, Employment and Society* 25, no. 3: 522–39. doi:10.1177/0950017011407971.

Hunter, D. J., J. Erskine, A. Small, T. McGovern, C. Hicks, P. Whitty, and E. Lugsden. 2015. "Doing Transformational Change in the English NHS in the Context of 'Big Bang' Redisorganisation." *Journal of Health Organization and Management* 29, no. 1: 10–24. doi:10.1108/jhom-01-2014-0019.

Iacobucci, G. 2013. "More Than a Third of GPs on Commissioning Groups Have Conflicts of Interest." *British Medical Journal* 346. doi:10.1136/bmj.f2043.

Iacobucci, G. 2014. "Private Companies Won 70% of Contracts Awarded by England's Commissioning Groups in Opening Months." *British Medical Journal* 348 doi:10.1136/bmj.g292.

Kings Fund. 2015a. "Quarterly Monitoring Report 17, October 2015." London, UK: The Kings Fund.

Kings Fund. 2015b. "NHS Staffing Numbers April 2015." London, UK: The Kings Fund. http://bit.ly/29illZe.

Klein, R. 2010. *The New Politics of the NHS* (6th edition). Oxford, UK: Radcliffe.

Krachler, N., and I. Greer. 2015. "When Does Marketisation Lead to Privatisation? Profit-Making in English Health Services after the 2012 Health and Social Care Act." *Social Science and Medicine* 124: 215–23. doi:10.1016/j.socscimed.2014.11.045.

Levitt, T. 2015 (Jan. 20). "Circle Was Not the Problem at Hinchingbrooke Hospital." *The Guardian*. http://bit.ly/2chsiDd.

Lintern, S. 2013 (Jun. 18). "NHS to Face Chronic Nurse Shortage by 2016." *Nursing Times Online.* http://bit.ly/29ioSAr.

Marchington, M., D. Grimshaw, J. Rubery, and H. Willmott, eds. 2005. *Fragmenting Work: Blurring Organizational Boundaries and Disordering Hierarchies.* Oxford, UK: Oxford University Press.

Matthews-King, A. 2015 (Aug. 17). "Largest GP Partnership in the UK to Launch with 'Nearly 200.'" *Pulse Today.* http://bit.ly/29ioqhb.

Millar, R., F. Lyon, and M. Gabriel. 2010. "Understanding the Programme Theory of the Social Enterprise Investment Fund in Health and Social Care: Analysis of 'Phase One' Stakeholder Interviews." Birmingham, UK: Third Sector Research Center, University of Birmingham Health Services Management Centre. http://bit.ly/29ip7XW.

NHS Support Federation. 2013. "Contract Alert: April–Dec 2013." London, UK: NHS Support Federation. http://bit.ly/29ipamH.

Noordegraaf, M. 2013 (Jun.). "Reconfiguring Professional Work: Changing Forms of Professionalism in Public Services." *Administration and Society.* doi:10.1177/0095399713509242.

Organisation for Economic Co-operation and Development. 2013. "Health at a Glance 2013: OECD Indicators." OECD Publishing. http://bit.ly/29L0ese.

Peckham, S., J. Falconer, S. Gillam, A. Hann, S. Kendall, K. Nanchahal, B. Ritchie, R. Rogers, and A. Wallace. 2015 (Jun.). "Impact of Changes in the Health and Social Care Act 2012 and Public Health White Paper." *Health Systems and Delivery Research* 3.29.

Peedell, C. 2011. "Further Privatisation Is Inevitable Under the Proposed NHS Reforms." *British Medical Journal* 342, no. 3: d2996–d2996. doi:10.1136/bmj.d2996.

Peel, E., and R. Harding. 2013. "'It's a Huge Maze, the System, It's a Terrible Maze': Dementia Carers' Constructions of Navigating Health and Social Care Services." *Dementia* 13, no. 5: 642–61. doi:10.1177/1471301213480514.

Plimmer, G. 2015a (Oct. 9). "Bupa Readies Sale of 200 UK Care Homes." *Financial Times.* http://on.ft.com/29uHvkf.

Plimmer, G. 2015b (Dec. 4). "Collapse of £1.2bn NHS Contract Raises Tendering Questions." *Financial Times.* http://on.ft.com/29is7YE.

Pollock, A. M., and G. Kirkwood. 2009. "Independent Sector Treatment Centres: Learning from a Scottish Case Study." *British Medical Journal* 338, no. 2. doi:10.1136/bmj.b1421.

Pollock, A., and C. Leys. 2005. *NHS Plc: The Privatisation of Our Health Care.* London, UK: Verso.

Pollock, A. M., A. MacFarlane, and S. Godden. 2012. "Dismantling the Signposts to Public Health? NHS Data Under the Health and Social Care Act 2012." *British Medical Journal* 344, no. 2. doi:10.1136/bmj.e2364.

Pollock, A. M., and D. Price. 2010. "The Private Finance Initiative: The Gift That Goes on Taking." *British Medical Journal* 341, no. 2: c7175–c7175. doi:10.1136/bmj.c7175.

Rivetts, G. 1998. "From Cradle to Grave: Fifty Years of the NHS." London, UK: The Kings Fund.

Robinson, A., T. Jones, R. Fevre, and D. Lewis. 2012. "Insight into Ill-Treatment in the Workplace: Patterns, Causes and Solutions." *Contemporary Readings in Law and Social Justice* 2: 246–77.

Rosen, R., and N. Mays. 1998. "The Impact of the UK NHS Purchaser–Provider Split on the 'Rational' Introduction of New Medical Technologies." *Health Policy* 43, no. 2: 103–23. doi:10.1016/s0168-8510(97)00091-2.

Royal College of Nursing. 2016. "Safe Staffing Review of 2015." London, UK: Royal College of Nursing. http://bit.ly/29isvC8.

Shaoul, J. 2005. "The Private Finance Initiative or the Public Funding of Private Profit?" In *The Challenge of Public-Private Partnerships: Learning from International Experience*, edited by G. A. Hodge and C. Greve, 190–208. Cheltenham, UK: Edward Elgar.

Sheaff, R. 2013. "Plural Provision of Primary Medical Care in England, 2002–2012." *Journal of Health Services Research and Policy* 18, 2 suppl: 20–28. doi:10.1177/1355819613489544.

Smith, A. 2012. "'Monday Will Never Be the Same Again': The Transformation of Employment and Work in a Public–Private Partnership." *Work, Employment and Society* 26, no. 1: 95–110. doi:10.1177/0950017011426319.

Speed, E., and J. Gabe. 2013. "The Health and Social Care Act for England 2012: The Extension of 'New Professionalism.'" *Critical Social Policy* 33, no. 3: 564–74. doi:10.1177/0261018313479010.

Stevens, S. 2014. *Five Year Forward View*. London, UK: NHS England.

Tallis, R., and J. Davis, eds. 2013. *NHS SOS: How the NHS Was Betrayed—And How We Can Save It*. London, UK: Oneworld.

Timmins, N. 2012. "Never Again. The Story of the Health and Social Care Act." London, UK: The Kings Fund.

Waring, J., and S. Bishop. 2011. "Healthcare Identities at the Crossroads of Service Modernisation: The Transfer of NHS Clinicians to the Independent Sector?" *Sociology of Health and Illness* 33, no. 5: 661–76. doi:10.1111/j.1467-9566.2010.01311.x.

Waring, J., G. Currie, and S. Bishop. 2013. "A Contingent Approach to the Organization and Management of Public–Private Partnerships: An Empirical Study of English Health Care." *Public Administration Review* 73, no. 2: 313–26. doi:10.1111/puar.12020.

Watt, N. 2014 (Aug. 19). "Income from Private Patients Soars at NHS Hospital Trusts." *The Guardian*. http://bit.ly/29itPVq.

Wenzl, M., S. McCuskee, and E. Mossialos. 2015. "Commissioning for Equity in the NHS: Rhetoric and Practice." *British Medical Bulletin* 115, no. 1: 5–17. doi:10.1093/bmb/ldv031.

Williams, D. 2015 (Oct. 6). "Former HEFT Chief to Lead Biggest Ever GP Partnership." *Health Service Journal*. http://bit.ly/29GZC3d.

World Health Organization. 2014. "Global Status Report on Alcohol and Health 2014." Geneva, Switzerland: World Health Organization. http://bit.ly/29ivhM2.

Chapter 10

Building Relational Coordination Across Front-Line Work Groups: A Case from Kaiser Permanente Northwest

Joan Resnick
Sarah Lax
Eliana Temkin
Kaiser Permanente Northwest

Jody Hoffer Gittell
Brandeis University

INTRODUCTION

Recent efforts to transform health care in the United States have focused on the transformation of primary care. New models stemming from the "medical home" or "patient-centered medical home" concept are expected to contribute to higher quality, more cost-effective care by moving resources from the treatment of illness in costly inpatient settings toward more comprehensive care coordination, care teams, and population health management in the community (Bitton, Martin, and Landon 2010). As in other industries, these fundamental changes in care delivery require fundamental changes in organizations themselves.

Some of these change efforts in the United States and abroad have been informed by the theory of relational coordination, which holds that highly interdependent, uncertain, and time-constrained work is most effectively coordinated through frequent, timely, accurate, problem-solving communication across work groups, supported by relationships of shared goals, shared knowledge, and mutual respect. Together these dynamics comprise relational coordination, which drives a range of performance outcomes and is shaped by organizational structures (Gittell 2003, 2009). The theory has evolved to include a dynamic change process that is driven by three types of interventions—relational, work process, and structural—as captured in the relational model of organizational change (Gittell 2016).

In this chapter, we analyze a local change initiative within Kaiser Permanente, the largest private health care system in the United States. In particular, we explore how relational coordination efforts were extended from the previous focus *within* departments, to include efforts *between* departments. As one vice president explained:

We have done great work within each department over the last few years to optimize our operations from a quality, service, and affordability standpoint. I believe it is the connections between the departments that offer us the opportunity to take our organization's performance to the next level.

We explore how administrative leaders, unionized staff, and clinicians became engaged in the change process, the methods they used, and the changes they achieved in four medical office buildings. We show a potential relationship between improved relational coordination across front-line work groups and a few key metrics, including quality of patient care and employee engagement. We discuss implications for practice, in particular suggesting guidance for change agents who seek to build relational coordination across boundaries. We develop new insights regarding the relational nature of the change process, contributing to relational theories of organizational change (e.g., Fletcher, Bailyn, and Blake-Beard 2009; Gittell 2016; Kellogg 2009; Kellogg, Orlikowski, and Yates 2006).

METHODS AND DATA

Our research questions are "How can an intentional effort to change culture and build coordination across work groups succeed, particularly in the midst of multiple organizational change initiatives?" and "How do change agents—formal leaders, co-workers, and clinicians—organize to enact those changes?" To answer these questions, we used a single case study methodology, appropriate for exploring research questions that ask how and for building theory.

Sample

For our case study we chose a site within Kaiser Permanente, founded in 1945 by industrialist Henry Kaiser and physician Sidney Garfield. As of January 2016, more than 10.2 million members have chosen Kaiser Permanente for their health care needs. Members are served in seven regions—Southern California, Northern California, Hawaii, Colorado, Northwest (Oregon and Southwest Washington), Mid-Atlantic, and Georgia. Because of its originating structure and philosophy as a self-insured health maintenance organization, Kaiser Permanente has a strong incentive to keep members healthy and keep them out of the hospital. Even so, like other health care organizations in the United States and elsewhere, the organization experiences pressures from evolving market demands and from its own internal drive to provide high-quality care at affordable prices.

We chose Kaiser Permanente for this case study for three important reasons. First, Kaiser Permanente's record of leadership and innovation made it attractive for study. Noted contributions included innovations in patient care delivery, health information systems, and labor–management relations (Kochan, Eaton, McKersie, and Adler 2009). Second, Kaiser Permanente's Northwest Region was already experienced in piloting basic relational coordination methodologies. Third, there were a number of leaders throughout the enterprise with growing interest in more fully exploring relational coordination's potential application. In other words, Kaiser Permanente was "ripe for change" in exactly the areas of focus for the relational model of organizational change (Gittell 2016). The Kaiser Permanente Northwest Region in particular was positioned for further exploration.

Kaiser Permanente's Northwest Region is a health system with 33 medical clinics, two hospitals, and 11,000 employees, of whom 1,200 are clinicians, providing care to more than 500,000 members in Oregon and Washington. The 33 medical clinics are spread over five service areas designated as North, Mid-Valley, East, West, and Eugene. The case study ultimately focuses on the East Service Area. The East Service Area serves the largest membership in the Kaiser Permanente Northwest Region, caring for approximately 204,000 members in four medical office buildings. Each medical office building is staffed by roughly 12 to 14 functional areas within primary care (i.e., physicians, nurses, clinicians, medical assistants), ancillary services (i.e., laboratory, pharmacy, and radiology), member services (i.e., registration representatives). A typical outpatient visit includes the call center, registration, primary care and/or specialty care, imaging, lab, pharmacy, and possibly member services. Clinic hours run from 7:00 A.M. to 6:00 P.M., with urgent care hours extended to 10:00 P.M.

Data

Three kinds of data were collected: (1) interviews of key stakeholders regarding the change process, (2) survey data gathered at two points in time to measure the quality of communicating and relating across all participating work groups, and (3) archival data gathered at two points in time to assess the quality of patient care and employee engagement.

Interviews

Interviews were conducted from June through November 2015 by the co-author designated to this role, using a loosely structured interview protocol developed jointly by the co-authors. Key stakeholder groups were identified by co-authors prior to the interview process, including all work groups surveyed in primary care in both management and front-line roles. Members of these groups were invited to participate in interviews that lasted from 30 to 60 minutes. A total of 17 interviews were conducted, taped, and transcribed, then analyzed by the co-authors to identify key events and themes. Two types of quotations—those that describe key events and represent common themes—are shared in the findings discussed in this chapter.

Survey Data

In addition to interview data, survey data were collected using the relational coordination survey (Gittell et al. 2000), a validated instrument developed for research purposes and more recently used to provide collective feedback in the form of a "boundary object" to participants engaged in improvement efforts (Carlile 2004). The relational coordination survey measures seven dimensions of communication and relationship quality among specific work groups involved in the target work process of interest. Survey questions are shown in Table 1.

The relational coordination survey is customized in two ways: (1) a target work process is inserted into each question, and (2) each question is asked about each of the work groups involved in that work process (Gittell 2016). In this case, the target work process for the relational coordination survey was "providing care and services for our patients." Up to approximately 150 employees in each of the four medical office buildings were invited to participate in the survey. Participants were asked to complete the survey through an e-mail invitation, with each participant receiving a unique survey link, and with three reminders also sent by

TABLE 1
Relational Coordination Survey Questions

RC Dimensions	Survey Questions
1. Frequent communication	How *frequently* do people in each of these groups communicate with you about [focal work process]?
2. Timely communication	How *timely* is their communication with you about [focal work process]?
3. Accurate communication	How *accurate* is their communication with you about [focal work process]?
4. Problem-solving communication	When there is a problem in [focal work process], do people in these groups blame others or try to *solve the problem*?
5. Shared goals	Do people in these groups *share your goals* for [focal work process]?
6. Shared knowledge	Do people in these groups *know* about the work you do with [focal work process]?
7. Mutual respect	Do people in these groups *respect* the work you do with [focal work process]?

e-mail. An overall response rate of 70% was achieved, with rates that varied by medical office building and by work group.

Archival Data

In addition, the co-authors had access to key performance outcomes for the East Service Area as a whole, for approximately the same two points in time that the relational coordination survey data were gathered. These performance outcomes were patient satisfaction and employee engagement.

FINDINGS

Background

The change effort we explore in this case was conceived in mid-2013, and we follow it through late 2015. Beginning with the 2013–2014 pilot relational coordination work in team-based care, a new concept emerged—that of *teamness*. Teamness is a colloquial word for those qualities that are exhibited by high-performing teams; at Kaiser Permanente Northwest, these qualities have become synonymous with the seven dimensions of relational coordination—frequent, timely, accurate, problem-solving communication supported by relationships of shared goals, shared knowledge, and mutual respect. The term was originally spread deliberately by change agents in the 17 primary care medical offices engaging in team-based care. In turn, the term resonated with staff, who then organically spread the concept by word of mouth. By the end of 2014, building and maintaining teamness became recognized among staff, clinicians, and administrative leaders for its critical role in developing new clinical processes.

Capitalizing on the teamness movement, leaders in the East Service Area sought to determine whether working within a relational coordination framework would help local teams quickly identify improvement opportunities while reinforcing a high-performance culture of teamness on behalf of members and patients. Several service area–wide changes were already under way as a result of various factors—movement and promotions among top leadership and physicians, relocation of a medical office building, and other regular operational change initiatives. Given those changes, East Service Area leaders wanted to implement relational coordination not to create more work but rather to focus or sustain work in progress. In short, they hoped to integrate relational coordination into everyday work processes and language.

Capacity Building and Engagement Strategy

Interviews revealed that regional leaders were seeking new ways to operate more efficiently across departmental lines to meet the next frontier of patient care and services. According to Wendy Watson, regional vice president for professional clinical and continuing care services:

> It is apparent to me that the only way to achieve our full value as an integrated delivery system is to operate more effectively across departmental lines. Our members don't care how we structure ourselves as departments; they only care that the services they receive are coordinated and delivered in a caring manner.

Ellie Godfrey, then vice president of quality and service and now retired, shared this perspective: "It's always been installed in my North Star that you have to bring people together who all touch the patient." Nevertheless, coordination was sometimes perceived to be a challenge because of the existing relational patterns and the reporting structures that reinforced them. According to Godfrey, "It's just that in our organization, and I think in all organizations, it's often easier for people to talk if they're within the same reporting structure. But if you get outside of that reporting structure, it becomes more difficult."

There had already been a great deal of focus on team building and intradepartmental communication in Kaiser Permanente Northwest. However, typical interventions were conducted with single teams in isolation or as "one-offs" in which consultants would work with one team at a time on their intragroup processes. Watson noted:

> We have done great work within each department over the last few years to optimize our operations from a quality, service, and affordability standpoint. I believe it is the connections between the departments that offer us the opportunity to take our organization's performance to the next level.

Several actions targeted at building the capacity for leaders and managers to understand the relational coordination survey and its value unfolded in the last few months of 2013 and continued throughout 2014. For the first time, regional administrative and physician leaders attended the annual Relational Coordination Roundtable in Berkeley, California, where they met with peers and heard success stories. Under the leadership of director Barbara Belk, the Learning and Organizational Effectiveness Department also produced two key educational opportunities for themselves and clients and leaders: (1) a seminar with a leading scholar and (2) a two-day training class where clients and consultants learned side by side about relational coordination from leading practitioners and in the company of another health system. These educational opportunities complemented the direct outreach conducted primarily by senior learning and organizational consultants Joan Resnick and Eliana Temkin, who gave a series of briefings and presentations and held one-on-one conversations. Additionally, Resnick presented the results of the earlier team-based care pilot at a national Kaiser Permanente conference, building additional support and interest.

Rahul Rastogi, medical director for continuing care services and a practicing Emergency Department doctor at the time, described how he learned about relational coordination:

> They said, "Hey, we have this thing we want to discuss with you and we really need some time with you." They gave me just enough detail to whet my appetite but not enough to sell the whole thing. Then [an academic researcher] came and presented. And when I listened to her presentation, my impression was this is the objective approach that would be a conversation changer with physician leaders needing to lead changes. It was the first time that I had seen a collective analysis of pulling together common business or team-building wisdom in a way that you can actually measure a pre- and post state.

Funding and commitment coalesced in fall 2014 with a modest investment. In her leadership role, vice president Godfrey provided the seed money and collaborative sponsorship from her physician partner, Dr. Tom Hickey, to begin work. Rahul Rastogi later became the chief operating officer of Northwest Permanente Medical Group, providing the initiative with the continued benefit of a top physician leader's support.

Where to Start? The East Service Area Engagement

With regional leadership support and resources in place, there was still the question of where to begin to use the relational coordination survey. The East Service Area was selected based primarily on its size and influence. Michelle Teeples of the East Service Area explained: "The East Service Area is so large that it basically moves the needle on all kinds of metrics. When it is doing well, everyone is doing well."

A typical medical office building in the East Service Area consisted of primary care, specialty care, and ancillary service departments in keeping with Kaiser Permanente's "all under one roof" philosophy. Most of the buildings provided a centralized check-in counter and functional modules in different hallways so that members might walk throughout the building to receive the whole suite of services, from primary care to pharmacy. While convenient, the layout also required staff to help members find their way to the next department and receive a warm hand-off to the next service.

Size and influence alone may have been sufficient motivations to pilot relational coordination in the East Service Area. Concurrently, there were several internal organizational changes that supported the pilot. One specific change included the appointment of Gena Bailey as the new senior service area department administrator, with leadership accountability for the entire East Service Area. Bailey also served as a champion on the Regional Primary Care Leadership Team to take the lead in promoting culture change in primary care throughout all 17 medical office buildings in the Northwest Region.

In both roles, Bailey sought ways to assess the culture and to fast-track identification of improvement opportunities. When Resnick and Temkin introduced relational coordination, Bailey was therefore eager to learn more. Bailey quickly perceived the potential of relational coordination to create interdepartmental dialogue and collaboration and to enhance focus on relationships. In her words:

> When I heard about relational coordination, I thought that it was exactly what we need and it's evidence-based. So, it will move quicker and move our work quicker. It would have taken me years to build cross-functional teams in the Portland metro area [compared to my previous work in a smaller area].

A close partnership between Learning and Organizational Excellence and the Operations group ensued. Bailey tapped her assistant department administrator Michelle Teeples to work closely with Resnick and Temkin and to be in effect the "face of relational coordination" for the East Service Area. Teeples brought her personal resonance with the importance of relationships to the partnership. Teeples saw the relational coordination approach as something different than "what we had already tried," while at the same time acknowledging that

> we tied the RC [relational coordination] work into patient care all around, so that it's not about doing more work but about bringing greater focus to the *ways we do our work.*

In partnership with Learning and Organizational Effectiveness, Bailey and Teeples began the process of engaging stakeholders at all levels of the organization to build awareness and prepare for the relational coordination survey. They engaged the East Service Area leadership team of clinic managers and assistant managers, physicians, and staff in all four East Service Area medical office buildings, senior leaders, and the designated labor leaders in primary care.

To secure physician engagement, Bailey enlisted the help of her physician partner Mark Harvey early on. "One of our biggest advantages was getting my physician partner on board because [our clinicians] are so scientific," said Bailey. However, it was not an easy task. By title, Dr. Harvey was the appropriate physician leader to engage. By temperament, he was skeptical. As Harvey explained: "I was skeptical and frankly thought it would be a big investment of time without any benefit." He came to believe that relational coordination was a great way to identify ways for the entire care team to have a better understanding of their roles and others' roles in the process of caring for patients. He added, "The part that it's evidence-based—and we could show that—was huge."

As it turned out, Dr. Harvey's early skepticism and later enthusiasm appeared to be another asset added to the resources Bailey had gathered.

He was able to meet other skeptics on an equal footing by explaining his own trajectory in learning about relational coordination. As a result of his experience, Dr. Harvey advised people who were first learning about relational coordination to "keep an open mind. Early skepticism is okay and in some cases good, as it assures that you are getting accurate results." Dr. Harvey's journey mirrored the same journey that several physicians and ancillary managers would take.

Bailey included the labor leaders from the primary care leadership team from the start, as well. Simultaneously, the department administrators responsible for leading relational coordination carried out their work within the Labor Management Partnership, working in particular with the care councils and unit-based teams (UBTs) in each medical office building. UBTs are natural work groups focused on performance improvement to achieve organizational goals. Managers and UBT co-leads, physicians, and union representatives, meet to report and share UBT projects, and best practices and to spark ideas in a collaborative environment in care councils. Figure 1 (on the following page) shows how communications about relational coordination were carried out through the Labor Management Partnership in an iterative fashion from the local Partnership in Action sponsor level through care council to the front line UBTs.

In describing the process of introducing relational coordination to an entire medical office building, department administrator Trevor Franklin explained:

> When I say what we've done in relational coordination and our role, I'm really talking about our leadership team, with labor and physician partners. So, a part of this is going back to our Care Council, and our Care Council will work with us and say, so what do we really need to do moving forward? What's the activity that will best help us be a better team to ultimately deliver better care and service?

The communication cascade focused on building awareness that relational coordination wasn't about more work, but about improving the *way work was done* through better communication and understanding of each other's work. Teeples explained:

> As we started to have different levels of engagement and conversations, and through the help of [Resnick] and [Temkin], we were able to very strategically map out a path in which we were going to help people understand that this was not extra work.

Teeples helped drive the survey process across all four medical office buildings in the East Service Area, checking in regularly with the managers (department administrators and assistant department administrators) and other staff to hear how things were going.

FIGURE 1
Relational Coordination Planning with the Labor Management Partnership

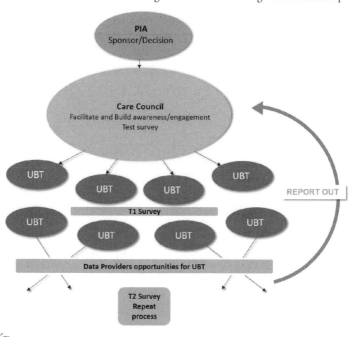

Key
PIA: Leadership team of physician-in-charge, labor partner, department administrator
Care Council: All UBT co-leads, physician UBT champions, managers
UBTs: All members of natural work group

Interviews with managers in the medical office buildings indicated that from multiple perspectives there was some resonance and enthusiasm for the relational coordination work, once understanding was in place. For example, Paula Edwards, an assistant department administrator, talked about how the Care Council in her medical office building began to see relational coordination as a value-added tool to the Labor Management Partnership:

> I think for me it [made sense] because we were doing Care Council anyway. I remember that we talked about relational coordination there and it seemed like a natural fit. That's the work we're doing in Care Council anyway, why wouldn't we roll this out? So, it was just a natural next step it seemed like.

A Laboratory Department manager agreed:

> You're looking at a really long-term employee, so I've seen a lot of initiatives come and go. I have to say that this is one of

the ones in which we could really sink our teeth into it, and we've seen results. And that's pretty awesome.

Gathering and Feeding Back Relational Coordination Data

The baseline surveys were deployed across all four East Service Area medical office buildings in roughly the same two-week period at the beginning of December 2014. Each building customized the survey slightly, allowing for slightly different configurations of functional roles, while consistently using the same survey questions. All four buildings logged sufficient response rates, ranging from 68% to 75%, to consider the results representative. Results were analyzed and compiled by Relational Coordination Analytics, a measurement organization engaged by KP Northwest to assess relational coordination, into four individual medical office building reports.

A best practice emerged with regard to how the data would be shared. Specifically, an informal but important agreement was made between the Learning and Organizational Effectiveness consultants (Resnick and Temkin) and operational leaders (Bailey and Teeples) about how to share the results. The agreement was that Learning and Organizational Effectiveness would hold the data and provide facilitated feedback sessions to the local leadership teams and Care Councils. They also agreed that the goal was to hand off report ownership to the local leaders once sufficient understanding of the relational coordination concept and data was demonstrated by the department administrators. This cautious approach ensured integrity of data and consistency in language and methods of interpretation, while simultaneously growing the expertise of the managers. In reality, there was much in the way of shared learning, especially given that no previous relational coordination surveys of this scale or scope had been attempted in Kaiser Permanente before.

Globally, two of the seven relational coordination dimensions were consistently weaker than the other dimensions across the East Service Area: "timely communication" and "shared knowledge." At the local site level, the data also identified communication gaps in specific cross-functional relationships via the relational coordination matrix. Relational coordination matrices are often considered by other practitioners to be highly sensitive information, given that each work group is rating each of the other work groups, including work groups that have hierarchical relationships such as physicians and medical assistants.

However, looking at data to highlight improvement opportunities was already a standard part of the Kaiser Permanente culture. Resnick and Temkin considered the potential risks, the culture, and the benefits of sharing data widely and transparently. They also judged the state of readiness and engagement to be sufficiently high in each medical office building to share the full matrix of relational coordination data in facilitated dialogue sessions. Figure 2 (following the next page) is a sample matrix for one medical office building, at baseline and at follow-up.

Specifically, Resnick and Temkin had each matrix blown up onto 11 × 14 sheets in color for a total of eight large posters printed per medical office building: one matrix [for overall relational coordination] and then one matrix for each dimension. Then results were presented to the various teams by taping the posters to the wall in a line and asking the group initially to stand back and observe from a distance. The facilitators gave the groups time to review and make meaning of the results and asked the groups a series of facilitative questions such as What do you notice? How does this relate to your experience? What stands out? Look at the colors in the matrices. Which dimensions are mostly green? Which dimensions are mostly gray? Once the group identified the strong dimensions and the weaker dimensions another facilitative conversation began: Why do you think this dimension is high? Why do you think this dimension is low? What are some interventions that could help to lift the results?

Jon Froeber, assistant department administrator, explained how the matrix showing the quality of specific interdepartmental relationships provided insight into the day-to-day experiences of himself and his colleagues:

> I think we hear it so often that we all want smoother communication between departments in order to provide a much better experience for our patients. The relational coordination data led us to an engaging and exciting conversation about how departments could better help each other.

Concerns and cautions about sharing data gave way to excitement as each data-sharing session opportunity seemed to become a positive intervention in and of itself. For example, in one medical office building, the UBT co-leads themselves facilitated the sharing of data at the Care Council. Remarking on the energy at that particular Care Council meeting, Business Office supervisor Cindy Kirk noted:

> I think the one thing where the timing was so perfect was when Kara [Wills, department administrator] had put this together with the Care Council which includes the unit-based team co-leads, managers and the Labor Improvement Advisor. In the past the meetings were good, but when this hit [the meetings] became dynamic. It was cross-unit-based team opportunities happening naturally. [Conversations became about such things as] "our two departments don't know enough about each other, so what are we going to do?" and solutions unfolded either instantly or as potential cross-UBT projects.

The relational coordination initiative was in effect creating a positive "vibe." The vibe became noticeable not just by employees but by patients and members walking through the medical office buildings. Momentum continued to build for the next stage of implementation.

Interventions at Four Levels

After the relational coordination data were shared back, several interventions emerged at multiple organizational levels. Interventions emerged from medical office building interventions, interdepartmental interventions at the unit-based team level, one-on-one interventions between individuals, and eventually at the entire service area level. The department administrators compiled an inventory of interventions, many of which supplemented or helped to focus existing work. The speed and ease with which these interventions occurred created further momentum and almost contagious spread. Below are examples from each level of intervention.

Level 1: Medical Office Buildingwide

Living-Room Huddles. One medical office building initiated an intervention called an all-office huddle or living-room huddle to bring people together, out of their natural department hallways, into one gathering space. The living-room huddle consisted of bringing all staff together for 30 to 45 minutes prior to opening the building for patient care. During the huddles, staff were provided a light breakfast and invited to participate in exercises to learn more about each other's roles and to understand the work of all the different departments within the building. Business Office supervisor Shannon Covington, who manages the front desk patient registration function, describes how to do a living-room huddle:

> For us, doing the living-room huddle was a huge change in terms of intentionally bringing people together for the primary purpose of connecting and getting to know each other and the different roles better. We lay the baseline far in advance—by having managers go around and talk up the huddle and exactly what's going to happen. And then when people arrive in the morning before the clinic is open, there is a lot of excitement and music is playing. We follow an agenda with the desired outcomes spelled out and make sure that the leaders acknowledge that people made the effort to come in early. Engaging people in activities like starter conversations helped our clinic team members connect in a new way. It's also important to follow up with staff after the huddle and ask, "How did that go?" "What did you think?" and then follow through in the next month with another huddle and so on to set a routine.

FIGURE 2

Baseline and Follow-Up Relational Coordination Matrix for One Medical Office Building

T1: Baseline

		Ratings of							
		LPNs	RNs	MAs	PCPs	MgrSp	Reps	Radio	Lab
Ratings by	Primary Care LPNs	4.52	4.48	4.24	4.29	4.38	4.00	3.95	4.14
	Primary Care RNs	4.06	4.08	3.67	4.06	4.14	3.67	3.73	3.65
	Primary Care MAs	3.56	3.89	4.13	4.27	3.68	2.78	3.62	3.40
	Primary Care Providers	4.10	4.25	4.20	4.32	4.02	3.54	3.79	3.56
	Managers and Supervisors	3.06	3.54	2.97	2.97	4.03	3.29	3.14	3.06
	Registration Representatives	4.14	4.14	4.29	4.14	4.93	4.50	4.21	4.14
	Radiology	3.93	3.96	4.00	3.96	3.86	3.36	4.46	3.75
	Laboratory	4.11	4.11	4.21	4.04	4.32	4.14	4.14	4.46

T2: Follow-Up

Ratings by		Ratings of								
		LPNs	RNs	MAs	PCPs	MgrSp	Reps	Radio	Lab	Pharm
	Primary Care LPNs	4.64	4.71	4.21	4.46	4.50	4.07	4.18	4.18	3.96
	Primary Care RNs	4.21	4.37	3.71	3.92	4.14	3.76	3.89	3.83	3.68
	Primary Care MAs	3.87	4.15	4.29	4.47	3.85	3.49	4.08	3.41	3.45
	Primary Care Providers	4.26	4.34	4.29	4.41	4.11	3.98	4.20	4.01	4.21
	Managers and Supervisors (PC/Lab/Rad/Reg)	4.20	4.31	3.86	4.14	4.57	4.06	4.09	4.09	3.83
	Registration Representatives	4.81	4.81	4.71	4.71	4.86	4.95	4.71	4.71	4.67
	Radiology	4.38	4.31	4.33	4.52	4.48	4.36	4.60	3.98	3.98
	Laboratory	4.12	4.12	4.08	4.04	4.35	4.20	3.86	4.33	3.88
	Pharmacy (Staff/Manager)	3.67	3.68	3.61	3.79	3.73	3.60	3.69	3.68	4.22

	Within Workgroups	Between Workgroups
Weak	<4.0	<3.5
Moderate	4.0-4.5	3.5-4.0
Strong	>4.5	>4.0

Response Rates
T1: 83%
T2: 85%

The relational coordination matrix shows how each work group rates the others (horizontal) and how it is rated by the others (vertical). The diagonal shows how each work group rates itself. Black shaded areas denote characteristics of high-performing teams; therefore, areas that are not black are potential targets for improvement.

The living-room huddles were perceived as a highly effective way to engage staff and for staff to learn more about the people they work with every day. People described how the vibe in the building was somehow different once the huddles started. People began to recognize each other by name. Voluntary by nature, participation in the huddles grew every month and people started coming in on their day off. According to department administrator Trevor Franklin people came "because they wanted to participate and saw the value in the huddles."

Starter Conversations. The first activity introduced at the initial living-room huddle was called a relational coordination starter conversation. The inspiration behind the starter conversation was an observation by one of the physician leaders who recognized that a change in building location and structure weakened connections between work groups that had been previously located closer together. In jest, the physician, Dr. Harburg, coined the hallways separating the various departments the "canyons that divide us." He acknowledged the challenge of making relational contact with people in different departments, given new physical barriers when electronic communication was seemingly faster. Dr. Harburg had an idea that small index cards with some initial facts about a person's name and role would be of use. Thus, the idea of connecting quickly using starter conversations was born.

The starter conversations were developed to help to close the gap of communication and shared knowledge between work groups. In practice, at a living-room huddle where the relational coordination survey had been deployed, the starter conversation typically began with the leaders (department administrator, physician lead, labor partner) introducing the purpose of gathering and reminding the group about the survey results, especially the shared knowledge dimension. Then each person was handed a card with three questions on it designed to spark a conversation about their respective roles:

- What do you want me to know about your role?
- What can I do to help us work together better?
- What is the best way for me to connect with you (e.g., voice mail, e-mail, chat etc.)?

The group was instructed to find a person they did not know, or did not know well, and ask each other the three questions during a seven-minute exchange. The facilitator marked time and then rang a bell and asked them to find a second partner to talk with. This was repeated one more time. After the rounds were completed the facilitator or leader asked, "What did you learn?" and "What was helpful about this exercise?"

Using this format, each participant could meet three new people from other functions in 30 minutes. According to Temkin: "It is an effective and efficient way to remove the shared knowledge mystery."

Afterward, these starter conversations were used in a wide array of settings, such as interdisciplinary meetings, trainings, national conferences, and a meeting with patient advisors. For the starter conversation with patients, the first question was changed to become "What do you want me to know about your care?" In a wide variety of settings, the starter conversation methodology produced dialogues that increased shared knowledge.

Job Shadowing. Upon review of the relational coordination survey data at several of the medical office buildings, an existing job-shadowing process called "Walk a Mile in My Shoes" was enhanced to have more structure and cross-functional exposure. For example, whereas it was typical for a new employee to be on-boarded to a medical office building by shadowing several different roles within his or her own department, there wasn't a systematic way to engage with other departments or for existing employees to participate. Those issues were resolved by the introduction of a nomination process. An employee interested in shadowing prepared a very brief summary of why he or she wanted to shadow a specific department. From the applications, the UBTs would nominate an employee to receive four hours of administrative time to shadow in a department of their choice. This practice allowed for staff and physicians to experience another department to learn the specific roles and duties of that department and how *that* department connects with or otherwise relies on other departments throughout the medical office building and the larger system.

There were plenty of local variations among UBTs that helped each medical office building develop its own customized experience and determine how to improve shared knowledge. For example, in one medical office building, a worksheet was filled out when employees shadowed another to capture key learnings that would be formally shared at the next UBT meeting. Another local variation included shadowing in teams. As Terri Imbach, assistant department administrator, explained:

> In one module we had teams go and interview another department for 20 minutes. For example, we had a dyad (a physician and medical assistant) who would go and shadow in registration for 20 minutes. It became standard to ask the question, "What can we do to work better together?" and that question then got shared at Care Council so that everyone used it when shadowing. So then there is sharing with every department about what we can do to work better together. It spread like that.

Level 2: Interdepartmental Interventions (UBT to UBT)

Specific department teams also used the relational coordination data to make an intentional effort to better know the roles of other departments. For example, in one medical office building, the matrix revealed a low level of relational coordination between patient registration representatives and the staff in Visual Essentials, the eyeglasses department. Although it would have been simple to assume no connection was needed (or using the language of the relational coordination survey, that "weak ties" were appropriate), the two staffs were curious to learn more about each other's roles. Once dialogue began, they realized that there were opportunities to improve revenue capture and the patients' experience of staff working as a team. The two teams used their existing UBT plan–do–study–act (PDSA) methodology to create a SMART goal (specific, measurable, achievable, results-focused, and time-bound) regarding missed co-pays. They soon realized that patient flow might bypass registration when directly accessing the Visual Essentials department, resulting in co-pay revenue loss. A very simple improvement was implemented and savings in one month on co-pays and post-service billing amounted to just over $1,000. When multiplied over time, the revenue gain became more significant.

A similar story unfolded between the laboratory and the back office nurses in another location. In this case, when the matrix revealed a relatively low level of relational coordination, the two departments had a conversation about what the data meant and what could be done to support each other. In short order, they discovered that on the occasions where lab orders were incomplete, the existing work flow did not adequately relieve the patient wait time while those orders were being confirmed. Although this was a common issue in health care systems and had been the subject of previous PDSAs, a very simple and durable solution ensued as the two departments made meaning of their relational coordination survey scores. As a result, patient wait time for orders in lab significantly decreased for several months in a row, then stabilized at the new level.

Many of the principals involved in the East Service Area work agreed that the informal improvements that came about from the focus on relational coordination were important for creating a positive culture and enhancing the "vibe." As the departments connected and more employees became engaged, relationships grew and performance improved. For example, lab technicians began a service to pick up specimens in a patient's room rather than having the practitioner delivering them to the lab, which directly improved the relationships between medical assistants and lab technicians. Staff soon began calling each other by name and in some cases by nickname. While they had previously extended professional courtesy to each other, they now offered camaraderie and mutual respect.

One of the stories to emerge about increased camaraderie centered on a seemingly small gesture when a group of registration representatives walked through the building delivering homemade brownies. Assistant department administrator Terri Imbach commented:

There's a gal in registration that decided to bake brownies for each department as a "thank you." Members of her team delivered them to other modules to say thank you for doing such a good job and we appreciate you. So you see that there's this camaraderie now happening between the departments that wasn't there before.

While they were delivering brownies the registration representatives also acquired a better understanding of daily operations in other areas of the medical office building. Interestingly, the brownie story jumped to an adjacent medical office building and was replicated with chocolate chip cookies.

Level 3: One-on-One Interventions

The relational coordination survey highlighted many improvement opportunities and existing strengths. It also focused awareness that though staff were naturally not as familiar with roles outside of their own department, there was potential benefit from increasing collaboration across department lines. People made deliberate efforts during the months of interventions to learn each other's names and create better relationships with co-workers in an effort to provide patients with better visits. For example, directions to patients regarding who they would next encounter (e.g., a radiology or pharmacy technician) were warmed by the increased positive regard among colleagues.

Level 4: Service Areawide Interventions (Across Medical Office Buildings)

As the interventions at each location started to take shape, operational leaders Bailey and Teeples sought to find a way to share experiences and best practices across the East Service Area. They wanted to increase collaboration among the leadership team to produce a more cohesive patient experience throughout the East Service Area. Teeples observed:

> Before relational coordination it was difficult to talk about best practices when each medical office building was so different. However, relational coordination helped the teams learn to appreciate the value of each other's experiences. They learned how to be different and how to leverage each other's strengths.

In partnership with their consultants, Resnick and Temkin, the leaders designed and hosted a series of relational coordination summits that brought all leaders, labor partners, and UBT co-leads together. The first summit used an existing East Service Area leadership team meeting time and extended attendance to ancillary managers and labor improvement advisors. This summit provided an opportunity for teams to make meaning of the baseline relational coordination data in an atmosphere of inclusion and problem solving. It was one of the first meetings in which ancillary department managers and primary care managers sat at the table together and took a broader perspective on their buildingwide coordination.

Based on the feedback from the first summit, a second summit was designed. The second summit focused on bringing teams together to share their learning from the survey and the interventions they had each developed. Rather than having individual teams report out their interventions one at a time, the second summit was organized to provide an opportunity for the teams to partner and present a composite of the best practices from each building. PowerPoint presentations were prohibited in order to make cross-team presentations more creative and spontaneous. According to participants, the summits helped create a more cohesive East Service Area as opposed to four independently strong medical office buildings. Department administrator Kara Willis explained:

> It was fun. We came prepared to talk about our own team's experience and then they (leaders and consultants) "relational coordinationed" us at the summit. We merged with another medical office building and came up with a larger view of RC. It was a good exercise. We felt like we learned new tactics that we hadn't thought of and that we could adopt. A lot of good positive energy came out of it and people seemed to respond well. It was like doing a large scale PDSA. It was positive.

The audience for the third summit grew as physician and UBT co-lead attendance was increased through advance scheduling. In addition, leaders from other Service Areas and the hospital attended to see the results of the East Service Area work. The third summit was designed to share the results of the follow-up relational coordination survey in real time and without prior cascading through structured rollout. By then the Learning and Organizational Excellence consultants, together with Bailey and Teeples, had enough confidence in the data and its use by the teams to share it widely with the teams who "owned" it.

In sum, relational coordination interventions in the East Service Area occurred at four different organizational levels, sometimes sequentially and sometimes in parallel. The interventions included quick fixes such as instant problem-solving communication, as well as more elaborate projects using the PDSA process. Figure 3 provides a high-level time line showing the sequencing of engagement, surveys, and summits.

FIGURE 3
Relational Coordination Implementation Plan for East Service Area

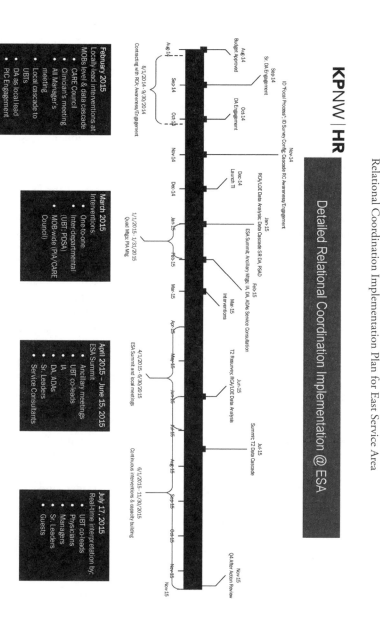

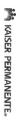

Changes in Relational Coordination Scores and Performance Outcomes

When the relational coordination approach was first introduced in the East Service Area, it was expected to improve cross-functional communication and relationships. At the same time, it was hoped that performance outcomes would improve accordingly. Because relational coordination was launched in the daily operational context of continual improvement, it was difficult to identify a causal relationship between interventions, relational coordination scores, and performance outcomes. Also, given the experimental nature of the implementation, no specific targets had been set proactively at a service area level. There were instances in which local UBTs chose interventions in accordance with their own local PDSA and SMART goal processes.

With these caveats, improvements in relational coordination scores as well as performance outcomes were observed. Data analyzed by Cadie Bennett, senior research consultant at Kaiser Permanente Northwest, revealed the following trends for employee engagement, measured by the People Pulse survey, and patient satisfaction:

- **Employee Engagement:** More People Pulse items for the four East Service Area medical offices showed annual improvements relative to the comparison group. For People Pulse items most aligned with the seven relational coordination elements, average scores were four points higher than the comparison group. The biggest gains were seen for frequent and timely communications along with shared goals.
- **Patient Satisfaction:** Average improvement levels at the four medical office buildings were one to two percentage points higher than the comparison group on several key aspects of the patient experience. Targeted interventions aimed at streamlining and making the care experience more efficient, such as reducing lab wait times, appeared to have a more immediate impact on the patient experience ratings.

In addition to Bennett's analyses, the operational leaders and consulting team noted the following:

- **Relational Coordination:** Two of four medical office buildings experienced improved relational coordination scores on all seven dimensions across all work groups, while the third showed relatively unchanged scores, and the fourth experienced gains and losses on various dimensions.

In addition to these quantitative improvements, East Service Area participants began referring to the "RC vibe" or "RC lifestyle." Senior leaders reported that they could tell when walking through a medical office building whether or not that building had engaged in relational coordination efforts. Assistant department administrator Hannah Austin explained:

> As you know, the story is not always just the numbers, it is how people feel when they walk through the clinic. We want to have a positive feeling and experience wherever our members are and there's not always a name for that. I feel that the overall pulse and the building has changed. You can really *feel* it.

In another medical office building, a team member offered the following observation:

> When I go into the break room now I know people by name whereas before, even though I worked here for two or three years, I hardly knew anybody. I look at that as a huge win-win because it translates when we interact with different departments. For example, now when the medical assistants bring something to the lab, they know each other by name and greet each other warmly. It's so different—the atmosphere and camaraderie—and it's awesome. I think the medical assistants actually now look forward to it when they have to bring something to the lab.

Trevor Franklin, department administrator at a third East Service Area site, noted the following:

> What RC really did for us was to identify those core dimensions that we could target as a team to make our teamness even better. Our teams moved from a small building to a larger building and in that transition, colleagues lost track of each other, and their patterns of interaction changed. People from different departments no longer had lunch together. It's a simple thing, right? But it mattered. So we promoted this idea of recognizing that we are a work family and need to connect in order to have seamless communication and teamwork. We focused our energies on activities that would promote getting to know each other, what each other did, and what each other needed in order to enhance the patient care and service experience. It really led to some good momentum.

There were some early indications of spread. In primary care operations, people began to hear stories about relational coordination and wanted to learn more. Some interventions were organically spread throughout the Northwest Region, and demand grew for the relational coordination survey. For busy operational leaders, physicians, and labor partners, a new tool or best practice has to be of high perceived value in order to get buy-in and engagement. The East Service Area relational coordination initiative laid the foundation for all of the criteria.

Best Practices, Lessons Learned, and Future Implications

After six months of gaining leadership support and one year of working with relational coordination, the Learning and Operational Excellence team and the East Service Area leaders came together to debrief their experiences. Prior to meeting, the leaders rounded with staff and physicians to gather their feedback. Consistent with Kaiser Permanente's process improvement culture, the leadership team produced a list of what worked well and what could be improved.

What Worked Well

Engagement

- It's important to engage the leadership team at each clinic early on so that labor, physicians, and management are on board and have ownership of the work.
- It's important to have RC as a standing agenda item in the medical office building leadership team meetings in order to support and sustain the work throughout the entire process.
- Rounding with staff before the survey is launched raises awareness and helps staff to understand the survey.
- Staff liked the concept behind RC and got excited about how to improve in areas of opportunity.
- It's extremely important to have someone in the role Michelle Teeples played [functioning as an operational champion for RC] to organize communications.
- Gena Bailey and Dr. Harvey, the senior primary care leaders, worked with other managers and influenced each medical office building to get engagement.

Launching the Survey

- Rounding with staff while the survey is active is important so that they complete the survey rather than opt out or exit before completing it.
- Be sure to have administrative support ready to manage the survey requirements such as supplying e-mail addresses and monitoring bounced e-mails.
- Monitor response rates every few days and make specific attempts to engage departments that have low response rates.
- Surveying all departments in the building at the same time is better than adding departments in the follow-up survey.
- Engaging the Care Council in the test survey to test language and survey configuration worked really well and engaged them even more.
- It was important to have a central support team from Leadership and Organizational Excellence to answer questions.

Interventions and Data Cascade; Involvement at Front Line

- It worked well for the Care Council and UBT co-leads to present the data once they learned how to use it and what it meant. They could figure out where to take it next.
- Care Council teams enjoyed the RC information and working in interdepartmental groups.
- It worked well to focus on opportunities for RC improvement instead of making negative references to survey results.
- UBTs developed improvement projects that mattered to them while using the RC data to improve RC between and within work groups.
- The living-room huddles worked well
- The job and department shadowing went really well.
- Finding ways to connect personally (like sharing brownies and baking for each other) makes a difference.
- The "Getting to Know You" picture game worked well to increase staff participation and cross-departmental knowledge.

What Could Be Improved

Engagement

- The timing in one clinic was difficult as it was a time with many leadership changes.
- There should be written information about the survey—what it is, what we are looking for, and where to find it—before the survey comes out. We spent a lot of time helping people look through their e-mails to find the survey when we didn't have a large-enough response rate initially.
- It is critical to formally schedule physician time to enable their engagement.
- Since the survey was initiated originally by primary care, it was challenging to engage the pharmacy and ancillary departments. Primary care response rates were higher as a result.

Launching the Survey

- Survey questions were confusing to some participants and required spending time on clarification.
- Participants needed much clarification on how to rate their RC with other roles when there was no interaction between those roles—they wanted a "not applicable" category in the survey to address those instances.
- Gathering e-mail addresses according to roles and monitoring e-mail bounces was challenging.
- For purposes of recording interventions, it would have been helpful to interview people while RC interventions were taking place rather than only afterward.

- Where leadership changes took place, we needed to provide more support and onboarding to the RC process. We needed a transition plan to bring new leaders up to speed on where the medical office building was relative to RC.

The Role of Leadership and Partnership

There was widespread agreement in this final reflection that leadership readiness had been critical to the success of the East Service Area's initiative. Several participants noted that relational coordination was a natural extension of Bailey's leadership style. According to Department Administrator Teeples:

> The way that [Bailey] brought RC to her leadership team was pivotal because she said, "Look, here's some amazing work, here's some information about it, and we're going to move forward with it." And I don't think without her support and guidance, letting people know that this is part of their work, I don't know that as many people would have glommed onto it as quickly as they did. They would have been like "I need some of that, give me some of that...." Her credibility is probably what surged it along.

Assistant department manager Hannah Austin agreed:

> It came at a good time, because when Gena first came to our region we started to do these "culture clouds." We asked, "What is our current culture?" and we drew the responses as a cloud on the whiteboard and then asked, "What do you want our culture to be?" And then we rolled out RC. So it was a really nice progression of changing culture in the region.

Regional vice president Wendy Watson pointed to the role of leadership as well:

> Capitalizing on the opportunity requires leadership that accepts the opportunity to be boundaryless and to focus on improving the care continuum versus departmental performance. And when you provide the leaders who are passionate about moving in that direction with a great tool like relational coordination, you have the ability to truly transform our culture and deliver even greater value for our members.

The East Service Area leaders also concluded in their final reflection that partnership with labor, management, and physicians was needed in order to use relational coordination effectively for performance improvement. In future work at Kaiser Permanente, readiness criteria for the relational coordination approach would therefore include management leadership, labor leadership, and physician leadership, as well as partnership among them. As department administrator Trevor Franklin explained: "I've been with KP for 12 or 13 years now and I think this is probably the best tool … that I've participated in. But I really think it takes a big group to move this, it's not just one person."

Leaders also noted the investment of time required to continually round with staff, provide reinforcement, and maintain enthusiasm and focus. The "operational champion" role fulfilled by department administrator Teeples in the East Service Area was estimated at about 20% FTE over the course of the year. Sustainability would also be a concern moving forward. Mark Harvey, the physician leader who had moved past initial skepticism to become supportive of relational coordination, wondered how they would sustain the culture of relational coordination that had developed in the East Service Area: "It is a concern, especially with turnover of staff. If it doesn't get ingrained into the culture, it may need to be repeated at intervals."

While the feedback of relational coordination data had helped participants identify opportunities for improvement, it was likely the successful execution of interventions that would determine sustained levels of improvement.

CONCLUSION

In this chapter, we analyzed a single case study in depth to explore how intentional efforts to change culture and build coordination across work groups can succeed in the midst of multiple organizational initiatives, and how change agents—formal leaders, co-workers, and clinicians—organize to enact these changes. We saw how change agents were able to address skepticism by (1) emphasizing the evidence base for the new initiative and (2) sharing with participants that the new initiative was not about *more work* but rather about improving the *way work was done* through better communication and understanding of each other's work.

We observed change agents organizing to form high-quality relationships across boundaries that were previously barriers to performance, using relational, work process, and structural interventions. *Relational interventions* included the measurement and sharing of baseline relational coordination data with participants, using these data in effect as a boundary object to create a common understanding across work groups to increase understanding of each other's work or alignment with each other's goals (Carlile 2004).

Relational interventions were paired with *work process interventions* to embed the new relationships into the work itself using the organization's existing PDSA methodology. These efforts were supported by *structural interventions*, including new structures such as living-room huddles and relational coordination summits, as well as existing structures such as job shadowing, unit-based teams, and care councils. These relational, work process, and structural interventions are key components of the relational model of organizational change (Figure 4).

In this case, we observed change agents engaging in relational interventions to improve relationships directly, while using new and existing structures to support these relationships. Our case study thus contributes to relational/structural theories of organizational change that feature dynamic iterations between relational and structural interventions (e.g., Barley and Tolbert 1997; Feldman 2003; Fletcher, Bailyn, and Blake-Beard 2009; Gittell 2016; Kellogg 2009; Kellogg, Orlikowski, and Yates 2006; Orlikowski and Yates 1994; Perlow, Gittell, and Katz 2004), moving beyond linear models in which structures shape relationships in a one-way causal flow (e.g., Gittell and Douglass 2012; Gittell, Seidner, and Wimbush 2010).

More generally, this case study provides insight into the complex process of intentional change for organizations that are facing pressures for performance, with multiple stakeholders at multiple levels who must be engaged in order to succeed.

FIGURE 4
Relational Model of Organizational Change

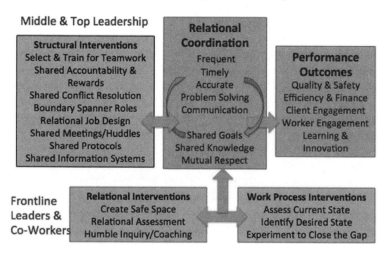

Source: Gittell 2016.

ACKNOWLEDGMENTS
We acknowledge the help of colleagues who made this study possible:

Alma Anaya, Administrative Assistant, Primary Care

Geri Auerbach, RN, Assistant Department Administrator, Primary Care

Hannah Austin, Assistant Department Administrator, Primary Care

Gena Bailey, Senior Administrator, East Service Area, Primary Care

Barbara Belk, PhD, Director, Learning and Organizational Development

Laura Billingsley, Medical Assistant, Primary Care

Karen Carter, RPh, Senior Administrator, Team-Based Care, Primary Care

Shannon Covington, Assistant Department Administrator, Primary Care

Paula Edwards, RN, Assistant Department Administrator, Primary Care

Ruth-Ann Erickson, RN, Nurse Team Lead, Primary Care

Brenton Farner, Assistant Department Administrator, Primary Care

Christina Fawcett, RN, Assistant Department Administrator, Primary Care

Trevor Franklin, Department Administrator, Primary Care

Jonathan Froeber, Assistant Department Administrator, Primary Care

Kathryn Glassberg, MD, Clinic Physician Lead, Primary Care

Ellie Godfrey, Former Vice President, Quality and Service

Mynell Harper, RN, Assistant Department Administrator, Primary Care

Mark Harvey, MD, Physician Leader, East Service Area, Primary Care

Jennifer Houten, RN, Director of Professional Practice

Marianne Bunce-Houston, RN, Consultant, Nursing Professional Development

Terri Imbach, RN, Assistant Department Administrator, Primary Care

Cindy Kirk, Supervisor, Business Office

Isha Leinow, Senior Consultant, Organizational Effectiveness

Sirena Long, Assistant Department Administrator, Primary Care

Mandi Marchek, Department Administrator, Primary Care

Maribeth Markeson, Assistant Department Administrator, Primary Care

Saleema Moore, PhD, Acting Chief Executive Officer, Relational Coordination Analytics

Sara Perkins, RN, Assistant Department Administrator, Primary Care

Barb Puckett, Lead Medical Assistant

Rahul Rastogi, MD, Chief Operating Officer

Joan Resnick, Senior Consultant, Organizational Effectiveness

Dylan Ross, PhD, Senior Manager, Integrated Behavioral Health Quality

Kurt Shusterich, Senior Consultant, Organizational Effectiveness

Michelle Teeples, Assistant Department Administrator, Primary Care

Eliana Temkin, Senior Consultant, Organizational Effectiveness

Nancy Louie Lee, RPh, Senior Director, Quality, Prevention, and Population Health

Wendy Watson, Executive Director, Ambulatory Care

Kate Willis, Senior Consultant, Organizational Effectiveness

Kara Wills, RN, Department Administrator, Primary Care

James Wood, MD, Associate Medical Director of Quality, Risk, Patient Safety and Peer Review

Leslie Mathies, Administrative Assistant, Learning and Organizational Effectiveness

William Weichmann, Vice President, Regional Counsel, Legal Department Northwest Region

Catherine Hernandez, Vice President, Brand Strategy

REFERENCES

Barley, S. R., and P. S. Tolbert. 1997. "Institutionalization and Structuration: Studying the Links Between Action and Institution." *Organization Studies* 18, no. 1: 93–117. doi:10.1177/017084069701800106.

Bitton, A., C. Martin, and B. E. Landon. 2010. "A Nationwide Survey of Patient Centered Medical Home Demonstration Projects." *Journal of General Internal Medicine* 25, no. 6: 584–92. doi:10.1007/s11606-010-1262-8.

Carlile, P. R. 2004. "Transferring, Translating, and Transforming: An Integrative Framework for Managing Knowledge Across Boundaries." *Organization Science* 15, no. 5: 555–68. doi:10.1287/orsc.1040.0094.

Feldman, M. S. 2003. "A Performative Perspective on Stability and Change in Organizational Routines." *Industrial and Corporate Change* 12, no. 4: 727–52. doi:10.1093/icc/12.4.727.

Fletcher, J. K., L. Bailyn, and S. Blake-Beard. 2009. "Practical Pushing: Creating Discursive Space in Organizational Narratives." In *Critical Management Studies at Work: Negotiating Tensions Between Theory and Practice*, edited by J. W. Cox, 82–93. Cheltenham, UK: Edward Elgar.

Gittell, J. H. 2003. *The Southwest Airlines Way: Using the Power of Relationships to Achieve High Performance.* New York, NY: McGraw-Hill.

Gittell, J. H. 2009. *High Performance Healthcare: Using the Power of Relationships to Achieve Quality, Efficiency and Resilience.* New York, NY: McGraw-Hill.

Gittell, J. H. 2016. *Transforming Relationships for High Performance: The Power of Relational Coordination.* Palo Alto, CA: Stanford University Press.

Gittell, J. H., and A. Douglass. 2012. "Relational Bureaucracy: Structuring Reciprocal Relationships into Roles." *Academy of Management Review* 37, no. 4: 709–33. doi:10.5465/amr.2010.0438.

Gittell, J. H., R. Seidner, and J. Wimbush. 2010. "A Relational Model of How High-Performance Work Systems Work." *Organization Science* 21, no. 2: 490–506. doi:10.1287/orsc.1090.0446.

Gittell, J. H., et al. 2000. "Impact of Relational Coordination on Quality of Care, Postoperative Pain and Functioning, and Length of Stay." *Medical Care* 38, no. 8: 807–19. doi:10.1097/00005650-200008000-00005.

Kellogg, K. C. 2009. "Operating Room: Relational Spaces and Microinstitutional Change in Surgery." *American Journal of Sociology* 115, no. 3: 657–711. doi:10.1086/603535.

Kellogg, K. C., W. J. Orlikowski, and J. Yates. 2006. "Life in the Trading Zone: Structuring Coordination Across Boundaries in Postbureaucratic Organizations." *Organization Science* 17 (1): 22–44. doi:10.1287/orsc.1050.0157.

Kochan, T. A., A. E. Eaton, R. B. McKersie, and P. S. Adler. 2009. *Healing Together: The Labor Management Partnership at Kaiser Permanente.* Ithaca, NY: ILR Press.

Orlikowski, W. J., and J. Yates. 1994. "Genre Repertoire: The Structuring of Communicative Practices in Organizations." *Administrative Science Quarterly* 39, no. 4: 541. doi:10.2307/2393771.

Perlow, L. A., J. H. Gittell, and N. Katz. 2004. "Contextualizing Patterns of Work Group Interaction: Toward a Nested Theory of Structuration." *Organization Science* 15, no. 5: 520–36. doi:10.1287/orsc.1040.0097.

CHAPTER 11

Impact of Electronic Health Records on Hospital Patient Satisfaction: What Is the Influence of Organizational Characteristics?

EDMUND R. BECKER

Department of Health Policy and Management
Rollins School of Public Health at Emory University

JAEYONG BAE

School of Health Studies
Northern Illinois University

INTRODUCTION

With recent regulatory changes in health care legislation, health information technology (HIT) is becoming essential in hospitals with the potential that it will reduce costs, eliminate waste, and improve the quality of care in the U.S. health care system (Blum 2011). In the health care industry, electronic health records (EHRs) specifically have been touted as improving quality and outcomes of health care by innovating the process of health care delivery (Chaudhry et al. 2006).

The improvements through EHRs come about by (1) providing clinicians timely and appropriate patient information, (2) enhancing care coordination, (3) increasing physician compliance to care guidelines, (4) facilitating clinical monitoring from large-scale screening and aggregation of data, (5) improving clinical workflow, (6) improving communication between clinicians and patients as well as among clinicians, and (7) decreasing medication errors (Appari, Johnson, and Anthony 2013; Bates and Gawande 2003; Chaudhry et al. 2006; Hillestad et al. 2005a; Quinn et al. 2012).

Nevertheless, despite these potential benefits, the overall rate of EHR adoption by U.S. hospitals has initially been quite slow, and the evidence of its performance benefits is unclear (Agarwal, Gao, DesRoches, and Jha 2010). EHRs that transmit information across care settings could facilitate speedy transmission of accurate and timely clinical data, especially where these EHR systems are integrated and fully implemented (Campbell et al. 2008; Cherouny, Haraden, Leavitt Gullo, and Resar 2005; Eden et al. 2008; McCartney 2006). Nevertheless, by 2008, only 11% of general acute-care hospitals had adopted a basic EHR system (Jha et al. 2009).

There are substantial barriers that interfere with implementing and using EHRs effectively to achieve improved quality and outcomes in health care. Among those barriers is the high acquisition and implementation cost of an EHR system (DesRoches et al. 2008; Hersh 2004; Hillestad et al. 2005b; Jha et al. 2009; Simon, Rundall, and Shortell 2005). Researchers have estimated that a fully wired National Health Information Network would cost $156 billion, but HIT could save $81 billion to $162 billion annually while reducing morbidity and mortality (Hillestad et al. 2005a; Kaushal et al. 2005; Taylor et al. 2005).

In addition to the financial burdens, lack of compatibility between various EHR components is another common barrier thought to impact the implementation of EHRs and their effective use (Hillestad et al. 2005b; Hersh 2004). Connectivity—the ability to share information from system to system—is poor. Although HIT implementation is growing, there is little sharing of health information between existing systems. There has also been little market pressure to develop HIT systems that are integrated and can communicate with each other. This piecemeal implementation approach may actually create additional barriers to the development of a viable HIT system because of the high costs of replacing or converting today's nonstandard systems.

Ominously, a study funded by the Robert Wood Johnson Foundation (RWJF) also cautions that while hospitals may be quick at adopting EHRs, they have not yet figured out how to use the new technology to improve patient safety and reduce health care costs. For example, the RWJF study found while 42% of hospitals now meet federal standards for one of the components—collecting electronic health data—only 5% also meet federal standards for exchanging that data with other providers to allow widespread physician access to a patient's records (DesRoches, Painter, and Jha 2013). Consequently, it is likely to take time for organizations to make the applicable adjustments and learning about HIT to fully demonstrate their effectiveness (Borzekowski 2009; Devaraj and Kohli 2000; Frisse et al. 2012; Garrido et al. 2005; Javitt, Rebitzer, and Reisman 2008).

Some of these barriers have become even more challenging for hospitals in the current environment as national health care regulations, implemented in 2009 and 2011, were designed to align financial incentives for EHR adoption in the nation's hospitals and improve patient value in their hospital experience (VanLare and Conway 2012). The emphasis on patient value and patient experience is an epic shift in the nation's health care paradigm because it moves the current payment paradigm away from a supply side–driven health care to paying for patient-centered health care services based on their value to the patient and the patient's experience with these services.

The impact of the adoption and use of information technology (IT) is of keen interest to organizational researchers and health policy investigators for a number of reasons. First, the dramatic shift in the payment paradigm in the hospital industry underscores the importance of questions about the influence of hospital structures and processes on patient satisfaction. Questions linking health care provider EHR responses to these initiatives in different markets with variations among hospitals' organizational characteristics provides a unique opportunity to test and evaluate specific organizational tenets that link organizational innovation and patient objectives. To date, very little empirical research has investigated the relationships between EHR implementation and hospital organizational characteristics and their influence on patient satisfaction under the new payment paradigm.

Second, substantial gains are seen for the nation's inpatients through EHR implementation. Related to both efficiency and effectiveness, increased patient value will be generated by the hospital's EHR adaptation and associated innovation because it will have a strong influence on the delivery process and enhance the actual service being delivered. EHRs will automate standard health procedures and routines and improve their outcomes, thereby leading to improved productivity. EHRs also help manage complexity and reduce uncertainty, and they allow more widespread sharing of critical information among health care professionals and patients. HIT permits hospitals to consider different—even conflicting outcomes—simultaneously. Hence, the dilemmas that face most hospital choices can be better anticipated, managed, and balanced through the use of EHRs.

Finally, organizational researchers have noted that innovation research has been dominated by two types of empirical studies: (1) cross-sectional studies aimed at identifying contextual, organizational, and individual predictors of innovativeness, which they argue are seen almost universally as the necessary characteristic of organizations, and (2) longitudinal event history studies aimed at predicting diffusion rates for specific innovations across organizational populations as a function of community, population, and organizational level variables (Drazin and Schoonhoven 1996). These researchers note that both approaches use coarse predictors to summarize the complexity of organizational processes thought to be relevant to innovation and outcomes. Some researchers have criticized this type of research for its lack of attention to the organizational processes by which individual innovations penetrate the organization. These researchers argue that traditional variance studies are weak because they jumble together a wide variety of innovations and eclectic organizational samples that are unlikely to produce cumulative knowledge or useful generalizations. Our research methodology seeks to address these concerns.

In this investigation, we sought to fill this void in two ways. Using data from approximately 1,200 short-term general hospitals (one fourth of the nation's acute-care hospitals, which typically have patient stays less than 30 days and, thus, similar patient care objectives), we first evaluate three years of variation in ten measures of patient satisfaction in relation to the presence of EHRs while controlling for relevant hospital characteristics, including environmental, structure, and process measures.

Building on organizational theory and research, the first phase of our analysis used variations in the extent of the implementation of EHRs in these acute-care hospitals (full implementation, partial implementation, and no EHR systems) to evaluate the influence of these differences on the variation in patients' hospital care experience. In the second phase of our investigation, we interacted these three levels of EHR implementation with four dimensions of the hospital's organizational milieu—their market (competitive, moderately competitive, or monopoly), ownership (government, for profit, or nongovernment, nonprofit), bedsize (<100, 100–249, 250–399, or 400+), and extent of health system membership (none, independent, decentralized, moderately centralized, or centralized).

To our knowledge, there are no comprehensive investigations that have evaluated patient satisfaction and organizational characteristics in the context of the variations in their EHR implementation while controlling for major dimensions of hospital services, including cost and quality.

BACKGROUND

Given the barriers to HIT adoption by hospitals discussed in our introduction, there were two recent major legislative efforts to incentivize hospitals to implement EHR systems in their hospitals. The Health Information Technology for Economic and Clinical Health (HITECH) Act, legislated as part of the American Recovery and Reinvestment Act of 2009, was signed into law in 2009 to promote the adoption and meaningful use of health information technology in the nation's health system. As part of the HITECH Act, there were strong incentive payments beginning in 2011 for eligible hospitals that adopt a certified EHR system and were meaningful users of certified EHR technology.

Coupled with the HITECH Act, the financial pressure on the nation's acute-care hospitals was intensified a year later with the passage of the Patient Protection and Affordable Care Act of 2010 (ACA) legislation (also commonly referred to as Obamacare), which was designed to improve patient quality and potentially lower costs. With the ACA legislation, the Medicare payment methodology for the nation's hospitals, referred to as value-based purchasing (VBP), shifted the current payment paradigm away from a supply side–driven health care system based on established provider arrangements to paying for patient-centered health care services based on a patient's needs and the value of those services to the patient.

To translate this shift from provider-centered to patient-centered care, the new Medicare VBP legislation links hospital payment levels, in part, to the hospital's scores on measures of clinical quality and patient satisfaction by rewarding quality health care providers through payment incentives and transparency regarding performance. Under this program, up to $30 billion in financial incentives were available to promote "meaningful use" of EHR over ten years (Buntin, Jain, and Blumenthal 2010). As of December 2014, more than 80% (4,740) of U.S. hospitals had received a total of $17.4 billion through the Centers for Medicare and Medicaid Services' (CMS) EHR incentive program (Centers for Medicare and Medicaid Services 2014).

Since its implementation, the incentive program has increased EHR adoption by hospitals. Between 2008 and 2012, the adoption rate of basic EHRs among general acute hospitals increased from 9% to 44% (DesRoches, Painter, and Jha 2013; Jha et al. 2009). The number of hospitals with a basic EHR system tripled from 2010 to 2012, with more than four of every ten hospitals now equipped with the new health information technology (Adler-Milstein and Jha 2012). The report also underscored that EHR adoption has increased throughout the American health care system. It's not just big hospitals in major metropolitan centers that are purchasing the new technology. The number of rural hospitals with an EHR system increased from about 10% to 33.5% between 2010 and 2012, while urban hospitals saw EHR adoption rates rise from 17% to nearly 48%.

Growing Emphasis on Patient-Centered Hospital Experience

Coinciding with the growing emphasis on health IT is the value of the patient's hospital experience, which is now embedded in national health care policy. In effect, with the passage of the 2010 ACA, most of the nation's acute Medicare hospitals are now competing against each other based, in part, on the value of the patient's assessment of their services (Goodrich, Garcia, and Conway 2012; VanLare and Conway 2012).

Starting on October 1, 2012, the CMS Hospital Readmissions Reduction Program (HRRP) reduced Medicare payments to all acute-care hospitals by 1% to create a funding pool of approximately $1 billion for incentive payments to U.S. hospitals. This pool was then used to distribute incentive payments to hospitals based on their patient performance scores linked to their clinical processes and patient satisfaction; this process will continue each year (Rau 2013). The following October, the CMS HRRP increased its penalty on excess hospital readmissions for low-performing hospitals from 1% to 2% of their total hospital Medicare reimbursement.

Consequently, in 2015, in the fourth year of this penalty, the majority of the nation's acute-care hospitals (2,592 hospitals) were penalized by Medicare for having patients return too quickly, within a month of discharge, losing a combined $420 million (Rau 2015).

Significantly, the HRRP program is just one part of the federal government's efforts to shift hospitals and providers toward VBPs. Coupled with the VBP program and the more recently introduced Hospital-Acquired Condition Reduction (HACR) program, most of the nation's acute-care hospitals became eligible in fiscal year 2015 to be penalized by all three programs, with Medicare hospital reimbursement rates to a specific hospital potentially cut by up to 5.5% (Figueroa, Wang, and Jha 2016).

THEORETICAL FRAMEWORK

Information technology is recognized by many researchers as process innovation that has improved productivity and efficiency across a variety of service industries (Brynjolfsson and Hitt 2003; Davenport 1993; Stiroh 2002). Here, process innovation means the implementation of a new or significantly improved production or delivery method, including significant changes in techniques, equipment, and/or software.

Our study built on the IT process–enabling innovation framework developed by Thomas Davenport (1993), which asserts that IT improves the productivity and performance of organizations through process improvement and innovations. We view the EHR system as a tool to innovate and improve processes of health care delivery to the patient, consistent with previous health IT studies by Dranove, Forman, Goldfarb, and Greenstein (2012) and McCullough, Parente, and Town (2013).

The process by which patient satisfaction is influenced by HIT is the service delivery triad model. Cowing, Davino-Ramaya, Ramaya, and Szmerikovsky (2009) tailored the triad to the health care delivery setting based on earlier work by Glickman and colleagues' (2007) adoption of the Donabedian (2005) health services delivery model, which links structure, process, and outcomes.

The idea that the way employees are managed and the way work is structured impacts organizational performance and client satisfaction is the foundation of human resource management. Researchers have documented that certain sets of human resource practices improve employee effectiveness and predict higher levels of organizational performance on efficiency outcomes (Arthur 1994; Bartel 1994, 2004; Collins and Smith 2006; Delery and Doty 1996; Gittell, Seidner, and Wimbush 2010; Huselid 1995; Ichniowski et al. 1996) and that differences in human resource practices can explain differences across many but not all settings (Batt 1999; Cappelli and Neumark 2004; Collins and Clark 2003; Gittell, Seidner, and Wimbush 2010; Ichniowski et al. 1996; Richard and Johnson 2004).

In the hospital setting, a wide variety of characteristics (Figure 1), which the patient may or may not be aware of, have a direct impact on the patient's experience. An extensive literature exists on factors relating to the hospital's environment, structure, and processes, all of which have been shown to significantly impact patient satisfaction (Cleary and McNeil 1988; Jha, Orav, Zheng, and Epstein 2008; Vahey et al. 2004; Young,

FIGURE 1

Conceptual Framework and Major Hospital Variables

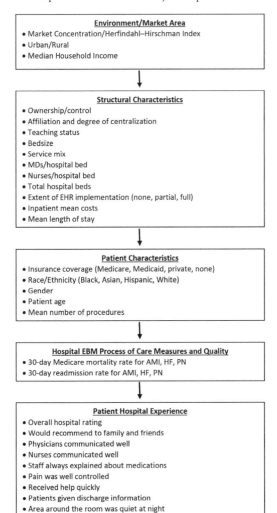

Environment/Market Area
- Market Concentration/Herfindahl–Hirschman Index
- Urban/Rural
- Median Household Income

Structural Characteristics
- Ownership/control
- Affiliation and degree of centralization
- Teaching status
- Bedsize
- Service mix
- MDs/hospital bed
- Nurses/hospital bed
- Total hospital beds
- Extent of EHR implementation (none, partial, full)
- Inpatient mean costs
- Mean length of stay

Patient Characteristics
- Insurance coverage (Medicare, Medicaid, private, none)
- Race/Ethnicity (Black, Asian, Hispanic, White)
- Gender
- Patient age
- Mean number of procedures

Hospital EBM Process of Care Measures and Quality
- 30-day Medicare mortality rate for AMI, HF, PN
- 30-day readmission rate for AMI, HF, PN

Patient Hospital Experience
- Overall hospital rating
- Would recommend to family and friends
- Physicians communicated well
- Nurses communicated well
- Staff always explained about medications
- Pain was well controlled
- Received help quickly
- Patients given discharge information
- Area around the room was quiet at night
- Rooms and bathrooms were clean

Meterko, and Desai 2000). A health care organization influences patient satisfaction indirectly through its relationship with its staff, which affects such characteristics as communication, culture, incentives, pressures, scheduling, and training. In this model, health care organizations employ clinicians (doctors, nurses, etc.), who are the hospital's front-line team for dealing with the patients' medical conditions, and make available to those clinicians the resources, such as EHRs, that serve to achieve the hospital's varied and competing goals—which are typically described as encompassing various degrees of clinical service, teaching, and research.

This direct contact and service to the patient means that the relationship between the clinical staff and the patient is key, and that essential aspects of the relationship—which are built on effective communication, competent service, and advocacy for the patient—will have important consequences for patient satisfaction. Health IT and, specifically, the extent of EHR implementation in the hospital, therefore, is expected to have a direct impact on the success of hospital providers and staff to provide proper services to patients and understand their needs.

Timely updates and reminders about the patient's medications and discharge protocols, along with relevant clinical and nonclinical information about the patient, can be coordinated through the EHR and, with a well-functioning EHR system, be effortlessly created and disseminated to patients. Health IT has the capacity to positively enhance the clinician–patient relationship, and we would expect major differences among the arrangements of EHR systems in a hospital to be a critical dimension of this relationship and one that will impact patient satisfaction.

Accordingly, we argue that HIT is expected to have a positive impact on organizational performance and organizations, with higher levels of HIT implementation producing better outcomes on performance measures than organizations with lower levels of HIT implementation. More specifically, we hypothesize that, *ceteris paribus*,

- H1: Hospitals with HIT systems will have higher levels of patient satisfaction than hospitals without such systems.
- H2: Hospitals with fully implemented HIT systems will have higher levels of patient satisfaction than hospitals with only partially implemented HIT systems.

Degree of EHR Implementation and Organizational Characteristics

Yet, as we noted previously, a health care organization influences patient satisfaction in complex ways through its relationship with staff and allocation of resources, which affect communication, culture, incentives, pressures, scheduling, training and, ultimately, the quality of care and level of service its patients receive. How do the potential advantages of

EHR systems impact patient satisfaction across variations in a hospital's environment and structure?

In the second part of our investigation, we sought to address this question by evaluating three levels of EHR implementation and interacting them with four dimensions of the hospital's organizational characteristics. To our knowledge, the importance of variations in the extent of implementation of EHRs in hospitals, coupled with these four organizational characteristics, has never been systematically examined (Chukmaitov et al. 2009).

Hospital Market

There has been a growing trend in hospital market consolidation for several decades, especially in rural areas (Luke, Ozcan, and Olden 1995). A more up-to-date study evaluating hospitals, market structure, and consolidation noted that, because of the incentives in the ACA and the declining use of inpatient services, there has been a significant increase in consolidation in the hospital industry in recent years. What was once a set of independent hospitals having limited relationships with physicians and clinicians who provided health services has become increasingly consolidated into a small number of locally integrated health systems, typically arranged around a large academic medical center (Cutler and Morton 2013).

An extensive empirical literature exists that examines the effects of hospital competition on the cost, access, patient satisfaction, and quality of hospital services. These studies typically find statistically significant effects (Federal Trade Commission and U.S. Department of Justice 2004; Gaynor and Town 2011; Pautler and Vita 1994). For example, several studies have examined the relationships between competition and quality of health care (Chassin 1997; Enthoven 1993; Kassirer 1995; Zwanziger and Melnick 1996); between competition and health care system costs (Robinson and Luft 1985, 1987, 1988; Zwanziger and Melnick 1988, 1996); and between competition and patient satisfaction (Brook and Kosecoff 1988; Miller 1996).

Those studies showed that improved efficiency, access to care, and quality of care, in theory, may lower costs because the more care a hospital provides, the more efficient and less expensive it should become. These studies reinforce the theory that competition is capable of increasing value for customers over time. Quality enhancements and process improvements should lead to decreased costs, which in turn, should result in increased customer/patient satisfaction.

In contrast, consolidation results in hospitals having considerable market power. Here, market power is characterized as approaching a monopoly and denotes an organization's ability to raise and maintain price above the level that would prevail under competition. The exercise of market power has been found to actually lead to reduced output and loss of economic welfare (Creswell and Abelson 2013; Federal Trade Commission and U.S. Department of Justice 2004). In the health care market, higher levels of hospital consolidation increase the market power for those hospitals because it becomes more difficult for insurers to bargain successfully with a limited number of health systems. Health systems that are more consolidated have greater market power, and this market power gives them the potential to more successfully influence prices but also to dominate and organize care across different practitioners and sites of care (Gawande 2012). As a result, we hypothesize that

- H3: Hospitals in more-competitive markets with higher levels of EHR implementation will have higher scores on patient satisfaction measures than those in less-competitive markets and lower levels of EHR implementation.

Hospital Ownership

There is a variety of ownership patterns among U.S. acute-care hospitals. In 2014, of the 4,926 short-term, community hospitals in the United States (which typically serve acute-care patients with lengths of stay fewer than 30 days and that are not federal or specialty hospitals—such as psychiatric or long-term care hospitals), the majority were nonprofit (58.3%). State and local government hospitals controlled 20.3% of these short-term community hospitals, while for-profit hospitals owned 21.4% (American Hospital Association 2015).

For-profit hospitals may have a greater propensity to adopt HIT than nonprofit hospitals because for-profit hospitals tend to be more sensitive to operational costs and efficiencies and are more likely to view HIT as a means of improving efficiency and reducing costs (Boardman and Vining 1989; De Alessi 1996; Hikmet et al. 2008). However, such cost reductions also influence eventual profitability and can impact shareholder returns in for-profit hospitals; therefore, over the long-term, the extent of EHR adoption may be uncertain. Related to patient care, some researchers find that the differences in patient quality (with quality measured in terms of survival, changes in functional and cognitive status, and living arrangements) resulted in no differences in outcomes on the basis of hospital ownership (Sloan, Picone, Taylor, and Chou 2001). However, there is also considerable literature suggesting that factors other than profit influence government and voluntary hospitals. Those studies argue that patient outcomes and patient satisfaction concerns are typically poorly aligned with the profit motive (Becker and Potter 2002; Devereaux et al. 2002; Rushing 1974).

Consequently, given the promise of EHRs for improved costs and increased effectiveness, we might expect for-profit hospitals to have a higher share of EHR systems that are partially or fully implemented, but it is uncertain whether their ownership imperatives related to the profit motive will translate into higher patient satisfaction scores. Therefore, we speculate as follows:

- H4: Hospital ownership status will not influence the relationship between EHR and patient satisfaction.
- H5: Regardless of ownership status, hospitals with higher levels of EHR implementation will have better patient scores than hospitals with lower levels of EHR implementation.

Hospital Size

More than half of U.S. hospitals are relatively small—fewer than 100 beds—but, as previously noted, hospital markets are dominated by large systems. At the center of these large systems are large hospitals that typically average more than 500 beds.

The organizational literature has consistently identified size as one of the most important organizational characteristics predicting innovation adoption among organizations (Aldrich and Auster 1986; Kimberly and Evanisko 1981). Larger organizations typically adopt IT more quickly and extensively than smaller organizations. Larger organizations tend to have more financial resources that they can devote to implementing new technologies, and their size often necessitates IT solutions to improve their operations. Conversely, lacking financial resources, smaller organizations are typically forced to make difficult trade-offs in their investment choices and often forgo implementation of expensive technologies. Similarly, we generally expect that larger hospitals—because of their need for and access to superior resources—will adopt greater levels of HIT than smaller hospitals.

Nevertheless, it is not clear that the potential positive qualities of HIT will offset the consequences of hospital size. As hospitals get larger, they typically become increasingly complex and bureaucratic in all stages of clinical service, teaching, and research. While we still anticipate that HIT will have a positive impact on their outcomes, the intensifying pressures of size could be expected to ameliorate the HIT advantages. Consequently, we hypothesize the following:

- H6: The size of hospitals will have a negative impact on patient satisfaction.
- H7: In larger hospitals, higher levels of EHR implementation will ameliorate the negative influence of size.

Hospital System Membership

The growing consolidation of hospitals in markets has been paralleled by rapid growth in hospital system membership (Cutler and Scott Morton 2013). Recent evidence indicates that the typical U.S. region has three to five consolidated health systems that span a wide range of care settings and a smaller fringe of health care centers outside those systems. On average, the top three market share leaders in an area accounted for 77% of hospital admissions, and the top five hospitals or systems accounted for 88% of the market share (Cutler and Scott Morton 2013).

Hospitals that are part of a hospital system or network are more likely than an independent hospital to adopt HIT. The reason for this is, unlike independent hospitals, system or network-connected hospitals can greatly benefit from economies of scale and scope in HIT adoption initiatives because the costs, risks, and management of these new technologies are spread over a bigger base of hospitals (Katz and Shapiro 1986). A health system can implement a common centralized infrastructure (purchasing cooperatives, shared databases and database services, HIT technologies and personnel, etc.) and leverage learning from one hospital to another. Other administrative processes such as insurance billing and physician integration also tend to benefit from system membership because these processes can be standardized and supported from a central location (Carey 2003). Absent such affiliation, independent hospitals must bear the entire costs and risks of HIT adoption and are more likely to be slower adopting new and unproven HIT.

An important qualification among system membership in the hospital industry is the nature of a hospital's membership in its health care system. Hospitals are assigned to one of five categories (centralized, centralized physician/insurance, moderately centralized, decentralized, and independent) based on the degree that they differentiate and centralize their hospital services, physician arrangements, and provider-based insurance products (Bazzoli et al. 1999). In this taxonomy, differentiation refers to the number of different products or services that the organization offers. A health system is assigned to one of five categories based on how much they differentiate and centralize their hospital services, physician arrangements, and provider-based insurance products. Here, differentiation refers to the number of different products or services that the organization offers. The taxonomy is widely used in the health care literature and is formally part of the American Hospital Association's (AHA) annual survey database (Bazzoli et al. 1999).

The centralized versus decentralized distinction offers a unique opportunity to investigate the influence of the health system on hospital performance. We are not familiar with any research that has linked system membership with EHR adoption and use and patient satisfaction while controlling for other significant aspects of the hospital's structure. Speculatively, we therefore propose the following:

- H8: Hospitals affiliated with a system will be more likely than independent hospitals to implement EHR.

- H9: The association of EHR implementation with patient satisfaction will be moderated by the level of centralization of a hospital's system.
- H10: Patient satisfaction will be highest with fully implemented EHR in decentralized hospital systems where products can be differentiated in accordance with local supply and demand factors.

DATABASE CONSTRUCTION, VARIABLES, AND METHODS

Our hospital database merged data from a number of sources. First, the core of the database was the inpatient satisfaction data from the Hospital Quality Alliance (HQA) collaboration. HQA is a public and private partnership that includes CMS and the Joint Commission and is leading the effort in the hospital sector to monitor and report on hospital quality from the patient's perspective. Referred to as the Hospital Consumer Assessment of Healthcare Providers and Hospital System Survey (HCAHPS), it is the first publicly available, standardized survey designed to gather information from adult inpatients about the degree of their inpatient centered care experiences. The U.S. Department of Health and Human Services, on the website Hospital Compare, currently reports hospital performance data collected from the over 4,000 participating hospitals on more than 2.1 million completed surveys. On average, every day more than 8,400 patients complete HCAHPS surveys (Centers for Medicare and Medicaid Services 2015).

The HCAHPS is administered to a random sample of patients 18 years old or older after an inpatient stay of at least one night for medical, surgical, or maternity care. Estimates indicate that 85% of inpatients at participating U.S. hospitals are eligible (Elliott et al. 2010). The number of hospitals that collected data qualifying them for public reporting of their survey scores for public reporting in March 2009 accounted for 97% of eligible inpatient stays (Elliott et al. 2010). The specific measures of the patient's hospital experience are noted below.

To augment the HCAHPS, we added data on the hospital's market area, structure, processes, and outcomes from a variety of data sources. The first, the Healthcare Cost and Utilization Project (HCUP), is a family of health care databases developed by the Agency for Healthcare Research and Quality (AHRQ) (Agency for Healthcare Quality and Research, "Healthcare Cost," no date). The HCUP State Inpatient Databases (HCUP-SIDs) (Agency for Healthcare Quality and Research, "SID Database," no date), a 100% discharge abstract data system, contains more than 100 clinical and nonclinical variables such as principal and secondary diagnoses, principal and secondary procedures, admission and discharge status, patient demographics (gender, age, and, for some states, race), expected payment source (Medicare, Medicaid, private insurance, self-pay), total charges, and length of stay.

Additional data come from the 2009 and 2010 AHA annual survey of hospitals, which contains more than 700 fields of data for over 6,000 hospitals representing 98% of all short-term general acute-care hospitals in the United States (American Hospital Association, "AHA Annual Survey Database," no date) and includes demographic information, organizational structure, facilities and services, utilization data, community orientation indicators, physician arrangements, managed care relationships, expenses, and staffing.

Another set of data came from the 2007 and 2011 AHA Electronic Health Record Database (American Hospital Association, "AHA Annual Survey IT Database," no date). These databases report data on the 2006 and 2009 EHR implementation statuses of the nation's hospitals and have data that illustrate the depth and level of technology integration.

Finally, we used a nonhospital source, the Area Health Resource File (AHRF), containing more than 6,000 variables for each of the nation's counties and available from the Health Resources and Services Administration (HRSA) to link data on health facilities, health professions, measures of resource scarcity, population health status, area economic activity, health training programs, and socioeconomic and environmental characteristics of the hospitals' county (Health Resources and Services Administration 2016).

Our unit of analysis was the hospital, and our resulting database represented approximately 25% of all hospitals nationally and 33% of inpatient discharges in 2009.

VARIABLE CONSTRUCTION

Dependent Variables

The ten measures of the patient's hospital experience collected in the HCAHPS survey were linked to each hospital: (1) patient's overall rating of the hospital, (2) willingness to recommend the hospital to family and friends, (3) communication with doctors, (4) communication with nurses, (5) responsiveness of hospital staff, (6) pain management, (7) communication about medicines, (8) discharge information, (9) cleanliness of the hospital environment, and (10) quietness of the hospital environment (Hospital Consumer Assessment of Healthcare Providers and Systems 2015).

Independent Variables

The key explanatory variable in our study was the extent of EHR implementation. An EHR, as defined by the AHA, integrates electronically originated and maintained patient-level clinical health information, derived from multiple sources, into one point of access. The AHA EHR data note the presence or absence of 32 clinical functionalities of an electronic record system and whether the hospital (1) had fully implemented these functionalities in all major clinical units, (2) had implemented them in one or more (but not all) major clinical units, or (3) had not begun implementation of an EHR. In our study, EHR was a dummy variable representing three different levels of EHR adoption: (1) no EHR, (2) partially implemented EHR, and (3) fully implemented EHR, with no EHR as the excluded dummy variable.

Market Structure and Concentration

We used three measures to capture hospital area characteristics. First, the Herfindahl–Hirschman Index (HHI) was used as a measure of market concentration, where the HHI was calculated as the sum of the squared market shares for all hospitals in the local market. Here, markets were defined by hospital referral regions (HRRs) that represent regional health care markets for tertiary medical care (Dartmouth Atlas of Health Care, no date). To define the nature of the hospital's market structure, we used the U.S. Department of Justice's definitions of competitive (HHI < 1,000), moderately competitive (HHI 1,000 to 1,800), and a highly concentrated marketplace (HHI > 1,800) (U.S. Department of Justice and Federal Trade Commission 2010).

Next, urban/rural was used as an area indicator reflecting population density and travel implications for patients. Finally, median population income level provided an indicator, consistent with the competitive market model of how "attractive" the patient population might be. Where hospital areas overlap several counties, we used the ZIP codes to weight median income by the population totals for the overlapping areas.

Hospital Structural Characteristics

Our definitions of ownership/control for short-term community hospitals were consistent with AHA definitions: (1) for-profit, private' (2) nonprofit, nongovernment; and (3) government controlled (American Hospital Association 2015).

Hospital teaching status was drawn from AHA data and described by three binary variables: (1) hospitals with at least one approved residency program but no medical school affiliation, (2) hospitals with a medical school but not a member of the Council of Teaching Hospitals, and (3) hospitals that are members of the Council of Teaching Hospitals. This construction expresses teaching in terms of the level of teaching commitment and has been used extensively and effectively in past research (Becker and Potter 2002; Becker and Sloan 1983, 1985).

Number of beds in a hospital (aka bedsize) is a continuous variable we used to capture differences in hospital scale and the importance and complexity that comes with size (Becker and Sloan 1983, 1985).

Hospital staffing may be critical to different aspects of patient satisfaction, and we included two measures of potential provider availability and accessibility for each hospital: (1) full-time equivalent (FTE) physician per hospital bed, and (2) FTE nurses per hospital bed.

Although most patients have some degree of insurance coverage, the cost of the hospitalization and the length of stay (LOS) may also influence patient satisfaction. To test for this effect, we included mean hospital costs per stay and the mean LOS after controlling for patient insurance status. The inpatient mean costs for each patient was calculated from hospital charges adjusted with the hospital's cost-charge ratio to develop an average cost (Healthcare Cost and Utilization Project 2016).

A number of variables were used to capture inpatient characteristics at the hospital level. Male and female inpatients were distinguished with the ratio of female inpatients included in the regression. Mean patient age was a continuous variable taken from the HCUP-SID files. The mean number of procedures per patient represented important information about the potential severity of the inpatient admission and the "case mix" of the hospital. The ratio of patients who were insured by Medicare, Medicaid, private/HMO insurance, self-pay, no insurance, or other insurers (e.g., workers compensation, CHAMPUS, and other government payers) provided another measure of patient mix and the potential financial health of the hospital. Five racial/ethnicity distinctions were included in percentage terms: (1) white, (2) black, (3) Hispanic, (4) Asian or Pacific Islander, (5) other races/ethnicities (Becker 2007; Becker and Rahimi 2006).

The quality of care at a hospital is likely to have an important impact on patient satisfaction and needs to be controlled. We included six measures to capture dimensions of the care quality delivered at the nation's acute-care hospitals. The inpatient 30-day Medicare mortality rates for acute myocardial infarction (AMI; heart attacks), heart failure (HF), and pneumonia (PN) were included, as well as the 30-day readmission rates for AMI, HF, and PN.

We included the five measures of system membership (centralized health system, centralized physician/insurance health system, moderately centralized health system, decentralized health system, and independent hospital system) developed by Bazzoli and colleagues, as previously described in this chapter (Bazzoli et al. 1999).

METHODS

Descriptive and multivariate regression results are reported. Multivariate regressions take two forms. Initially, consistent with our model in Figure 1, we estimated the impact of all environmental, structural, and process variables on the ten patient satisfaction measures shown in Table 1* using partial and fully implemented EHR dummy variables in the regression (using hospitals with no EHRs as the reference category) to assess the overall impact of EHRs on each patient satisfaction measure.

Next, we interacted the three levels of EHR implementation with each dimension of the hospital's organizational milieu—its market (competitive, moderately competitive, or monopoly), ownership (government; for-profit; or nongovernment, nonprofit), bedsize (<100, 100–249, 250–399, or 400+), and extent of health system membership (none, independent, decentralized, moderately centralized, or centralized). Each of these interaction variables were included in the regression. To be judicious with space, only the significant regression results for these interacted variables are reported in Table 2.

RESULTS

Descriptive Results

Table 3 reports means and standard deviations for dependent and independent variables in our study (other statistical characteristics—medians, minimums, and maximums—were sometimes reported but are not shown in the table).

For the ten patient satisfaction scores, hospitals ranged from a high of 81.4% for the satisfaction measure "patients were given info about what to do during their recovery at home" to a low of 53% for the "area around the hospital always kept quiet at night." For the overall satisfaction measures—"patient overall rating of the hospital is high" and "patient would definitely recommend hospital to family and friends," about two thirds of patients in our sample hospitals reported that they were highly satisfied or would definitely recommend—64.8% and 68%, respectively. Both measures showed a maximum of 94% for those two measures, while the minimums were 41% and 36.2%, respectively.

Staffing satisfaction for hospital patients progressively declined for physicians, nurses, and staff. Among the Table 3 satisfaction measures, physicians had the highest level of patient satisfaction, 77.5% (for "always communicated well with patients"), while nurses followed closely with a 73.7% level of patients always satisfied. Staff received lower scores for instructions about medicines always being well explained (58.5%) and patients always receiving assistance quickly (59.9%). The greatest source of patients' dissatisfaction with their hospital stay involved the noise level of their room environment at night. Only 53% of patients said their hospital surroundings at night were quiet; that satisfaction measure also had the lowest median (53%) and minimum score (34%) among all ten satisfaction measures.

---

*The sizes of the Tables 1, 2, and 3 precluded their inclusion in this publication. They may be accessed online at http://bit.ly/2efXSoS.

Notably, many hospital characteristics in Table 3 show a very diverse range of structural, patient, and area characteristics among our sample hospitals. Table 3 shows that hospitals averaged 257 hospital beds, with a median of 167, and ranging from just four beds to 2,258. On average, clinical staffing levels indicated a physician for every ten beds and two nurses per bed. The typical patient in our sample hospitals had 1.48 procedures, with a mean cost per patient of $9,456 and a mean length of stay of 4.46 days.

For our variable of interest—the extent of EHR development—the majority of hospitals in our sample (37.5%) had partial EHR systems in place, just slightly ahead of hospitals without any EHR (35.1%). Only 27.5% of hospitals reported a fully implemented EHR.

A full 61% of the hospitals were in an urban area, with an average median household income of $57,716. The vast majority of acute-care hospitals (57.6%) were classified as nonprofit, nongovernment, while the other three classifications—government owned, for-profit, and religiously affiliated—ranged between 12.4% and 16.7%.

Most study hospitals (67.5%) had no teaching affiliation, while 15.7% had only interns and residents. Around 11% of our sample hospitals had the highest level of teaching affiliation recognized by AHA—a Council of Teaching Hospital (COTH). A little more than one third (37.8%) of hospitals in the study had no affiliation with an organized health system, but 24.7% were associated with a decentralized health system and 21% were associated with a moderately centralized health system.

The majority of patients (57.6%) were females, and the typical patient was 53 years old, white (69.1%), and had Medicare coverage (42.3%). For AMI, HF, and PN 30-day mortality rates, hospitals averaged between 11% and 16%, while 30-day readmission rates averaged between 18.7% and 24.9%. Interestingly, the standard deviations for these six hospital quality measures were small, all below 1.5%.

Multivariate Results

Multivariate results for the ten patient satisfaction measures and all independent variables are reported in Table 1. All regressions are statistically significant, with an R^2 ranging from 0.249 to 0.399.

EHR Effects

For the primary variable of interest, either partial or full implementation of EHRs, 17 of the 20 coefficients on patient satisfaction were positive and statistically significant at a 0.05 level or less. In all other cases but one ("physicians always communicated well"), when both EHR coefficients were statistically significant, the "full EHR" coefficient was greater than the "partial EHR"—indicating that, *ceteris paribus*, a fully implemented EHR had a higher impact on patient satisfaction than a partially implemented EHR.

The three variables with coefficients that were not significant were both EHR coefficients for the patient satisfaction variable "recommend the hospital to family and friends" when compared with the excluded reference category "no EHR." The coefficient for "partial EHR" for the satisfaction measure "pain was well controlled" was the third one that was statistically insignificant.

The greatest impact of the fully implemented EHR on patient satisfaction measures (+1.875) was for the variable "area around the room quiet at night," while for the partially implemented EHR, the patient satisfaction measure with the greatest impact was "nurses communicated well" (+1.139). Alternatively, the EHR patient coefficients that were statistically significant but had the lowest impact on patient satisfaction measures were "pain being well controlled" (+0.609) for the fully implemented EHR and "physician always communicated well" (+0.285) for the partially implemented EHR coefficient. Interestingly, for the patient satisfaction measure "physician always communicated well," the coefficient for the fully implement EHR was only slightly above (+0.668) the "pain being well controlled variable"—suggesting that physician communication may not be as essential as some of the other variables, such as nursing communication and staffing involvement with the patient, in terms of their contribution to patient satisfaction.

Several other independent variables in the regression showed interesting patterns in their impact on patient satisfaction. Among the hospital characteristics, hospital bedsize and mean length of stay in the hospital had negative impacts on patient satisfaction. Nine of the ten bedsize variables were negative, with seven of the ten being statistically significant at the 0.05 level or lower, while six of the ten length-of-stay variables were negative and statistically significant. Perhaps, not surprisingly, seven of the ten nursing staff ratios were also statistically significant at the 0.05 level or lower but, in that case, all ten variables had positive coefficients, indicating that nursing care is an important ingredient in creating patient satisfaction.

Teaching status shows a unique but mixed pattern. A full 19 of the 20 coefficients for the variables "hospitals with interns and residents" and a hospital being a COTH were positive, with four and nine, respectively, and statistically significant at the ≤0.05 level. In contrast, all ten of the coefficient signs for the "medical school" variable were negative, although only one was statistically significant. Only one variable among the hospital categories for the "degree of centralization" showed a consistent impact—a moderately centralized health system. Nine of the ten patient satisfaction variables were statistically significant, while all ten were positive when compared with the reference category "not part of a hospital system."

Among the patient characteristics, gender was statistically insignificant for all ten measures. Age was always negative, with eight of the ten revealing statistical significance. When compared with Medicare patients, the excluded category (patients with Medicaid insurance coverage) had negative coefficients for patient satisfaction for all ten measures, but were statistically significant on six measures. In contrast, patients with private insurance all had positive patient satisfaction scores, although just two were statistically significant. Patient race and ethnicity also showed a distinct pattern for several groups. When compared with white patients, Hispanic and Asian patients all had negative patient satisfaction scores, with eight and nine, respectively, and being statistically significant at the ≤0.05 level.

EHR and Organizational Variable Interaction Effects
Table 2 reports the regression results for the organizational characteristics interacted with three different levels of EHR implementation. In this section, we discuss those results.

Market Competition
With respect to the level of market competition, Table 2 shows that 18 of the 20 patient satisfaction coefficients in the partial or fully implemented EHR were positive (p < 0.05) and higher in market structures that are monopolistic rather than in more competitive markets. While for the moderately competitive market, 14 of the coefficients were positive and statistically significant at the 5% level, for only one measure of satisfaction ("room quiet") was the effect larger for hospitals with more competition. Interestingly, patient satisfaction on this measure is actually highest in hospitals with no EHR and in more competitive markets.

Hospital Size
In Table 2, we continue to see the negative effect of larger bedsize on satisfaction. For the categories of 100 to 249 beds, 250 to 399 beds, and 400+ beds, of the 90 potential coefficients, 60 were negative and statistically significant, with 23, 25, and 12 significant negative variables, respectively, for the three bedsize categories. Our hypothesis that EHR will moderate this effect held for eight of the ten measures of satisfaction for hospitals in the bedsize range of 100 to 249, where the negative effect of bedsize was lower with either a partial or full EHR system compared to none—including the "rate high" and "would recommend" measures. While there were mixed results for hospitals in the bedsize range 250 to 399, the negative effect of larger size was reduced for seven of the satisfaction measures with the presence of a full, versus partial, EHR system.

Ownership

Hospital ownership variables indicated a marked difference in patient satisfaction scores between the nonprofit and for-profit hospitals. All the significant coefficients for the two nonprofit hospital groups were positive, while all the coefficients but two ("room quiet") for the for-profit hospitals were negative, although six of the eight negative coefficients for the for-profits were significant only at the 10% level. Implementing a partial or full EHR system improved satisfaction scores for the nongovernment, nonprofit hospitals; in such cases, those coefficients were significant. Among for-profit hospitals, the implementation of a full EHR system appeared to reduce patient satisfaction scores; the effect (–2.403) was large for "would you recommend" and "room quiet" (–2.531) or "room clean" (–2.570), although only the latter was significant at $p < 0.05$.

Teaching

Among the teaching status measures, nearly all the significant coefficients for the patient satisfaction measures were positive when compared to the reference—no teaching, no EHR hospital—with the exception of hospitals affiliated with a medical school, although most coefficients were insignificant for those hospitals. Hospitals without any teaching programs or with a COTH membership appeared to have a clear advantage in their patient satisfaction scores, with 16 of the 20 potential coefficients being significant and positive for the no teaching hospitals at the 5% level and two more significant at the 10% level. Having a COTH membership indicated a strong positive association with satisfaction when compared with the excluded reference category; implementation of either a partial or full EHR resulted in effects generally larger than 2.0 percentage points, including "rate high" and "would recommend." There were also large effects for the group of hospitals with either partial or full EHR for "help quickly," "staff explain well," and "room clean."

Health System Structure

Table 2 shows that more decentralized hospital systems were associated with higher satisfaction, even without the implementation of EHR. The largest positive effect across all organization characteristics on "rate high" and "would you recommend" was decentralized hospitals with no EHR; there were also large effects for "help quickly," and "room clean" for this category. The effect for decentralized systems on "rate high" was slightly higher for full versus partial EHR but was still lower than seen for no EHR.

Hospitals that were part of a moderately centralized health system also showed positive and strong impacts on patient satisfaction among the health system structure variables. Of the 20 potential significant coefficients in the partial or fully implemented EHR status, when compared with the excluded reference category (hospitals that are not part of any health system or independent), 18 were significant and positive in these two EHR categories. Hospitals in moderately centralized hospital systems benefited from full versus partial implementation of EHR in the "rate high" and "would recommend" measures.

DISCUSSION

Recent changes in health care policy and regulations aimed at reforming the nation's payment and delivery models to better coordinate care, improve outcomes, and lower costs have put hospitals under considerable pressure to change. Combined with the record-low annual growth of 3.9% in U.S. health spending, hospitals have been forced to accelerate their efforts to initiate new systems to become more efficient and effective. Those pressures, along with substantial financial incentives in federal legislation to support purchase of EHR systems (and future penalties under the ACA that will be assessed against hospitals who do not use EHRs), have driven hospitals to employ new information technology solutions such as EHRs.

These rapid changes in the hospital industry—including incentives to expand use of EHRs—raise important questions about the impact of such systems on patient satisfaction. In other industries, it can take a decade or more after a particular technology is developed to diffuse and be integrated into broad use (Ortt and Schoormans 2004; Thompson 2012). In the hospital industry, however, the changes have come about quickly. What has been the impact of EHR on patient satisfaction, and what role do organizational characteristics play?

Our investigation posited ten hypotheses. Two of the hypotheses related to the overall impact of different levels of EHR implementation (none, partial, or full) on patient satisfaction. The eight remaining hypotheses tested additional questions about the extent of the interactions among these three levels of EHR implementation and selected organizational features of the hospital (market structure, ownership, teaching status, size, and system membership) on patient satisfaction. Our multivariate analyses included measures of cost and quality to further control for potential differences among hospitals as we tested these hypotheses within the complex reality of the hospital industry.

Our study's multivariate results indicated strong support for our first and second hypotheses regarding the overall impact of EHRs on patient satisfaction. All things being equal, EHR systems have a positive impact on patient satisfaction, and fully implemented EHR systems have a greater impact than partially implemented EHRs when compared with hospitals without EHRs. These results stay consistent across all ten patient satisfaction measures and underscore the impact that EHR and IT can have on the patient experience.

For our remaining hypotheses on market competition, bedsize, ownership, and centralization of the hospitals' system, we had mixed results. Regarding market share and EHR implementation, we postulated that hospitals in more competitive markets and with higher levels of EHR implementation will have higher scores on patient satisfaction measures than those in less competitive markets and with lower levels of EHR implementation. This hypothesis found no support. In fact, the strongest support for the hypothesis appears to be the opposite case—that hospitals in monopolistic markets with higher levels of EHR implementation will have higher scores on patient satisfaction measures than those in less competitive markets and with lower levels of EHR implementation. The recent merger activity in the hospital sector has been of concern because the economies of scale with such mergers may not be reflected in lower prices because hospitals are faced with less competitive market pressure. The findings here may reduce the level of concern with hospital mergers because it appears that patient satisfaction, as hospitals invest in EHR systems, can actually be higher in those markets.

With respect to ownership, from our descriptive data it appears that nonprofit hospitals, whether government owned or nongovernment, have adopted EHR systems quicker than for-profit hospitals. The percentages of for-profit hospitals with partial or fully implemented EHRs were always lower—generally, by several percentage points—than the adoption rates by government and nonprofit hospitals.

The fifth hypothesis, which predicted that hospitals with higher levels of EHR implementation (regardless of their ownership status) would have better patient satisfaction scores than those with lower levels of EHR implementation found strong support overall for either level of EHR implementation in the two forms of nonprofit hospital ownership but not for-profit hospitals. In contrast, for-profit hospitals had statistically significant negative scores on several patient satisfaction measures, although most coefficients for the patient satisfaction measures were not statistically significant.

With respect to hospital size, larger hospitals had a negative impact on patient satisfaction. Compared with smaller hospitals (<100 beds), larger hospitals had a negative influence on all patient satisfaction measures. This negative relationship between hospital bedsize and EHR implementation held true for all coefficients for the larger hospital categories, even those not statistically significant and not shown. Interestingly, this negative relationship held for the larger hospitals even when they had no EHR implementation.

Our findings on the effects of bedsize and implementation of EHRs tended to support our hypothesis that EHR implementation will ameliorate the negative influence of size. This finding was supported largely for the bedsize range of 100–249 and in part for the 250–399 bedsize range. As hospitals get larger, the partial and fully implemented coefficients, where comparisons can be made across the EHR implementation levels, are all negative and typically smaller than the coefficients in the no EHR category, although there were several instances where that was not the case. However, for most of these counterintuitive findings, the differences among the three levels of EHR implementation were small.

Our next hypothesis, that hospitals affiliated with a system will be more likely to adopt EHR than independent hospitals, found strong support. As hospitals became part of a system, the likelihood of their implementing a partial or fully implemented EHR was substantially higher.

Our ninth hypothesis, that the level of EHR implementation was higher in centralized than decentralized and independent hospitals, was not supported. Decentralized hospitals had the highest levels of EHR implementation regardless of whether it was partial or full implementation. Centralized health system hospitals ranked below moderately centralized health system hospitals, but above independent hospital systems, in the percentage of hospitals that had partial and fully implemented EHRs.

Our final hypothesis, that patient satisfaction will be highest in fully implemented EHR systems within each system membership distinction, found support only among moderately centralized health system hospitals. In all eight of the ten patient satisfaction categories where significant positive comparisons could be made between the fully implemented and partially implemented EHR category, the fully implemented EHR category for hospitals in moderately centralized systems had higher scores.

CONCLUDING COMMENTS

What do these findings mean, especially as they pertain to organizational theory and practice? We offer a number of observations.

Size matters, and its influence permeates much of our analysis. Beginning in earnest with the contingency theorists such as Burns and Stalker (1961), Lawrence and Lorsch (1967), and Woodward (1965), interest in the influence of size on design and the way that organizations use management systems has been extensive. Increased size poses major communication and control problems and, as organizations increase in size, accounting and control processes tend to become more specialized and sophisticated (Bruns and Waterhouse 1975; Ezzamel 1990; Libby and Waterhouse 1996).

While the influence of size is certainly not new, in our study of hospitals, its impact cannot be underrated. Although the mean bedsize of our sampled hospitals was 257 beds, it ranged from fewer than 20 beds to more than 2,000 beds. Also, hospital characteristics such as increased teaching commitment and system membership are tied to problems associated with increasing levels of bureaucracy, complexity, and integration. As hospitals get larger and become more complex, the need for HIT and EHR systems to control and manage complex goals such as patient care, teaching, and research becomes essential.

However, clearly acquiring EHR is not enough. As we noted earlier, many hospitals have been slow and unwilling accomplices in the recent HIT trends, and until the financial penalties that accompanied the regulatory pressures started to "bite," they had been slow to implement. Consequently, the challenges of not only implementing but managing, maintaining, and operating the new technologies are intense at this point in the IT revolution in the health care industry.

Critically important, while hospitals may be adopting EHRs, they have not yet figured out how to use the new technology to improve patient satisfaction, improve patient safety, and reduce health care costs. As the RWJF study noted, while 42% of hospitals now meet federal standards for collecting electronic health data, only 5% also meet federal standards for exchanging that data with other providers to allow widespread physician access to a patient's records (DesRoches, Painter, and Jha 2013). This challenge underscores the importance of the "learning curve"—the idea that the cost of doing most tasks decreases as the experience of doing those tasks increases (Bartel and Lichtenberg 1987). In the hospital industry, it is not clear how steep the learning curve will be—especially across different organizational characteristics like those of market structure, ownership, and system membership. Moreover, it is not clear how success will be defined in such a dynamic and competitive environment like health care. However, our early investigation suggests that many hospitals will continue to experience the problems associated with HIT growing pains, and those differences in experience likely strongly influence our results.

A related influence of size, growth, and the implementation of decision-making processes and performance control systems on hospitals is that these organizations may not be well suited for these types of processes or systems. Chandler (1962) and Mintzberg (1981) have both commented on the development and implementation of decision-making processes and performance control systems in organizations as they have evolved and grown larger.

Chandler analyzed and documented the evolution of large-scale organizations that came to dominate their environments and the accompanying changes in their structure and processes. Of particular interest are the changes in the economic control systems—the financial accounting and information control systems—that were necessary to permit these organizations to develop new administrative structures that could adapt and easily change as the organization grew into a more diversified and decentralized multidivisional structure.

Mintzberg articulated these changes in some critical aspects of decentralized multidivisional structures or divisionalized form, as he terms it. The divisionalized form, he noted, was created to solve the problem of adaptability in bureaucratic organizations. By overlaying another level of administrative structure (corporate level), the organization could add and subtract organizations and quickly adapt to new conditions and spread the risk of failure over a broader range of business units. Moreover, with the corporate level administrating the various units, the new entity could grow substantially larger and more diversified than the earlier types of organizational structure.

However, to maintain control over the divisionalized organizations, Mintzberg argued that performance control systems are put into place that standardize the outputs of the divisionalized organizations. Such performance control systems rely heavily on formal rationality. In fact, performance criteria are typically established, and the success or failure of the organizational unit is judged by its ability to meet or exceed these goals.

Here, rationality is viewed through the Weberian conceptual framework. Weber identified two types of rationality associated with economic action: formal and substantive. Formal rationality, according to Weber, is the extent to which quantitative calculation or accounting is applied—that is, a system of "economic activity (was) called 'formally' rational according to the degree in which the provision for needs … is capable of being expressed in numerical, calculable terms, and is so expressed" (Weber 1947: 185). For Weber, formal rationality was unambiguous in the sense that expression, in monetary terms, yielded the highest degree of formal calculability.

On the other hand, substantive rationality exists when the process of developing a plan of action is not entirely based on market calculations. For substantive rationality, Weber observed:

> It is not sufficient to consider only the purely formal fact that calculations are being made on grounds of expediency by the methods which are, among those available, technically the most nearly adequate. In addition, it is necessary to take account of the fact that economic activity is oriented to ultimate ends (*Forderungen*) of some kind, whether they be ethical, political, utilitarian, hedonistic, the attainment of social equality or of anything else. Substantive rationality cannot be measured in terms of formal calculation alone, but also involves a relation to the absolute values or to the content of the particular given ends to which it is oriented. In principle,

there is an indefinite number of possible standards of value
which are "rational" in this sense. (Weber 1947: 185)

Because of the indefinite number of possible standards of value, Weber
viewed actions based on substantive rationality as full of difficulties. There
were numerous standards that were of potential "substantive" significance.
In his formative article using Weber's framework and a sample of
Tennessee hospitals, Rushing (1976) argued that rational calculations are
facilitated if economic criteria are the basis for the calculation. For the
profit-making enterprise, market pressures generate the need for cost calculations and for the pricing of various inputs. For the nonprofit enterprise, market pressure is of less concern; rather, calculations and decisions
are made relative to the values or ideals of the enterprise and the related
tax obligation. Various inputs and strategies are priced in relation to the
value or ideal of the enterprise instead of in relation to market demands.

Rushing noted the importance of formal and substantive rationality
when he summarizes their impact on organizations, in general, and on
hospitals in particular:

> [F]or most organizations, "formal" or economic assessments
> are easier to make than "substantive" assessments. The eco-
> nomic costs and the expected economic price are easier to as-
> sess than is the relationship between the economic costs and
> the extent to which operations contribute to some absolute
> ideal or meet some social need. For example, it is far easier
> to measure the extent to which a hospital's income exceeds
> its economic costs than it is to measure the extent to which
> hospital operations have had an impact on the medical welfare
> of a target population. And the net balance between economic
> costs and expected economic return is far easier to quantify
> than the net balance between economic costs and social ben-
> efit derived from hospital operations. Moreover, the optimum
> or even reasonable balance will vary widely when "substan-
> tive" matters are central, depending on value preferences in
> respect to economic outcomes and the medical welfare of
> the community. Thus, in comparison to "substantive" crite-
> ria, economic criteria provide a much clearer framework for
> the rational calculation of costs and organizational return for
> those costs and, thus, they provide a less ambiguous basis for
> decision-making. (Rushing 1976: 678).

Formal rationality, more so than substantive rationality, provides a
lucid and easier framework for decision making, but formal rationality
also lends itself more readily to organizational situations in which
managers are evaluating economic assessments such as efficiency and/or

profitability more than situations that involve substantive matters or activities such as social responsibility or social performance. For this reason, as Weber suggested, organizations prefer to use criteria of formal rationality in their decision-making process.

By emphasizing the measurement of performance as a means of control, Mintzberg extended this difference and argued that a bias arises in favor of those organizational goals that can be operationalized, which usually means goals that are economic in nature and not social. As a consequence, by focusing on economic measures, Mintzberg argued that the diversified form of organization is driven "to act in ways that are, at best, socially unresponsive, at worst, socially irresponsible" (Mintzberg 1989: 170).

There is some evidence to support this concern. Ackerman (1975) found social benefits that could not be easily measured and could not be plugged into performance control systems. As a result, he concluded, the financial reporting system may actually inhibit the organization's social responsiveness. By focusing on economic performance, even with safeguards to protect against sacrificing long-term benefits, Ackerman concluded, the performance control system directs energy and resources to results measured in financial expression.

Becker and Potter (2002) in their study of 4,705 of the nation's short-term general hospitals using two measures of hospital efficiency and four measures of social responsibility confirmed that for-profit hospitals managed stakeholder relationships in ways that increased efficiency but decreased their social responsiveness. The authors' findings suggested that major measures of hospital efficiency and social responsibility show that these goals are inversely related (Becker and Potter 2002).

This discussion raises the question of the relationship between organizational performance and social responsibility and suggests they may be opposite sides of the same coin—when one goes up, the other goes down. More specifically, consistent with Weber's and Rushing's context, the greater the extent to which values or ideals shape the organizational decision-making process (i.e., instead of market demands), the more likely the organization is to excel on these "substantive" criteria and the more difficult it will be for the organization to be efficient.

This discussion underscores the importance of the hospital ownership variables in our study and, in fact, some of the specific concerns expressed by Weber and Rushing go to the heart of the debate on efficiency versus patient-centered care. As hospitals strive to become more efficient and control resources and costs, do these pressures clash with patient needs? Specifically, for example, we might ask "Does the profit/nonprofit status of a hospital clash with patient needs?" The subtle implication is that nonprofit hospitals are disadvantaged by their need to use some degree of substantive rationality in their decision-making process, and that disadvantage results in decisions that are not as certain, decisive, and precise as those made by for-profit hospitals—and, consequently, the nonprofit hospitals will never achieve the same degree of economic success as for-profit hospitals.

Similar questions might be raised about markets and hospital system membership. How do more competitive markets influence hospital patient care, or how does hospital system membership impact patient satisfaction and outcomes? Overall, our study shows strong positive impacts of EHR systems on patient satisfaction, but when we analyzed the interaction among different levels of EHR implementation and major hospital characteristics on patient satisfaction, large disparities in patient satisfaction appeared.

Certainly it is too early in the evolution of the recent and ongoing regulatory changes in the health care market to fully assess the impact of the new patient-centered paradigm, but these are critical and viable research questions that require further investigation.

ACKNOWLEDGMENTS

This work was supported through a Patient-Centered Outcomes Research Institute (PCORI) Pilot Project Program Award (1IP2PI000167-01). All statements in this report, including its findings and conclusions, are solely those of the authors and do not necessarily represent the views of the Patient-Centered Outcomes Research Institute (PCORI), its Board of Governors or Methodology Committee.

REFERENCES

Ackerman, R. W. 1975. *The Social Challenge to Business.* Cambridge, MA: Harvard University Press.

Adler-Milstein, J., and A. K. Jha. 2012. "Sharing Clinical Data Electronically." *Journal of the American Medical Association* 307, no. 16: 1695–96. doi:10.1001/jama.2012.525.

Agarwal, R., G. Gao, C. DesRoches, and A. K. Jha. 2010. "Research Commentary—The Digital Transformation of Healthcare: Current Status and the Road Ahead." *Information Systems Research* 21, no. 4: 796–809. doi:10.1287/isre.1100.0327.

Agency for Healthcare Quality and Research. No date. "Healthcare Cost and Utilization Project (HCUP)." http://bit.ly/2aGLYhd.

Agency for Healthcare Quality and Research. No date. "SID Database Documentation." http://bit.ly/2aGM2xE.

Aldrich, H., and E. R. Auster. 1986. "Even Dwarfs Started Small: Liabilities of Age and Size and Their Strategic Implications." *Research in Organizational Behavior* 8: 165–86.

American Hospital Association. No date. "AHA Annual Survey Database." http://bit.ly/2alM95a.

American Hospital Association. No date. "AHA Annual Survey IT Database." http://bit.ly/2alMzZc.

American Hospital Association. 2015. "Fast Facts on US Hospitals." http://bit.ly/2alNyIX.

Appari, A., M. E. Johnson, and D. L. Anthony. 2013. "Meaningful Use of Electronic Health Record Systems and Process Quality of Care: Evidence from a Panel Data Analysis of U.S. Acute-Care Hospitals." *Health Services Research* 48, no. 2, part 1: 354–75. doi:10.1111/j.1475-6773.2012.01448.x.

Arthur, J. B. 1994. "Effects of Human Resource Systems on Manufacturing Performance and Turnover." *Academy of Management Journal* 37, no. 3: 670–87. doi:10.2307/256705.

Bartel, A. P. 1994. "Productivity Gains from the Implementation of Employee Training Programs." *Industrial Relations* 33, no. 4: 411–25. doi:10.1111/j.1468-232x.1994.tb00349.x.

Bartel, A. P. 2004. "Human Resource Management and Organizational Performance: Evidence from Retail Banking." *Industrial and Labor Relations Review* 57, no. 2: 181–203. doi:10.2307/4126616.

Bartel, A. P., and F. R. Lichtenberg. 1987. "The Comparative Advantage of Educated Workers in Implementing New Technology." *The Review of Economics and Statistics* 69, no. 1: 1–11. doi:10.2307/1937894.

Bates, D. W., and A. A. Gawande. 2003. "Improving Safety with Information Technology." *New England Journal of Medicine* 348, no. 25: 2526–34. doi:10.1056/nejmsa020847.

Batt, R. 1999. "Work Organization, Technology, and Performance in Customer Service and Sales." *Industrial and Labor Relations Review* 52, no. 4: 539–64. doi:10.2307/2525063.

Bazzoli, G. J., S. M. Shortell, N. Dubbs, C. Chan, and P. Kralovec. 1999. "A Taxonomy of Health Networks and Systems: Bringing Order Out of Chaos." *Health Services Research* 33, no. 6: 1683–1717.

Becker, E. R. 2007. "National Trends and Determinants of Hospitalization Costs and Lengths-of-Stay for Uterine Fibroids Procedures." *Journal of Health Care Finance* 33, no. 3: 1–16.

Becker, E. R., and S. J. Potter. 2002. "Organizational Rationality, Performance, and Social Responsibility." *Journal of Health Care Finance* 29, no. 1: 23–48.

Becker, E. R., and A. Rahimi. 2006. "Disparities in Race/Ethnicity and Gender in In-Hospital Mortality Rates for Coronary Artery Bypass Surgery Patients." *Journal of the American Medical Association* 98, no. 11: 1729–39.

Becker, E. R., and F. A. Sloan. 1983. "Utilization of Hospital Services: The Roles of Teaching, Case Mix, and Reimbursement." *Inquiry: The Journal of Health Care Organization, Provision, and Financing* 20, no. 3: 248–57.

Becker, E. R., and F. A. Sloan. 1985. "Hospital Ownership and Performance." *Economic Inquiry* 23, no. 1: 21–36.

Blum, J. 2011. "Improving Quality, Lowering Costs: The Role of Health Care Delivery System." http://bit.ly/2aU5tGA.

Boardman, A. E., and A. R. Vining. 1989. "Ownership and Performance in Competitive Environments: A Comparison of the Performance of Private, Mixed, and State-Owned Enterprises." *The Journal of Law and Economics* 32, no. 1: 1–33. doi:10.1086/467167.

Borzekowski, R. 2009. "Measuring the Cost Impact of Hospital Information Systems: 1987–1994." *Journal of Health Economics* 28, no. 5: 938–49. doi:10.1016/j.jhealeco.2009.06.004.

Brook, R. H., and J. B. Kosecoff. 1988. "Competition and Quality." *Health Affairs* 7, no. 3: 150–61. doi:10.1377/hlthaff.7.3.150.

Bruns, W. J., and J. H. Waterhouse. 1975. "Budgetary Control and Organization Structure." *Journal of Accounting Research* 13, no. 2: 177–203. doi:10.2307/2490360.

Brynjolfsson, E., and L. M. Hitt. 2003. "Computing Productivity: Firm-Level Evidence." *Review of Economics and Statistics* 85, no. 4: 793–808. doi:10.1162/003465303772815736.

Buntin, M. B., S. H. Jain, and D. Blumenthal. 2010. "Health Information Technology: Laying the Infrastructure for National Health Reform." *Health Affairs* 29, no. 6: 1214–19. doi:10.1377/hlthaff.2010.0503.

Burns, T. E., and G. M. Stalker. 1961. "The Management of Innovation." University of Illinois at Urbana-Champaign's Academy for Entrepreneurial Leadership Historical Research Reference in Entrepreneurship.

Campbell, E. M., H. Li, T. Mori, P. Osterweil, and Jeanne-Marie Guise. 2008. "The Impact of Health Information Technology on Work Process and Patient Care in Labor and Delivery." In *Advances in Patient Safety: From Research to Implementation (Volume 4: Programs, Tools, and Products)*. http://bit.ly/2aGPFn7.

Cappelli, P., and D. Neumark. 2004. "External Churning and Internal Flexibility: Evidence on the Functional Flexibility and Core-Periphery Hypotheses." *Industrial Relations* 43, no. 1: 148–82. doi:10.1111/j.0019-8676.2004.00322.x.

Carey, K. 2003. "Hospital Cost Efficiency and System Membership." *Inquiry: The Journal of Health Care Organization, Provision, and Financing* 40, no. 1: 25–38. doi:10.5034/inquiryjrnl_40.1.25.

Centers for Medicare and Medicaid Services. 2014. "EHR Incentive Program: Active Registrations." http://go.cms.gov/2aGPlVl.

Centers for Medicare and Medicaid Services. 2015. "Spring 2015 HCAHPS Executive Insight Letter." http://bit.ly/2aGPzfb.

Chandler, A. D. 1962. *Strategy and Structure: Chapters in the History of the Industrial Enterprise*. Cambridge, MA: MIT Press.

Chassin, M. R. 1997. "Assessing Strategies for Quality Improvement." *Health Affairs* 16, no. 3: 151–61. doi:10.1377/hlthaff.16.3.151.

Chaudhry, B., J. Wang, S. Wu, M. Maglione, W. Mojica, E. Roth, S. C. Morton, and P. G. Shekelle. 2006. "Systematic Review: Impact of Health Information Technology on Quality, Efficiency, and Costs of Medical Care." *Annals of Internal Medicine* 144, no. 10: 742–52. doi:10.7326/0003-4819-144-10-200605160-00125.

Cherouny, P., F. Federico, C. Haraden, S. Leavitt Gullo, and R. Resar. 2005. "Idealized Design of Perinatal Care." IHI Innovation Series white paper. Cambridge, MA: Institute for Healthcare Improvement.

Chukmaitov, A. S., G. J. Bazzoli, D. W. Harless, R. E. Hurley, K. J. Devers, and M. Zhao. 2009. "Variations in Inpatient Mortality Among Hospitals in Different System Types, 1995 to 2000." *Medical Care* 47, no. 4: 466–73. doi:10.1097/mlr.0b013e31818dcdf0.

Cleary, P. D., and B. J. McNeil. 1988. "Patient Satisfaction as an Indicator of Quality Care." *Inquiry: The Journal of Health Care Organization, Provision, and Financing* 25, no. 1: 25–36.

Collins, C. J., and K. D. Clark. 2003. "Strategic Human Resource Practices, Top Management Team Social Networks, and Firm Performance: The Role of Human Resource Practices in Creating Organizational Competitive Advantage." *Academy of Management Journal* 46, no. 6: 740–51. doi:10.2307/30040665.

Collins, C. J., and K. G. Smith. 2006. "Knowledge Exchange and Combination: The Role of Human Resource Practices in the Performance of High-Technology Firms." *Academy of Management Journal* 49, no. 3: 544–60. doi:10.5465/amj.2006.21794671.

Cowing, M., C. M. Davino-Ramaya, K. Ramaya, and J. Szmerekovsky. 2009. "Health Care Delivery Performance: Service, Outcomes, and Resource Stewardship." *The Permanente Journal* 13, no. 4: 72–78. doi:10.7812/tpp/08-100.

Creswell, J., and R. Abelson. 2013 (Aug. 12). "New Laws and Rising Costs Create a Surge of Supersizing Hospitals." *New York Times*. http://nyti.ms/2aGPgBg.

Cutler, D. M., and F. Scott Morton. 2013. "Hospitals, Market Share, and Consolidation." *Journal of the American Medical Association* 310, no. 18: 1964–70. doi:10.1001/jama.2013.281675.

Dartmouth Atlas of Health Care. No date. "Research Methods." http://bit.ly/2aGQk88.

Davenport, T. H. 1993. *Process Innovation: Reengineering Work Through Information Technology*. Boston, MA: Harvard Business School Press.

De Alessi, L. 1996. "The Economics of Property Rights: A Review of the Evidence." *Privatization: Critical Perspectives on the World Economy* 1: 233–380.

Delery, J. E., and D. H. Doty. 1996. "Modes of Theorizing in Strategic Human Resource Management: Tests of Universalistic, Contingency, and Configurations. Performance Predictions." *Academy of Management Journal* 39, no. 4: 802–35. doi:10.2307/256713.

DesRoches, C. M., E. G. Campbell, S. R. Rao, K. Donelan, T. G. Ferris, A. Jha, R. Kaushal, et al. 2008. "Electronic Health Records in Ambulatory Care—A National Survey of Physicians." *New England Journal of Medicine* 359, no. 1: 50–60. doi:10.1056/nejmsa0802005.

DesRoches, C. M., M. W. Painter, and A. K. Jha. 2013. "Health Information Technology in the United States 2013: Better Information Systems for Better Care." Mathematica Policy Research, Harvard School of Public Healthy, and the Robert Wood Johnson Foundation. http://rwjf.ws/2aGRekZ.

Devaraj, S., and R. Kohli. 2000. "Information Technology Payoff in the Health-Care Industry: A Longitudinal Study." *Journal of Management Information Systems* 16, no. 4: 41–67. doi:10.1080/07421222.2000.11518265.

Devereaux, P. J., P. T. L. Choi, C. Lacchetti, B. Weaver, H. J. Schunemann, T. Haines, J. N. Lavis, et al. 2002. "A Systematic Review and Meta-Analysis of Studies Comparing Mortality Rates of Private For-Profit and Private Not-for-Profit Hospitals." *Canadian Medical Association Journal* 166, no. 11: 1399–1406.

Donabedian, A. 2005. "Evaluating the Quality of Medical Care." *Milbank Quarterly* 83, no. 4: 691–729. doi:10.1111/j.1468-0009.2005.00397.x.

Dranove, D., C. Forman, A. Goldfarb, and S. Greenstein. 2012. "The Trillion Dollar Conundrum: Complementarities and Health Information Technology." *American Economic Journal: Economic Policy* 6, no. 4. doi:10.1257/pol.6.4.239.

Drazin, R., and C. B. Schoonhoven. 1996. "Community, Population, and Organization Effects on Innovation: A Multilevel Perspective." *Academy of Management Journal* 39, no. 5: 1065–83. doi:10.2307/256992.

Eden, K. B., R. Messina, H. Li, P. Osterweil, C. R. Henderson, and J.-M. Guise. 2008. "Examining the Value of Electronic Health Records on Labor and Delivery." *American Journal of Obstetrics and Gynecology* 199, no. 3: 307e1-307e9. doi:10.1016/j.ajog.2008.07.004.

Elliott, M. N., W. G. Lehrman, E. H. Goldstein, L. A. Giordano, M. K. Beckett, C. W. Cohea, and P. D. Cleary. 2010. "Hospital Survey Shows Improvements in Patient Experience." *Health Affairs* 29, no. 11: 2061–67. doi:10.1377/hlthaff.2009.0876.

Enthoven, A. C. 1993. "Why Managed Care Has Failed to Contain Health Costs." *Health Affairs* 12, no. 3: 27–43. doi:10.1377/hlthaff.12.3.27.

Ezzamel, M. 1990. "The Impact of Environmental Uncertainty, Managerial Autonomy and Size on Budget Characteristics." *Management Accounting Research* 1, no. 3: 181–97. doi:10.1016/s1044-5005(90)70057-1.

Federal Trade Commission and U.S. Department of Justice. 2004. "Improving Health Care: A Dose of Competition." http://bit.ly/2aGRsIS.

Figueroa, J. F., D. E. Wang, and A. K. Jha. 2016 (Mar.). "Characteristics of Hospitals Receiving the Largest Penalties by US Pay-for-Performance Programmes." *BMJ Quality and Safety.* doi:10.1136/bmjqs-2015-005040.

Frisse, M. E., K. B. Johnson, H. Nian, C. L. Davison, C. S. Gadd, K. M. Unertl, P. A. Turri, and Q. Chen. 2012. "The Financial Impact of Health Information Exchange on Emergency Department Care." *Journal of the American Medical Informatics Association* 19, no. 3: 328–33. doi:10.1136/amiajnl-2011-000394.

Garrido, T., L. Jamieson, Y. Zhou, A. Wiesenthal, and L. Liang. 2005. "Effect of Electronic Health Records in Ambulatory Care: Retrospective, Serial, Cross Sectional Study." *British Medical Journal* 330, no. 7491: 581. doi:10.1136/bmj.330.7491.581.

Gawande, A. 2012 (Aug. 3). "Big Med: Restaurant Chains Have Managed to Combine Quality Control, Cost Control, and Innovation. Can Health Care?" *The New Yorker.* http://bit.ly/2aGRSz1.

Gaynor, M., and R. J. Town. 2011. "Competition in Health Care Markets." In *Handbook of Health Economics*, edited by P. Borras, T. McGuire, and M. Pauly, 2: 499–637. Amsterdam, Netherlands: Elsevier.

Gittell, J. Hoffer, R. Seidner, and J. Wimbush. 2010. "A Relational Model of How High-Performance Work Systems Work." *Organization Science* 21, no. 2: 490–506. doi:10.1287/orsc.1090.0446.

Glickman, S. W., K. A. Baggett, C. G. Krubert, E. D. Peterson, and K. A. Schulman. 2007. "Promoting Quality: The Health-Care Organization from a Management Perspective." *International Journal for Quality in Health Care* 19, no. 6: 341–48. doi:10.1093/intqhc/mzm047.

Goodrich, K., E. Garcia, and P. H. Conway. 2012. "A History of and a Vision for CMS Quality Measurement Programs." *Joint Commission Journal on Quality and Patient Safety* 38, no. 10: 465–70.

Health Resources and Services Administration. 2016. "Area Health Resources Files." http://ahrf.hrsa.gov.

Healthcare Cost and Utilization Project. 2016. "Cost-to-Charge Ratio Files." http://bit.ly/2anUFAI.

Hersh, W. 2004. "Health Care Information Technology." *Journal of the American Medical Association* 292, no. 18: 2273–74. doi:10.1001/jama.292.18.2273.

Hikmet, N., A. Bhattacherjee, N. Menachemi, V. O. Kayhan, and R. G. Brooks. 2008. "The Role of Organizational Factors in the Adoption of Healthcare Information Technology in Florida Hospitals." *Health Care Management Science* 11, no. 1: 1–9. doi:10.1007/s10729-007-9036-5.

Hillestad, R., J. Bigelow, A. Bower, F. Girosi, R. Meili, R. Scoville, and R. Taylor. 2005a. "Can Electronic Medical Record Systems Transform Health Care? Potential Health Benefits, Savings, and Costs." *Health Affairs* 24, no. 5: 1103–17. doi:10.1377/hlthaff.24.5.1103.

Hillestad, R., J. H. Bigelow, K. Fonkych, A. G. Bower, C. Fung, J. Wang, R. Taylor, et al. 2005b. "Health Information Technology: Can HIT Lower Costs and Improve Quality?" Santa Monica, CA: RAND Corporation. http://bit.ly/2anV1Hq.

Hospital Consumer Assessment of Healthcare Providers and Systems. 2015 (Jun.). "HCAHPS Fact Sheet." http://bit.ly/2anUeq7.

Huselid, M. A. 1995. "The Impact of Human Resource Management Practices on Turnover, Productivity, and Corporate Financial Performance." *Academy of Management Journal* 38, no. 3: 635–72. doi:10.2307/256741.

Ichniowski, C., T. A. Kochan, D. Levine, C. Olson, and G. Strauss. 1996. "What Works at Work: Overview and Assessment." *Industrial Relations* 35, no. 3: 299–333. doi:10.1111/j.1468-232x.1996.tb00409.x.

Javitt, J. C., J. B. Rebitzer, and L. Reisman. 2008. "Information Technology and Medical Missteps: Evidence from a Randomized Trial." *Journal of Health Economics* 27, no. 3: 585–602. doi:10.1016/j.jhealeco.2007.10.008.

Jha, A. K., C. M. DesRoches, E. G. Campbell, K. Donelan, S. R. Rao, T. G. Ferris, A. Shields, S. Rosenbaum, and D. Blumenthal. 2009. "Use of Electronic Health Records in U.S. Hospitals." *New England Journal of Medicine* 360, no. 16: 1628–38. doi:10.1056/nejmsa0900592.

Jha, A. K., E. J. Orav, J. Zheng, and A. M. Epstein. 2008. "Patients' Perception of Hospital Care in the United States." *New England Journal of Medicine* 359, no. 18: 1921–31. doi:10.1056/nejmsa0804116.

Kassirer, J. P. 1995. "Managed Care and the Morality of the Marketplace." *New England Journal of Medicine* 333, no. 1: 50–52. doi:10.1056/nejm199507063330110.

Katz, M. L., and C. Shapiro. 1986. "Technology Adoption in the Presence of Network Externalities." *Journal of Political Economy* 94, no. 4: 822–41. doi:10.1086/261409.

Kaushal, R., D. Blumenthal, E. G. Poon, A. K. Jha, C. Franz, B. Middleton, J. Glaser, et al. 2005. "The Costs of a National Health Information Network." *Annals of Internal Medicine* 143, no. 3: 165. doi:10.7326/0003-4819-143-3-200508020-00002.

Kimberly, J. R., and M. J. Evanisko. 1981. "Organizational Innovation: The Influence of Individual, Organizational, and Contextual Factors on Hospital Adoption of Technological and Administrative Innovations." *Academy of Management Journal* 24, no. 4: 689–713. doi:10.2307/256170.

Lawrence, P. R., and J. W. Lorsch. 1967. "Differentiation and Integration in Complex Organizations." *Administrative Science Quarterly* 12, no. 1: 1–30. doi:10.2307/2391211.

Libby, T., and J. H. Waterhouse. 1996. "Predicting Change in Management Accounting Systems." *Journal of Management Accounting Research* 8: 137–50.

Luke, R. D., Y. A. Ozcan, and P. C. Olden. 1995. "Local Markets and Systems: Hospital Consolidations in Metropolitan Areas." *Health Services Research* 30, no. 4: 555–75.

McCartney, P. R. 2006. "Using Technology to Promote Perinatal Patient Safety." *Journal of Obstetric, Gynecologic and Neonatal Nursing* 35, no. 3: 424–31. doi:10.1111/j.1552-6909.2006.00059.x.

McCullough, J. S., S. Parente, and R. Town. 2013. *Health Information Technology and Patient Outcomes: The Role of Organizational and Informational Complementarities.* Cambridge, MA: National Bureau of Economic Research.

Miller, R. H. 1996. "Competition in the Health System: Good News and Bad News." *Health Affairs* 15, no. 2: 107–20. doi:10.1377/hlthaff.15.2.107.

Mintzberg, H. 1981. "Organizational Design: Fashion or Fit?" *Harvard Business Review* 31: 103–16.

Mintzberg, H. 1989. *Mintzberg on Management*. New York, NY: Free Press.

Ortt, J. R., and J. P. L. Schoormans. 2004. "The Pattern of Development and Diffusion of Breakthrough Communication Technologies." *European Journal of Innovation Management* 7, no. 4: 292–302. doi:10.1108/14601060410565047.

Pautler, P. A., and M. G. Vita. 1994. "Hospital Market Structure, Hospital Competition, and Consumer Welfare: What Can the Evidence Tell Us?" *Journal of Contemporary Health Law and Policy* 10, no. 1: 117–68.

Quinn, M. A., A. M. Kats, K. Kleinman, D. W. Bates, and S. R. Simon. 2012. "The Relationship Between Electronic Health Records and Malpractice Claims." *Archives of Internal Medicine* 172, no. 15: 1187–89. doi:10.1001/archinternmed.2012.2371.

Rau, J. 2013 (Nov. 14). Nearly 1,500 Hospitals Penalized Under Medicare Program Rating Quality." *Kaiser Health News*. http://bit.ly/2anW2PY.

Rau, J. 2015 (Aug. 3). "Half of Nation's Hospitals Fail Again to Escape Medicare's Readmission Penalties." *Kaiser Health News*. http://bit.ly/2anW6iF.

Richard, O. C., and N. B. Johnson. 2004. "High Performance Work Practices and Human Resource Management Effectiveness: Substitutes or Complements?" *Journal of Business Strategies* 21, no. 2: 133–48.

Robinson, J. C., and H. S. Luft. 1985. "The Impact of Hospital Market Structure on Patient Volume, Average Length of Stay, and the Cost of Care." *Journal of Health Economics* 4, no. 4: 333–56. doi:10.1016/0167-6296(85)90012-8.

Robinson, J. C., and H. S. Luft. 1987. "Competition and the Cost of Hospital Care, 1972 to 1982." *Journal of the American Medical Association* 257, no. 23: 3241–45. doi:10.1001/jama.1987.03390230077028.

Robinson, J. C., and H. S. Luft. 1988. "Competition, Regulation, and Hospital Costs, 1982 to 1986." *Journal of the American Medical Association* 260, no. 18: 2676–81.

Rushing, W. 1974. "Differences in Profit and Nonprofit Organizations: A Study of Effectiveness and Efficiency in General Short-Stay Hospitals." *Administrative Science Quarterly* 19, no. 4: 474–84. doi:10.2307/2391804.

Rushing, W. A. 1976. "Profit and Nonprofit Orientations and the Differentiations–Coordination Hypothesis for Organizations: A Study of Small General Hospitals." *American Sociological Review* 41, no. 4: 676–91. doi:10.2307/2094843.

Simon, J. S., T. G. Rundall, and S. M. Shortell. 2005. "Drivers of Electronic Medical Record Adoption Among Medical Groups." *Joint Commission Journal on Quality and Patient Safety* 31, no. 11: 631–39.

Sloan, F. A., G. A. Picone, D. H. Taylor, and S.-Y. Chou. 2001. "Hospital Ownership and Cost and Quality of Care: Is There a Dime's Worth of Difference?" *Journal of Health Economics* 20, no. 1: 1–21. doi:10.3386/w6706.

Stiroh, K. J. 2002. "Information Technology and the U.S. Productivity Revival: What Do the Industry Data Say?" *American Economic Review* 92, no. 5: 1559–76. doi:10.2139/ssrn.923623.

Taylor, R., A. Bower, F. Girosi, J. Bigelow, K. Fonkych, and R. Hillestad. 2005. "Promoting Health Information Technology: Is There a Case for More-Aggressive Government Action?" *Health Affairs* 24, no. 5: 1234–45. doi:10.1377/hlthaff.24.5.1234.

Thompson, D. 2012 (Apr. 7). "The 100 Year March of Technology in 1 Graph." *The Atlantic*. http://theatln.tc/2anVHMR.

U.S. Department of Justice and Federal Trade Commission. 2010 (Aug. 19). "Horizontal Merger Guidelines." http://bit.ly/2anVLMX.

Vahey, D. C., L. H. Aiken, D. M. Sloane, S. P. Clarke, and D. Vargas. 2004. "Nurse Burnout and Patient Satisfaction." *Medical Care* 42, no. 2 suppl.: II57–II66. doi:10.1097/01.mlr.0000109126.50398.5a.

VanLare, J. M., and P. H. Conway. 2012. "Value-Based Purchasing—National Programs to Move from Volume to Value." *New England Journal of Medicine* 367, no. 21: 2060 doi:10.1056/nejmx120083.

Weber, M. 1947. *The Theory of Social and Economic Organizations*. Translated by A. M. Henderson and T. Parsons. New York, NY: Free Press.

Woodward, J. 1965. *Industrial Organization: Theory and Practice*. Oxford, UK: Oxford University Press.

Young, G. J., M. Meterko, and K. R. Desai. 2000. "Patient Satisfaction with Hospital Care: Effects of Demographic and Institutional Characteristics." *Medical Care* 38, no. 3: 325–34. doi:10.1097/00005650-200003000-00009.

Zwanziger, J., and G. A. Melnick. 1988. "The Effects of Hospital Competition and the Medicare PPS Program on Hospital Cost Behavior in California." *Journal of Health Economics* 7, no. 4: 301–20. doi:10.1016/0167-6296(88)90018-5.

Zwanziger, J., and G. A. Melnick. 1996. "Can Managed Care Plans Control Health Care Costs?" *Health Affairs* 15, no. 2: 185–99. doi:10.1377/hlthaff.15.2.185.

CHAPTER 12

A New Perspective on Organizational Climate as a Boundary Spanner: Integrating a Fragmented Health Care System

TAL KATZ-NAVON

Arison School of Business
The Interdisciplinary Center, Herzliya, Israel

EITAN NAVEH

Faculty of Industrial Engineering and Management
Technion—Israel Institute of Technology, Haifa, Israel

INTRODUCTION

Integrated health care systems are considered part of the solution to the challenge of achieving high-quality and low-cost health care services. Integrated systems provide and coordinate all core services along a continuum of health for the population served (e.g., in the United States, it takes the form of accountable care organizations that attempt to enhance care delivery across the continuum of care). This includes services from primary through tertiary care as well as cooperation between health and social care organizations. Although initiatives to improve integration are already in place, health care delivery is still structurally fragmented, and often the provision of care is not continuous but punctuated. This means that the financing and delivery of care is distributed across a variety of distinct and often competing entities, each with its own objectives, obligations, and capabilities. The following examples illustrate this point:

- Services of individual health care agencies do not cover all multi-condition patients' demands. For example, older patients with coronary heart disease, diabetes, or psychogeriatric problems have long-term needs for a coherent set of products and services delivered by collaborating local and regional health care agencies, such as in- or outpatient hospital care, district nursing, domiciliary care, physiotherapy, and social support (Coburn 2001; Hardy, Mur-Veeman, Steenbergen, and Wistow 1999).

- Medical care is delivered both inside the hospital (inpatient care) and outside the hospital (outpatient or ambulatory care). Some physicians spend their time at more than one hospital or practice, while many more split their time and attention between hospital inpatient care and their office-based practices (Fisher, Staiger, Bynum, and Gottlieb 2006). Therefore, the same physicians provide services in different entities and locations.
- The majority of physicians work in small, single-specialty groups, although some large multi-specialty group practices do exist (Wilensky, Wolter, and Fischer 2006).
- A physician might work in a hospital and in addition spend part of her time in a tertiary care community clinic, or a community clinic physician might also have a private clinic.
- Structural fragmentation is also present within hospitals because physicians are central to resource allocation and care processes in the hospital, yet they are largely independent of hospital management. The principle of physician autonomy is deeply embedded in the laws and regulations governing hospitals. As Harris stated in his article on the internal organization of hospitals, "The net result is one organization split into two disjoint pieces, each with its own objectives, managers, pricing strategy, and constraints" (1977: 468).

These fragmented organizational structures lead to patients obtaining care from multiple entities (e.g., primary care, clinics, hospitals) in a variety of settings, disrupted relationships among physicians and patients, poor information flows, and misaligned incentives that combine to reduce care quality and increase costs (Cebul, Rebitzer, Taylor, and Votruba 2008). In light of the dispersed nature of the health care system and the structural fragmentation of health care organizations, the system needs to focus on integration of the entities—that is, adapt and innovate in order to integrate across the continuum of entities that have entered into formal relationships, but where boundaries still exist.

Organizational climate is simultaneously the source of and solution to integration problems; past research found organizational culture and climate to be barriers to integration (Suter, Oelke, Adair, and Armitage 2009). Clashing organizational cultures were found to be one of the reasons for failed integration efforts because they create a specific mindset that may run counter to the concept of integration. For example, a physician may have a mindset that places the hospital at the center of the process of care; this mindset may run counter to a population-based health care delivery system (Shortell, Gillies, and Anderson 1994). However, organizational culture is conceptually different from organizational climate. While organizational climate refers to the shared meanings people attach to interrelated experiences they have at work, organizational culture is concerned with the basic assumptions about the world and the values that guide life in organizations. It includes the concepts of beliefs, ideology, language, rituals, and myths—and how they could be applied to understanding organizations (Schneider, Ehrhart, and Macey 2013). A number of essays on the qualitative difference between organizational climate and culture (e.g., Schneider, Ehrhart, and Macey 2013) are available to the interested reader. In this chapter, we discuss organizational climate as a mechanism that serves as an "organizational canopy" to integrate dispersed organizational structures. We develop the concept of climate to demonstrate how health care organizations may use it to adapt to new organizational structures and better integrate a dispersed system.

Organizational climate conceptualizes the way people experience and describe their work settings. It represents the sense employees make out of their organization and the essential meaning employees attach to what is the essence of their workplaces. As such, climate touches nearly every aspect of organizational life (Kuenzi and Schminke 2009; Schneider and Barbera 2014). Climate research examines the subjective perceptions of individuals regarding their work environment and how these perceptions drive their behaviors and attitudes (Schneider 2000), as well as their broader work outcomes such as safety (Katz-Navon, Naveh, and Stern 2005) and team performance (Colquitt, Noe, and Jackson 2002).

We discuss the complexities associated with the concept of climate, specifically in the context of a dispersed health care system, and we suggest that climate is an essential tool for integration because it is through shared understandings that integration occurs. Climate can serve as one mechanism that health care organizations need to consider when adopting innovations in response to changes in work organization and care delivery.

We organize the chapter around the two main definitions of the concept of climate. One leading definition describes climate in terms of perceived organizational priorities (Katz-Navon, Naveh, and Stern 2005; Zohar 2000). In a context of scare resources, the climate emphasizes the importance of certain employee behaviors and outcomes over others, such as emphasizing safety over productivity. The core assumption of this definition is the need to prioritize one behavior over others (an "either/or" concept). However, within and between organizations, employees need to balance several priorities, especially when the organization is dispersed and each fragment has different priorities. Examples of this situation may be found in the differences between the priorities of providers of medical services—for example, hospitals that prioritize fast response and lifesaving treatments versus long-term care services such as nursing homes that prioritize long-term individual human relationships with the patients, or between physicians who prioritize the best interests of the individual patient and thus prescribe specific expensive medication versus health maintenance organizations (HMOs) that prioritize economic efficiency. Thus, we suggest expanding the concept of climate into an "and" concept in which employees learn how to balance several priorities.

The second definition refers to climate in terms of shared employee perceptions regarding the practices, procedures, and behaviors that are expected and rewarded by management (Schneider 1990). This definition is transactional in nature (i.e., employees behave according to what they perceive to be management expectations in order to gain rewards). However, we suggest that when organizations are dispersed, a more transformational meaning of climate must be created so that this concept spans organizational boundaries and influences employee behaviors outside any specific organization. Given the reality of simultaneous priorities, for a climate to truly characterize an organization and shape the thoughts and actions of its members, managers and researchers alike need to recognize its transactional and transformational aspects.

UNDERSTANDING CLIMATE AND ITS APPLICATIONS IN HEALTH CARE

The literature suggests two main approaches to the exertion of influence on employee behaviors in organizations. The first approach concentrates on changing the formal organization. For example, in regard to safety behaviors, health care organizations traditionally implement safety procedures and standards to ensure safety performance. The premise behind this approach is that to ensure safety and avoid the costs of adverse events, organizations must invest in the implementation of formal safety programs and risk management systems. In addition, organizations also develop practical interventions to implement safety practices, such as performing routine equipment maintenance and introducing technological safety features that enhance safety.

The second approach to influencing employee behavior is the behavioral approach, which aims to influence behaviors through formal tools, such as training and compensation and informal tools, such as changing the organizational climate. Climate is the employees' informal interpretations of the meaning of a particular form of training, compensation, and other formal tools and leader actions. Management strives to improve and change behaviors by influencing the perceptions of employees. For example, because many patient safety incidents have a behavioral component, management may try to modify safety behaviors by creating a high-safety climate that emphasizes the importance of patient safety—and thus influences employee behaviors and provides an important control mechanism that improves safety performance.

Organizational climate is a complex concept for several reasons. First, climate is a multilevel concept that simultaneously implicates the individual, team, and organizational levels. The concept of climate is qualitatively different at different levels (Chan 1998): psychological climate at the individual level (e.g., Brown, and Leigh 1996; Burke, Borucki, and Kaufman 2002; Glick 1985), as a shared team-level concept (e.g., Baer and Frese 2002; Dragoni 2005; Smith-Jentsch, Salas, and Brannick 2001), and as an organizational-level concept (Denison 1996; Turnipseed and Turnipseed 2013).

At the individual level, psychological climate refers to an employee's perceptions and interpretations of his or her work environment (James, Hater, Gent, and Bruni 1978; James and James 1989). An individual's values influence his or her perceptions of the organizational environment, and the environment takes on a personal meaning and motivational or emotional significance for employees. Psychological climate is an individual rather than an organizational attribute, measured in terms of perceptions that are psychologically meaningful to the individual rather than in terms of concrete organizational features (James, Hater, Gent, and Bruni 1978). When employees perceive the organizational environment positively (i.e., as consistent with their own values and self-interests), they are likely to identify their personal goals with those of the organization and to invest greater effort pursuing them (Brown and Leigh 1996).

Climate as a team-level concept is qualitatively similar to psychological climate; however, it represents the team's shared perceptions. As a team-level concept, climate refers to how organizational environments are collectively perceived and interpreted by team members. Team members come to share similar perceptions because of the similar social and organizational conditions they experience. Thus, they share meaning, motivations, emotions, and cognitive representations and interpretations of the features of the team's work environment. Hence, different teams within the organization may have different levels of climate (Schneider 1990).

Similarly, on the organizational level, perceptions, meaning, motivations, emotions, and interpretations are shared by all members of the organization (although researchers rarely measure hospital/organizational-level climate in health care). Thus, different entities within the same health care organization may have different levels of climate (Wallace et al. 2013).

Second, climate is typically a facet-specific concept and thus is best regarded as a specific construct having a referent; that is, a climate is a climate of something, such as a climate of safety (Katz-Navon, Naveh, and Stern 2005; Naveh, Katz-Navon, and Stern 2005; Zohar 2000), of learning (Katz-Navon, Naveh, and Stern 2009), of innovation (Miron-Spektor, Erez, and Naveh 2011), or of service (Schneider, White, and Paul 1998). For the sake of simplicity and clarity, we use the term "organizational climate" as shorthand for the varied facet-specific climates that exist in organizations. Most of the health care literature on climate focuses on safety climate. Safety in organizations is generally defined as freedom from accidental injury (Perrow 1984; Roberts 1990) and is related to the safety of employees and other organizational stakeholders, such as the organization's customers. In health care, patients are the customers, and patient safety refers to the avoidance, prevention, and amelioration of adverse outcomes or injuries stemming from the processes of health care. These adverse outcomes include errors and accidents caused by medical actions (in contrast to disease complications), events that result from equipment failure, failure to complete a planned action as intended (e.g., surgical events; events involving devices, patient protection, and care), or the use of the wrong plan to achieve an aim (Gaba 2000; Leape 2002).

The informal aspects of the work environment (i.e., safety climate) play an important role in affecting safety (Katz-Navon, Naveh, and Stern 2005; Zohar 2000). Traditionally, safety climate has been studied in industries such as steel mills (Brown, Willis, and Prussia 2000; Zohar 2000), offshore environments (Mearns, Whitaker, and Flin 2003), and highly regulated industries such as nuclear power generation (Carroll, Hatakenaka, and Rudolph 2006). Over the past decade, safety climate has been considered a key organizational variable for understanding the level of patient safety in health care (Katz-Navon, Naveh, and Stern 2005; Naveh, Katz-Navon, and Stern 2006).

To achieve safe patient care, operations require a strong safety climate. A safety climate is necessary to encourage uniformly appropriate responses by staff members. Indeed, a growing body of studies demonstrates that safety climate is positively associated with safe work practices (Gershon et al. 2000) and hospital safety performance (e.g., Singer et al. 2009; Wu, Chen, and Li 2008), while it is negatively associated with medical treatment errors by physicians and nurses (Katz-Navon, Naveh, and Stern 2005; Naveh, Katz-Navon, and Stern 2005, 2006) and with hospital mortality and length of stay (Huang et al. 2010). However, although there is a widespread belief among health care practitioners and managers that safety climate improves safety performance, and numerous studies have been undertaken to develop valid and reliable safety climate scales relevant to health care, only a few studies have demonstrated a relationship between safety climate and positive safety outcomes in health care.

THE CHALLENGES OF BALANCING MULTIPLE CLIMATES

Health care organizations and staff members need to maintain some balance among several—often competing—goals, such as quality, productivity, costs, and innovation. Furthermore, keeping this balance among competing goals is even more challenging in a structurally fragmented system because different components along the continuum of care or different service providers may have different goals. For example, an HMO may prioritize efficiency and productivity, while the health care professionals focus on quality and what they think is the correct treatment for a specific patient. Moreover, hospitals may focus on new, innovative medical equipment and treatments, whereas community clinics may focus on developing relationships with the community in order to prevent illness.

Indeed, one of the agreed-upon definitions of climate refers to it as shared perceived relational priorities assigned to (sometimes competing) goals within an organization and between organizations. This means that the concept of climate represents shared employee perceptions of the priority of specific goals within (or between) the organization(s) over other competing goals. Because multiple goals and climates exist simultaneously within a single organization and between organizations, employees need to balance among priorities, especially in certain situations in which the required performance competes with other performance facets. Furthermore, in fragmented systems, employees need also to balance the priorities of different components of the system, and the literature insufficiently reflects this reality.

Competing priorities may intensify the system's fragmentation, and staff members may need to find ways to integrate those competing priorities. Here are several examples of potentially competing priorities within the fragmented health care system and how staff members may cope with them:

- Staff members perceive the degree of priority assigned to safety within their organization. However, when they share their time between several organizations, they may perceive different levels of priority attributed to safety within these organizations. Such priority refers to employee expectations and daily behaviors regarding the balance maintained among work pace, workload, and pressures for productivity and safety (Zohar 2000). Maintaining patient safety often entails working at a slower pace, investing extra effort, or operating under less comfortable conditions such as wearing gloves and safety glasses. Consequently, whenever work pressure increases, staff members should understand the organizational priorities for safety versus speed or productivity (Katz-Navon, Naveh, and Stern 2005; Stern, Naveh, and Katz-Navon 2008; Zohar 2000). The medical profession's rules and ethics guide the professional behaviors of physicians and help them set their priorities (Naveh, Katz-Navon, and Stern 2005). Physicians, as a group, view their profession's rules and ethics as superseding their organization's requirements. Thus, for instance, when the professional doctrine dictates safety more than the organization does, the organizational intent may receive a lower priority. In such a case, the medical profession's rules and ethics themselves serve as an integration mechanism—that is, physicians behave according to what their profession dictates wherever they are and potentially regardless of management priorities.

• Another priority that is vital for health care professionals in general—and novice professionals in particular, as well as for other professionals in high-reliability industries such as pilots and air traffic controllers or engineers in nuclear power plants—is learning new skills and improving acquired skills. Because the health care industry is characterized by high uncertainty, highly complex tasks, and nonroutine activities, traditional classroom learning cannot encompass all possible daily work situations, and on the job learning, experimentation, and exploration are necessary (Argote 1999; Bell and Kozlowski 2008). However, as learners actively explore the environment, patient safety may be compromised (Katz-Navon, Naveh, and Stern 2009).

This problem may be even more serious in the case of resident physicians. Residents are the front-line providers of the majority of inpatient medical care in teaching hospitals. Residency is a stressful and overwhelming period during which residents work long hours and take responsibility for the lives of the patients in their care. Residents have tremendous responsibility, but at the same time, they are novice practitioners in the process of learning and mastering their profession. Hence, residents may face a dilemma between two important priorities: on the one hand, their need to actively learn and explore, which is at the core of high-quality medicine and, on the other hand, the need to keep patients safe. These contradictory requirements are inherent in such a situation: the learning climate prioritizes exploration, risk taking, and tolerance of mistakes, whereas the safety climate emphasizes control and requires working through acceptable channels, planning, procedures, and rules. Thus, safety may be compromised when learning is prioritized, and learning may be compromised when safety receives high priority (Katz-Navon, Naveh, and Stern 2009).

• Another type of priority gap within an organization can appear between the enacted and espoused priorities of managers—that is, the extent of convergence or divergence between managers' words and deeds. In particular, managers' rhetoric on the importance of safety without actual safety behaviors may be perceived by staff members as nothing more than an empty declaration of intentions, and managers' actual safety behaviors without clear messages of management support of safety would probably not be fully executed. For example, declaring patient safety to be a high priority yet showing a reluctance to purchase safety equipment, or implementing strict patient safety procedures that limit resident working hours while expecting residents to meet high patient quotas may send a message to residents that the procedures could be ignored without consequences.

So how do staff members decide how to behave? From an employee standpoint, the overall pattern and signals sent by this complex web of activities across competing domains and within and between a fragmented system ultimately must be sorted out to discern what behavior is expected, rewarded, and supported (Naveh and Katz-Navon 2014) within a component of the system that he or she works in at a certain point in time. Staff members may react to such conflicting priorities in one of two ways. The first way a staff member may react to this competing priorities dilemma within or among the fragmented parts of the system is by experiencing an intra-role conflict. When the priorities of several conflicting demands or goals are high, there is a "simultaneous occurrence of two or more role expectations such that compliance with one would make compliance with the other more difficult" (Katz and Kahn 1978: 204), which results in an intra-role conflict. Experienced role conflict is negatively associated with employee performance (Katz and Kahn 1978). Thus, for example, linking a conflicting high climate of active learning with a high priority of safety will result in employees experiencing a role conflict, and the result might be low safety performance (Katz-Navon, Naveh, and Stern 2009).

The second way a staff member may react to such a dilemma is by using a complex system of considerations to balance competing priorities. This is a type of contextual ambidexterity (Gibson and Birkinshaw 2004) at the individual level. Contextual ambidexterity is the behavioral capacity to simultaneously demonstrate alignment and adaptability to specific features of the organizational context (e.g., the specific patient's condition, specific bed occupancy in the department, the senior physician who works with the resident at the time, and more). Alignment refers to the ability to integrate differing priorities, while adaptability refers to the capacity to reconfigure activities quickly to meet changing demands in the task. Specifically, a physician who shares her time between a hospital and community clinic may align to the different priorities of each facility by finding a common denominator for both facilities and integrating the different priorities, or she may adapt by changing her behavior according to the specific facility's priorities whenever she is in the hospital or in the clinic.

CLIMATE AS A BOUNDARY SPANNER

Fragmented organizational contexts challenge current organization theory. They call for a broadening of intra-organizational concepts traditionally studied within one organization's boundaries to the inter-organizational level to illustrate their possible influence on employees who transfer among the different system components. Thus, we now relate to why and how climate may span organizational boundaries to influence employee behaviors across organizations.

Climate research has already established the influence of climate on employee behaviors and performance within an organization's physical boundaries. We now propose to study the conditions under which a climate's influence may span organizational boundaries. Would a climate originating within one organization influence the behaviors of employees when they are outside that organization's physical boundaries? This is especially relevant today because the work environment of the 21st century is undergoing major changes in organization and technology, with significant effects on work arrangements (Heydebrand 1989; Hsu and Hannan 2005). Specifically, in health care, many physicians share their time between working in the hospital and working in private or community clinics or other remote institutions. Furthermore, in contemporary work arrangements, employees may work in various environments, such as client organizations, telecommuting, in alternative locations within the customer's organizations, or in international settings in which employees need to cooperate with peers across long geographic distances.

In these examples, how far does the influence of a climate originating within one organization go? To answer this question, we suggest that the influence of climate expands like ripples across the organization's boundaries to reach targets (employees) far removed from its intended or original purpose. We develop five arguments that expand the existing conceptualization of organizational climate to include its influence on employee behaviors when they are outside the organization's physical boundaries. We will do that by integrating climate theory with other topics in management literature, such as leadership and the work–family interface, to better understand the potential impact of climate on staff performance.

Postmodern Organizations

New bodies of knowledge that describe new organizational forms (Heydebrand 1989; Palmer, Benveniste, and Dunford 2007) suggest explanations for climate-spanning organizational boundaries. Specifically, neoclassical organizational theories claim that the traditional characteristics of the formal organization (Weber 1979)—hierarchy, formality, supervision, and boundaries—continue to be central concepts for understanding organizations but are expressed differently in new organizational forms. For example, structures shift from hierarchical to flat (Pettigrew and Fanton 2000), from highly centralized to decentralized management, and from formal rational control that builds on procedures and rules to normative control that builds on organizational culture and climate (Daft and Lewin 1993). This means the boundaries that once confined and defined organizations have eroded and become permeable (e.g., Smith, Carroll, and Ashford 1995). Because the organizations' boundaries are now permeable, a climate that was originated in one organization can transfer to another.

Similarly, postmodern organizational theories suggest that the traditional characteristics of the formal organization can no longer explain a significant portion of work processes today (e.g., Ahrne and Brunsson 2011), and researchers have proposed new work processes for the new era. For example, Barley and Kunda (2001) suggest a new definition of organization as a group of people who share a common professional identity and work together in the same geographic area or when there is no formal organization that controls them.

Other postmodern theories claim that the three main practices that define an organization are learning, common professional identity, and coordination, while a common geographical area is not necessary (Kogut and Zander 1996). Similarly, Mackenzie (2008) posits that a common work process exists whenever there is a common economic interest and a common organizational culture, even in the absence of any other formal organizational characteristics. Wenger, McDermott, and Snyder (2002) define the community of practice as a professional community that operates within and outside work organizations and whose members share knowledge and professional identity.

The main idea in these postmodern theories is that traditional formal organizational controls—structure, hierarchy, and boundaries—are no longer relevant in today's fragmented organizations, and that social mechanisms such as community, culture, ethos, and identity replace them. Hence, climate may span the components of a fragmented system because of permeable organizational boundaries. In particular, the medical profession's rules and ethics, not the formal organization's boundaries, guide physicians' professional behaviors wherever they work (Hekman, Steensma, Bigley, and Hereford 2009).

Perceptions of Organizational Boundaries

The fragmented health care system creates potential barriers to climate-spanning organizational boundaries. The many different types of hospitals—not-for-profit or for-profit, academic (i.e., a research or teaching mission and close associations with research universities and medical schools) or community, and specialty (i.e., focusing on the treatment of a specific disease) or general—may all lead staff members to perceive organizational boundaries as highly salient. In such a case, when organizational boundaries are salient, they may hinder climate from spanning and thus deepen fragmentation. However, these organizational boundaries are real to the individual in the sense that the individual perceives them as such and acts as though they are real (Weick 1979). Therefore, climate perceptions may be especially likely to span perceived organizational boundaries and operate as an integrating mechanism.

Boundary theory (Ashforth, Kreiner, and Fugate 2000) refers to employees' boundary-crossing activity as micro-transitions, or frequent and usually recurring transitions such as work–work (e.g., seeing patients at the hospital and in the community clinic) or work–home (e.g., between the roles of being an employee and being a family member, which is beyond the scope of this chapter). In work–work transitions, individuals may perceive one organization as their home organization and other organizations, outside the home organization's boundaries, as host organizations. Individual perceptions of one organization as the home organization may depend on different considerations. For example, the home organization may be the one in which the employee spends more hours or the one with which the employee identifies more, or it may relate to the way in which the home or host organization tries to define and influence employee identification. A host organization may formally define an employee as external to the organization; however, it also tries to increase the employee's identification with it and make the employee feel as if it were his or her home organization by using different activities.

Psychologically, employees may still perceive that they are within the boundaries of the home organization (Ashforth, Kreiner, and Fugate 2000), especially when the required behaviors in the host organization are part of the employees' jobs, if the employees perform similar roles in the home and host organizations, or when employees act as representatives or members of the organization. Specifically, in the case of health care, a physician is a physician both in the hospital and in the clinic, and thus, psychologically, the physician perceives continuity between what happens in the hospital and in the clinic. In this case, the physician will behave in the host organization according to the climate of the home organization. For example, if the safety climate is high in the hospital, it will influence the physician's safety behavior in the hospital and in the clinic.

The subjective perception of the permeability of the boundaries may also depend on how employees define "self" in relation to the home and to the host organizations. When identification with the home organization is high, employees perceive the boundaries between the home and the host organizations as salient. However, when identification with the home organization is low, employees perceive the boundaries between the home and the host organizations as more permeable (Korschun 2015). A high level of identification with the organization may increase both behaviors based on the climate and perceptions of salient boundaries. Employees will behave according to the home organization climate wherever they are because they see themselves as part of the home organization.

From Transactional to Transformational Influences of Climate

Climate has traditionally been defined as the shared perceptions of employees concerning the kind of behaviors that get rewarded, supported, and expected within the organization (Schneider 1990). According to this definition, employees abide by management expectations in order to gain rewards. This traditional definition of climate is basically transactional in nature—that is, employees conform to the induced behaviors because they understand from the climate that they will receive rewards for specific behaviors or suffer undesirable consequences for deviant behaviors.

However, when organizations are dispersed (e.g., units within a hospital) or when entities along the continuum of care are geographically dispersed, in order for the climate to span unit or organizational boundaries and influence employee behaviors outside a specific organization, climate needs to have a more transformational meaning. By definition, a climate's implicit expectations are shared and thus often socially translated into shared norms (Van Maanen and Barley 1984). Norms are informal rules and codes of behaviors that create pressures for conformity through a decentralized enforcement process in which noncompliance is penalized with social or economic sanctions (North 1990).

Changes in individual behaviors produced by social norms may be a result of two processes whereby the individual accepts influence: compliance and internalization (Kelman 1958). Compliance occurs when individuals behave according to the norm because they hope to achieve a favorable reaction from others. They adopt the induced behavior not because they necessarily believe in it but because they expect to gain specific rewards or approval and avoid specific punishment or disapproval. This is in accordance with the definition of climate in terms of the behaviors that are expected and rewarded within the organization (Schneider 1990). Employees comply with the induced behaviors within the home organization to get rewarded and may conform to the induced behaviors when they are outside the physical boundaries of the home organization only if they believe that they will suffer undesirable consequences or, conversely, receive rewards for specific behaviors that will be known to their home organization manager.

However, unlike this traditional transactional definition of climate, we suggest a definition in which climate has a *transformational* influence on employees, and they internalize the organization's values and norms.

This definition treats the climate as valuable by itself, separately from instrumental benefits. Climate within the organization signals the expected behaviors and priorities of the organization to the employees; as a result, employees internalize the organization's values. Indeed, values are susceptible to change in response to changes in business ideology (Rokeach 1979; Schwartz 1992), such as a change in organizational priorities.

Such changes in value and internalization occur when individuals behave according to what is supported and expected within the organization because the content of the induced behavior—the ideas and actions of which it is composed—is intrinsically rewarding. Individuals adopt the induced behavior because it becomes congruent with their value system and they truly believe in its merit (Kelman 1958). When a value becomes "part of an employee's DNA," it directs not only the way the employee behaves in the home organization but also the way he or she behaves in the host organization (Berry and Seltman 2014).

Hence, the transformational explanation of the influence of climate on employee behaviors is that the climate within the organization transforms employees' values, and they behave in the expected way both inside and outside the organization's physical boundaries because they truly believe that the priorities set by the organization are sound. This type of climate may be more durable and sustainable than the more extrinsic/transactional approach to climate.

Climate as a Control Mechanism

In traditional organizational structures and processes, employees work within the organization's boundaries and are in physical proximity to managers and peers. In such structures, most employees' behaviors are visible to managers and peers, who can supervise or control these behaviors (Erev, Ingram, Raz, and Shany 2010; Ostrom 2000). Particularly in hospitals, most of the time, the work of physicians and nurses is supervised and monitored by managers and peers who work in physical proximity to them inside the hospital.

However, in fragmented organizational structures, the organization's boundaries are permeable, and employees constantly transfer across boundaries and many times are outside the sight of managers and peers—for example, staff members work in shifts around the clock while managers are on the premises only part of the time, or employees work outside the hospital's physical boundaries. In situations such as these, managers have less control over employee behaviors and thus need a substitute for direct supervision (Avolio, Walumbwa, and Weber 2009) that can control employee behavior even when the employees are out of their sight.

Climate may serve as an informal mechanism for such control. For example, an important part of a health care practitioner's work is service.

The service behavior of employees largely occurs outside the direct control of managers; service is co-created between the health care practitioner and the patients, and the many contingencies that influence the way a service experience unfolds cannot easily be predicted. Thus, it is important for health care organizations to cultivate a strong service climate so that staff members understand what is expected of them during contact with patients (Schneider and Bowen 2010; Schneider, White, and Paul 1998). Hence, in the health care context, where a large part of clinical work is executed outside the physical boundaries of the hospital (e.g., clinics and physician practices), in settings where the proximity of the manager and peers is low or even entirely absent—and thus outside the direct control of managers and peers—climate may serve as a control mechanism and as an integrator across a fragmented system.

Spillover and Crossover of Climate

To capture potential transference of climate among the dispersed parts of the systems and between contexts of work, our fifth explanation of the influence of climate across organizational boundaries incorporates the concepts of spillover and crossover from the work–family literature (Edwards and Rothbard 2000; Kanter 1977). *Spillover* refers to an intra-individual contagion process by which cognitions (such as knowledge, values, and attitudes), skills, and behaviors carry over from one context to another for the same individual (Brummelhuis and Bakker 2012; Westman 2001). We suggest that through climate, individuals acquire such cognitions, which spill over from work across the organization's boundaries to other work contexts. By rewarding and supporting specific behaviors, the organization creates a climate that sets specific priorities and importance, as well as values and norms, and provides employees with information and skills. These values, norms, and priorities in turn may spill over or carry over from one work context to another (e.g., from a hospital to a community clinic).

Furthermore, the employee who spans boundaries may diffuse the climate from one context to another. *Crossover* is an inter-individual contagion process in which experiences of one person are transferred to another person; it occurs across contexts and generates similar reactions in another individual (Greenhaus and Powell 2006; Westman 2001). There is a conceptual difference between spillover and crossover: experiences in one domain can be transferred for the same employee from one domain to another domain (i.e., spillover), yet these experiences may not cross over to employees in another domain (Masuda, McNall, Allen, and Nicklin 2012; Westman, Etzion, and Chen 2009).

Experiences following job events in one organization may cross over and have an effect on employees in the other organization. Specifically, the priorities, values, norms, attitudes, and behaviors within a home organization as a result of a climate may be transferred across organizational boundaries (by an employee who crosses those boundaries) and influence the priorities, values, norms, attitudes, and behaviors in a host organization. For example, safety, ethical medicine, and high-quality patient care are behaviors that are encouraged within a hospital by the creation of certain climates (i.e., safety climate, ethical climate, service climate). Those climates are important and should be conducted similarly at the hospital and the community clinic. Specific climates created within a hospital influence the hospital staff members, who spill these behaviors over when they work in the community clinic; these behaviors then cross over to staff members of the community clinic, who adapt behaviors that support safety, ethics, and service.

Another potential crossover is from health care staff to patients—for example, a climate of fitness and healthy lifestyle within the health care facility may cross over to influence patients to improve their fitness and lifestyle. Another example is safety climate: in medical facilities where staff members had positive perceptions of their safety climate, patients also assessed patient safety positively. This suggests that safety climate and patient safety as perceived by the patients are mutually reinforcing and that investments and improvements in one domain positively influence the other (Mohr, Eaton, McPhaul, and Hodgson 2015).

CONCLUSION

Limited resources, continuing cost inflation, and service demand have intensified the need for more effective and efficient use of available resources through integrated service delivery models. We believe that this chapter has significant and viable implications for a broad audience in the organizational and health care management research regarding one potential mechanism to integrate a dispersed system, make integration work for newly merged entities, and aid the implementation of new collaborative organizational forms. Managers and practitioners in the health care system are encouraged to pay attention to how they can use climate to influence staff members' behaviors across structurally fragmented systems.

REFERENCES

Ahrne, G., and N. Brunsson. 2011. "Organization Outside Organizations: The Significance of Partial Organization." *Organization* 18, no. 1: 83–104. doi:10.1177/1350508410376256.

Argote, L. 1999. *Organizational Learning: Creating, Retaining, and Transferring Knowledge.* Boston, MA: Kluwer Academic.

Ashforth, B. E., G. E. Kreiner, and M. Fugate. 2000. "All in a Day's Work: Boundaries and Micro Role Transitions." *Academy of Management Review* 25, no. 3: 472–91. doi:10.5465/amr.2000.3363315.

Avolio, B. J., F. O. Walumbwa, and T. J. Weber. 2009. "Leadership: Current Theories, Research, and Future Directions." *Annual Review of Psychology* 60, no. 1: 421–49. doi:10.1146/annurev.psych.60.110707.163621.

Baer, M., and M. Frese. 2002. "Innovation Is Not Enough: Climates for Initiative and Psychological Safety, Process Innovations, and Firm Performance." *Journal of Organizational Behavior* 24, no. 1: 45–68. doi:10.1002/job.179.

Barley, S. R., and G. Kunda. 2001. "Bringing Work Back In." *Organization Science* 12, no. 1: 76–95. doi:10.1287/orsc.12.1.76.10122.

Bell, B. S., and S. W. J. Kozlowski. 2008. "Active Learning: Effects of Core Training Design Elements on Self-Regulatory Processes, Learning, and Adaptability." *Journal of Applied Psychology* 93, no. 2: 296–316. doi:10.1037/0021-9010.93.2.296.

Berry, L. M., and K. E. Seltman. 2014. "The Mayo Clinic Way: A Story of Cultural Strength and Sustainability." In *The Oxford Handbook of Organizational Climate and Culture*, edited by B. Schneider and K. M. Barbera, 603–19. Oxford, UK: Oxford University Press.

Brown, K. A., P. G. Willis, and G. E. Prussia. 2000. "Predicting Safe Employee Behavior in the Steel Industry: Development and Test of a Sociotechnical Model." *Journal of Operations Management* 18, no. 4: 445–65. doi:10.1016/s0272-6963(00)00033-4.

Brown, S. P., and T. W. Leigh. 1996. "A New Look at Psychological Climate and Its Relationship to Job Involvement, Effort, and Performance." *Journal of Applied Psychology* 81, no. 4: 358–68. doi:10.1037/0021-9010.81.4.358.

Brummelhuis, L. L. T., and A. B. Bakker. 2012. "A Resource Perspective on the Work–Home Interface: The Work–Home Resources Model." *American Psychologist* 67, no. 7: 545–56. doi:10.1037/a0027974.

Burke, M. J., C. C. Borucki, and J. D. Kaufman. 2002. "Contemporary Perspectives on the Study of Psychological Climate: A Commentary." *European Journal of Work and Organizational Psychology* 11, no. 3: 325–40. doi:10.1080/13594320244000210.

Carroll, J. S., S. Hatakenaka, and J. W. Rudolph. 2006. "Naturalistic Decision Making and Organizational Learning in Nuclear Power Plants: Negotiating Meaning Between Managers and Problem Investigation Teams." *Organization Studies* 27, no. 7: 1037–57. doi:10.1177/0170840606065709.

Cebul, R. D., J. B. Rebitzer, L. J. Taylor, and M. E. Votruba. 2008. "Organizational Fragmentation and Care Quality in the U.S. Healthcare System." *Journal of Economic Perspectives* 22, no. 4: 93–113. doi:10.1257/jep.22.4.93.

Chan, D. 1998. "Functional Relations Among Constructs in the Same Content Domain at Different Levels of Analysis: A Typology of Composition Models." *Journal of Applied Psychology* 83, no. 2: 234–46. doi:10.1037/0021-9010.83.2.234.

Coburn, A. F. 2001. "Models for Integrating and Managing Acute and Long-Term Care Services in Rural Areas." *Journal of Applied Gerontology* 20, no. 4: 386–408. doi:10.1177/073346480102000402.

Colquitt, J. A., R. A. Noe, and C. L. Jackson. 2002. "Justice in Teams: Antecedents and Consequences of Procedural Justice Climate." *Personnel Psychology* 55, no. 1: 83–109. doi:10.1111/j.1744-6570.2002.tb00104.x.

Daft, R. L., and A. Y. Lewin. 1993. "Where Are the Theories for the New Organizational Forms?" *Organization Science* 4, no. 4: 1–6.

Denison, D. R. 1996. "What Is the Difference Between Organizational Culture and Organizational Climate? A Native's Point of View on a Decade of Paradigm Wars." *Academy of Management Review* 21, no. 3: 619–54.

Dragoni, L. 2005. "Understanding the Emergence of State Goal Orientation in Organizational Work Groups: The Role of Leadership and Multilevel Climate Perceptions." *Journal of Applied Psychology* 90, no. 6: 1084–95. doi:10.1037/0021-9010.90.6.1084.

Edwards, J. R., and N. P. Rothbard. 2000. "Mechanisms Linking Work and Family: Clarifying the Relationship Between Work and Family Constructs." *Academy of Management Review* 25, no. 1: 178–99. doi:10.5465/amr.2000.2791609.

Erev, I., P. Ingram, O. Raz, and D. Shany. 2010. "Continuous Punishment and the Potential of Gentle Rule Enforcement." *Behavioural Processes* 84, no. 1: 366–71. doi:10.1016/j.beproc.2010.01.008.

Fisher, E. S., D. O. Staiger, J. P. W. Bynum, and D. J. Gottlieb. 2006. "Creating Accountable Care Organizations: The Extended Hospital Medical Staff." *Health Affairs* 26, no. 1: w44–w57. doi:10.1377/hlthaff.26.1.w44.

Gaba, D. M. 2000. "Structural and Organizational Issues in Patient Safety: A Comparison of Health Care to Other High-Hazard Industries." *California Management Review* 43, no. 1: 83–102. doi:10.2307/41166067.

Gershon, R. R., C. D. Karkashian, J. W. Grosch, L. R. Murphy, A. Escamilla-Cejudo, P. A. Flanagan, E. Bernacki, C. Kasting, and L. Martin. 2000. "Hospital Safety Climate and Its Relationship with Safe Work Practices and Workplace Exposure Incidents." *American Journal of Infection Control* 28, no. 3: 211–21. doi:10.1067/mic.2000.105288.

Gibson, C. B., and J. Birkinshaw. 2004. "The Antecedents, Consequences, and Mediating Role of Organizational Ambidexterity." *Academy of Management Journal* 47, no. 2: 209–26. doi:10.2307/20159573.

Glick, W. H. 1985. "Conceptualizing and Measuring Organizational and Psychological Climate: Pitfalls in Multilevel Research." *Academy of Management Review* 10, no. 2: 601–16. doi:10.5465/amr.1985.4279045.

Greenhaus, J. H., and G. N. Powell. 2006. "When Work and Family Are Allies: A Theory of Work-Family Enrichment." *Academy of Management Review* 31, no. 1: 72–92. doi: 10.5465/amr.2006.19379625.

Hardy, B., I. Mur-Veeman, M. Steenbergen, and G. Wistow. 1999. "Inter-Agency Services in England and The Netherlands: A Comparative Study of Integrated Care Development and Delivery." *Health Policy* 48, no. 2: 87–105. doi:10.1016/s0168-8510(99)00037-8.

Harris, J. E. 1977. "The Internal Organization of Hospitals: Some Economic Implications." *The Bell Journal of Economics* 8, no. 2: 467. doi:10.2307/3003297.

Hekman, D. R., H. K. Steensma, G. A. Bigley, and J. F. Hereford. 2009. "Effects of Organizational and Professional Identification on the Relationship Between Administrators' Social Influence and Professional Employees' Adoption of New Work Behavior." *Journal of Applied Psychology* 94, no. 5: 1325–35. doi:10.1037/a0015315.

Heydebrand, W. V. 1989. "New Organizational Forms." *Work and Occupations* 16, no. 3: 323–57. doi:10.1177/0730888489016003004.

Hsu, G., and M. T. Hannan. 2005. "Identities, Genres, and Organizational Forms." *Organization Science* 16, no. 5: 474–90. doi:10.1287/orsc.1050.0151.

Huang, D. T., G. Clermont, L. Kong, L. A. Weissfeld, J. B. Sexton, K. M. Rowan, and D. C. Angus. 2010. "Intensive Care Unit Safety Culture and Outcomes: A US Multicenter Study." *International Journal for Quality in Health Care* 22, no. 3: 151–61. doi:10.1093/intqhc/mzq017.

James, L. A., and L. R. James. 1989. "Integrating Work Environment Perceptions: Explorations into the Measurement of Meaning." *Journal of Applied Psychology* 74, no. 5: 739–51. doi:10.1037/0021-9010.74.5.739.

James, L. R., J. J. Hater, M. J. Gent, and J. R. Bruni. 1978. "Psychological Climate: Implications from Cognitive Social Learning Theory and Interactional Psychology." *Personnel Psychology* 31, no. 4: 783–813. doi:10.1111/j.1744-6570.1978.tb02124.x.

Kanter, R. M. 1977. *Men and Women of the Corporation.* Vol. 5049. New York, NY: Basic Books.

Katz, D., and R. L. Kahn. 1978. *The Social Psychology of Organizations.* New York, NY: Wiley.

Katz-Navon, T., E. Naveh, and Z. Stern. 2005. "Safety Climate in Health Care Organizations: A Multidimensional Approach." *Academy of Management Journal* 48, no. 6: 1075–89. doi:10.5465/amj.2005.19573110.

Katz-Navon, T., E. Naveh, and Z. Stern. 2009. "Active Learning: When Is More Better? The Case of Resident Physicians' Medical Errors." *Journal of Applied Psychology* 94, no. 5: 1200–1209. doi:10.1037/a0015979.

Kelman, H. C. 1958. "Compliance, Identification, and Internalization: Three Processes of Attitude Change." *Journal of Conflict Resolution* 2, no. 1: 51–60. doi:10.1177/002200275800200106.

Kogut, B., and U. Zander. 1996. "What Firms Do? Coordination, Identity, and Learning." *Organization Science* 7, no. 5: 502–18. doi:10.1287/orsc.7.5.502.

Korschun, D. 2015. "Boundary-Spanning Employees and Relationships with External Stakeholders: A Social Identity Approach." *Academy of Management Review* 40, no. 4: 611–29. doi:10.5465/amr.2012.0398.

Kuenzi, M., and M. Schminke. 2009. "Assembling Fragments into a Lens: A Review, Critique, and Proposed Research Agenda for the Organizational Work Climate Literature." *Journal of Management* 35, no. 3: 634–717. doi:10.1177/0149206308330559.

Leape, L. L. 2002. "Reporting of Adverse Events." *New England Journal of Medicine* 347, no. 20: 1633–38. doi:10.1056/nejmnejmhpr011493.

Mackenzie, R. 2008. "From Networks to Hierarchies: The Construction of a Subcontracting Regime in the Irish Telecommunications Industry." *Organization Studies* 29, no. 6: 867–86. doi:10.1177/0170840608088706.

Masuda, A. D., L. A. McNall, T. D. Allen, and J. M. Nicklin. 2012. "Examining the Constructs of Work-to-Family Enrichment and Positive Spillover." *Journal of Vocational Behavior* 80, no. 1: 197–210. doi:10.1016/j.jvb.2011.06.002.

Mearns, K., S. M. Whitaker, and R. Flin. 2003. "Safety Climate, Safety Management Practice and Safety Performance in Offshore Environments." *Safety Science* 41, no. 8: 641–80. doi:10.1016/s0925-7535(02)00011-5.

Miron-Spektor, E., M. Erez, and E. Naveh. 2011. "The Effect of Conformist and Attentive-to-Detail Members on Team Innovation: Reconciling the Innovation Paradox." *Academy of Management Journal* 54, no. 4: 740–60. doi:10.5465/amj.2011.64870100.

Mohr, D. C., J. L. Eaton, K. M. McPhaul, and M. J. Hodgson. 2015. "Does Employee Safety Matter for Patients Too? Employee Safety Climate and Patient Safety Culture in Health Care." *Journal of Patient Safety* (e-pub). doi:10.1097/pts.0000000000000186.

Naveh, E., and T. Katz-Navon. 2014. "Longitudinal Study of Road Safety Climate Intervention: Climate as Organizational Boundary Spanner." *Academy of Management Proceedings* 2014, no. 1: 12762. doi:10.5465/ambpp.2014.12762abstract.

Naveh, E., T. Katz-Navon, and Z. Stern. 2005. "Treatment Errors in Healthcare: A Safety Climate Approach." *Management Science* 51, no. 6: 948–60. doi:10.1287/mnsc.1050.0372.

Naveh, E., T. Katz-Navon, and Z. Stern. 2006. "Readiness to Report Medical Treatment Errors: The Effects of Safety Procedures, Safety Information, and Priority of Safety." *Medical Care* 44, no. 2: 117–23. doi:10.1097/01.mlr.0000197035.12311.88.

North, D. C. 1990. *Institutions, Institutional Change, and Economic Performance.* Cambridge, UK: Cambridge University Press.

Ostrom, E. 2000. "Collective Action and the Evolution of Social Norms." *Journal of Economic Perspectives* 14, no. 3: 137–58. doi:10.1257/jep.14.3.137.

Palmer, I., J. Benveniste, and R. Dunford. 2007. "New Organizational Forms: Towards a Generative Dialogue." *Organization Studies* 28, no. 12: 1829–47. doi:10.1177/0170840607079531.

Perrow, C. 1984. *Normal Accidents: Living with High-Risk Technologies.* New York, NY: Basic Books.

Pettigrew, A. M., and E. M. Fanton. 2000. *The Innovating Organization.* London, UK: Sage.

Roberts, K. H. 1990. "Managing High Reliability Organizations." *California Management Review* 32, no. 4: 101–13. doi:10.2307/41166631.

Rokeach, M. 1979. *Understanding Human Values: Individual and Societal.* New York, NY: Free Press.

Schneider, B., ed. 1990. *Organizational Climate and Culture.* San Francisco, CA: Jossey-Bass.

Schneider, B. 2000. "The Psychological Life of Organizations." In *Handbook of Organizational Culture and Climate*, edited by N. M. Ashkanasy, C. P. M. Wilderom, and M. F. Peterson, xvii-xxi. Thousand Oaks, CA: Sage.

Schneider, B., and K. M. Barbera. 2014. "Introduction." In *The Oxford Handbook of Organizational Climate and Culture*, edited by B. Schneider and K. M. Barbera, 3–22. Oxford, UK: Oxford University Press.

Schneider, B., and D. E. Bowen. 2010. *Winning the Service Game.* New York, NY: Springer U.S.

Schneider, B., M. G. Ehrhart, and W. H. Macey. 2013. "Organizational Climate and Culture." *Annual Review of Psychology* 64: 361–88.

Schneider, B., S. S. White, and M. C. Paul. 1998. "Linking Service Climate and Customer Perceptions of Service Quality: Tests of a Causal Model." *Journal of Applied Psychology* 83, no. 2: 150–63. doi:10.1037/0021-9010.83.2.150.

Schwartz, S. H. 1992. "Universals in the Content and Structure of Values: Theoretical Advances and Empirical Tests in 20 Countries." *Advances in Experimental Social Psychology* 25, no. 1: 1–65. doi:10.1016/s0065-2601(08)60281-6.

Shortell, S. M., R. R. Gillies, and D. A. Anderson. 1994. "The New World of Managed Care: Creating Organized Delivery Systems." *Health Affairs* 13, no. 5: 46–64. doi:10.1377/hlthaff.13.5.46.

Singer, S., S. Lin, A. Falwell, D. Gaba, and L. Baker. 2009. "Relationship of Safety Climate and Safety Performance in Hospitals." *Health Services Research* 44, no. 2p1: 399–421. doi:10.1111/j.1475-6773.2008.00918.x.

Smith, K. G., S. J. Carroll, and S. J. Ashford. 1995. "Intra- and Interorganizational Cooperation: Toward a Research Agenda." *Academy of Management Journal* 38, no. 4: 7–23. doi:10.2307/256726.

Smith-Jentsch, K. A., E. Salas, and M. T. Brannick. 2001. "To Transfer or Not to Transfer? Investigating the Combined Effects of Trainee Characteristics, Team Leader Support, and Team Climate." *Journal of Applied Psychology* 86, no. 2: 279–92. doi:10.1037/0021-9010.86.2.279.

Stern, Z., T. Katz-Navon, and E. Naveh. 2008. "The Influence of Situational Learning Orientation, Autonomy, and Voice on Error Making: The Case of Resident Physicians." *Management Science* 54, no. 9: 1553–64. doi:10.1287/mnsc.1080.0862.

Suter, E., N. Oelke, C. Adair, and G. Armitage. 2009. "Ten Key Principles for Successful Health Systems Integration." *Healthcare Quarterly* 13, Spec. No.: 16–23. doi:10.12927/hcq.2009.21092.

Turnipseed, P. H., and D. L. Turnipseed. 2013. "Testing the Proposed Linkage Between Organizational Citizenship Behaviours and an Innovative Organizational Climate." *Creativity and Innovation Management* 22, no. 4: 209–16. doi:10.1111/caim.12027.

Van Maanen, J., and S. Barley. 1984. "Occupational Communities: Culture and Control in Organizations." *Research in Organizational Behavior* 6: 287–365.

Wallace, J. C., B. D. Edwards, J. Paul, M. Burke, M. Christian, and G. Eissa. 2013. "Change the Referent? A Meta-Analytic Investigation of Direct and Referent-Shift Consensus Models for Organizational Climate." *Journal of Management* 39, no. 1: 1–24. doi:10.1177/0149206313484520.

Weber, M. 1979. *From Max Weber: Essays in Sociology*. Abingdon, UK: Routledge.

Weick, K. E. 1979. *The Social Psychology of Organizing* (2nd edition). Reading, MA: Addison-Wesley.

Wenger, E., R. A. McDermott, and W. Snyder. 2002. *Cultivating Communities of Practice: A Guide to Managing Knowledge*. Boston, MA: Harvard Business School Press.

Westman, M. 2001. "Stress and Strain Crossover." *Human Relations* 54, no. 6: 717–51. doi:10.1177/0018726701546002.

Westman, M., D. Etzion, and S. Chen. 2009. "Crossover of Positive Experiences from Business Travelers to Their Spouses." *Journal of Managerial Psychology* 24, no. 3: 269–84. doi:10.1108/02683940910939340.

Wilensky, G. R., N. Wolter, and M. M. Fischer. 2006. "Gain Sharing: A Good Concept Getting a Bad Name?" *Health Affairs* 26, no. 1: w58–w67. doi:10.1377/hlthaff.26.1.w58.

Wu, T.-C., C.-H. Chen, and C.-C. Li. 2008. "A Correlation Among Safety Leadership, Safety Climate and Safety Performance." *Journal of Loss Prevention in the Process Industries* 21, no. 3: 307–18. doi:10.1016/j.jlp.2007.11.001.

Zohar, D. 2000. "A Group-Level Model of Safety Climate: Testing the Effect of Group Climate on Microaccidents in Manufacturing Jobs." *Journal of Applied Psychology* 85, no. 4: 587–96. doi:10.1037/0021-9010.85.4.587.

Health Care Providers and Patients in Sync: Antecedents for Optimizing Provider and Patient Safety Outcomes

DEIRDRE MCCAUGHEY

Department of Health Services Administration
University of Alabama at Birmingham

GWEN MCGHAN

School of Nursing
University of Alabama at Birmingham

BACKGROUND

November 1999 saw the first definitive movement toward specifically pursuing better health care outcomes through the release of the Institute of Medicine's (IOM) seminal report on health care quality, *To Err Is Human* (Institute of Medicine 1999). The report focused attention on the estimated number of annual deaths attributable to preventable lapses in safety and served as a catalyst in driving patient safety to the forefront of industry focus.

Three salient facts emerged from the IOM (1999) report: first, safety lapses were ranked as the eighth leading cause of death in the United States; second, the estimated cost of these lapses was approximately $29 billion annually; and third, most of these preventable errors derived from systemic errors rather than being the "fault" of a care provider (Gandhi 2015). Driven by these three important issues, the IOM (1999) report launched a robust and continually evolving patient safety movement that has witnessed the emergence of think tanks and institutions devoted to improving processes and systems in pursuit of error-free patient care.

Simultaneously, the rate of employee injury and illness in the health care sector in United States rose substantially. Currently, and reflecting this trend over the past decade, the reported number of work-derived illnesses and injuries in health care is among the highest rates of all industries in the United States. Shockingly, the health care sector accounts for the greatest percentage (20.7%) of private industry nonfatal occupational injuries among all industry sectors (Gomaa et al. 2015). For example, in 2013, nurses and nursing assistants in federal and state government institutions had occupational injury rates of 13.6 cases and 19.2 cases per 100 workers, respectively, while the national average across all industries was 3.7 per 100 workers (U.S. Bureau of Labor Statistics 2013). Particularly concerning are the high rates of injuries requiring work absences. For example, musculoskeletal injuries, a key source of injuries requiring absences, represent approximately 34% of all worker absences and occur frequently among nurses and nursing aides (U.S. Bureau of Labor Statistics 2013). Nursing aides have the fifth highest rate of musculoskeletal injuries among U.S. workers, while nurses have the sixth highest rate (U.S. Bureau of Labor Statistics 2013). Given these numbers, it is not surprising that a recent U.S. Department of Labor Secretary identified the health care industry as a major source of all U.S. workplace injuries: "We remain concerned that more workers are injured in the health care and social assistance industry sector[s] than in any other, including construction and manufacturing" (U.S. Department of Labor Occupational Safety and Health Administration 2011).

Workplace-related injuries and illnesses also impose staggering financial costs. According to the Liberty Mutual Workplace Safety Index (2016), worker injury in the United States led to $61.88 billion in direct worker compensation costs, which equates to over $1 billion per week. Including the injury costs paid by private and employer insurance, in addition to those covered by worker compensation, studies estimate the total economic impact of occupational injury to be approximately $250 billion (Leigh 2011; Leigh and Marcin 2012).

While it is difficult to determine exact compensation costs by industry-specific titles, one study found injuries experienced by direct care workers (i.e., nursing assistants, home health aides) account for approximately 11.5% of all worker injury costs in the United States (Waehrer, Leigh, and Miller 2005). Another study estimated the direct and indirect costs associated with back injuries in the health care industry are approximately $20 billion annually (Collins, Nelson, and Sublet 2006).

These statistics offer evidence that working within the health care industry is inherently dangerous. Despite the enormous cost to the health care industry and the staggering rate of injuries and illnesses, no report about the occupational wellness of the health care workforce has catalyzed an industry response to occupational injury and illness in the health care industry as *To Err Is Human* (Institute of Medicine 1999) did for patient safety. As such, the purpose of this paper is to propose an overarching model to integrate research on patient safety and employee safety so that both might be addressed simultaneously. Achieving this integration will provide health care organizations with the tools by which they may better optimize safety outcomes for their patients while simultaneously improving workplace injury and illness incident rates.

THE PATIENT SAFETY MOVEMENT

Following the release of the IOM's *To Err Is Human* (1999) report, health care organizations were encouraged to develop an organizational environment that would support the definition and creation of a culture in which patient safety was a critical organizational priority (Sammer et al. 2010). This safety movement was further bolstered by government agencies and health care organizations demanding that patient safety become a key indicator of health care quality. The Joint Commission led this undertaking in establishing the National Patient Safety Goals and promoting systematic tools, such as Failure Mode and Effects Analysis, to promote proactive examinations of systems and processes that contribute to safety failure (Joint Commission Resources 2010).

Public reporting of patient safety incidents became widespread. In 2002, the National Quality Forum identified 27 serious, adverse events as being largely preventable. Concurrently, the Centers for Medicare and Medicaid Services (CMS) launched a series of quality measurement and quality reporting initiatives for nursing homes, home health agencies, and hospitals, including metrics measuring safety event frequency and degree of harm (Colmers 2007).

A further implementation of Medicare payment reductions for non-reporting resulted in hospitals submitting the required quality (safety) outcomes data. Private organizations also joined in the drive toward public access to health care outcome accountability through the creation of subscription-based (e.g., Consumer Reports) and free websites (e.g., HealthGrades, Leapfrog Hospital Safety Score) that provide data on patient outcome reporting by hospitals, physicians, nursing homes, and home health agencies (Colmers 2007).

The Agency for Healthcare Research and Quality (AHRQ) adopted a definition of patient safety culture that remains widely used throughout the industry (Sammer et al. 2010):

> The safety culture of an organization is the product of individual and group values, attitudes, perceptions, competencies, and patterns of behavior that determine the commitment to, and the style and proficiency of, an organization's health and safety management. (Health and Safety Commission Advisory Committee on the Safety of Nuclear Installations 1993)

Using this foundational definition, AHRQ developed and launched its patient safety measurement tool, Hospital Survey on Patient Safety Culture, in 2004. Since then, it has continually adapted the tool in an attempt to measure the safety culture within organizations including hospitals, medical offices, ambulatory surgery centers, and nursing homes. The patient safety culture tool measures a variety of subareas and helps health care organizations understand what their employees believe about the culture of safety that interacts with patient care.

While there are a number of safety culture tools and components, Sammer and colleagues' (2010) literature review of patient safety culture helps to categorize the general properties that contribute to creating a robust patient safety culture: leadership, teamwork, evidence-based (care practices), communication (e.g., speaking up), learning (the organization's learning capacity), just (errors are recognized as system rather than individual failures), and patient-centered. These factors are found to be critical to organizations' (or units) creating an optimal patient safety culture in which preventable adverse patient safety events are reduced and outcomes are optimized (Sammer et al. 2010).

As a result of these surveys, an entire body of literature emerged examining the relationship between perceptions of safety culture and patient outcomes. In general, organizations and units that score high on patient safety culture surveys tend to have lower rates of patient safety adverse events and higher patient satisfaction (Aiken et al. 2012; Hoff, Jameson, Hannan, and Flink 2004; Singer, Lin et al. 2009). Clearly, health care organizations can benefit by investing resources and energy into strengthening their patient safety culture.

EMPLOYEE SAFETY CLIMATE

As previously noted, safety in the realm of patient outcomes and care is delineated by the term "safety culture." Safety culture is meant to describe the values, norms, and assumptions held by employees regarding the safety in an organization (Reiman and Rollenhagen 2014; Sammer et al. 2010). The deeper values are often reflected in and measured by shared perceptions of existing safety policies, procedures, and practices and are referred to as safety climate (Flin 2007). In other words, safety climate is a snapshot in time of employee beliefs about safety, linked to specific and identifiable policies and practices (Flin 2007). Thus, in this chapter we use the term "patient safety climate" when we refer to facets of both patient safety and employee safety.

A separate yet similar climate exists within organizations and reflects employee perceptions of the organizational climate and leadership, as well as experiential factors (e.g., being injured at work) that foster individual opinions of the workplace as potentially harmful or safe for the individual (Carr, Schmidt, Ford, and DeShon 2003; Parker et al. 2003). Referred to as "employee safety climate" in the occupational health and safety literature, it reflects a broad concept encompassing employee perceptions of safety practices, safety knowledge, organizational safety policies, and safety training, among other factors (McCaughey, DelliFraine, McGhan, and Bruning 2013; Neal, Griffin, and Hart 2000). In keeping with the established norms of the extant occupational health and safety literature, in this chapter we use the term "employee safety climate" when we refer to facets of employee health and safety.

A substantial body of research examining employee safety climate has established that individuals who perceive their organization as valuing safety are more likely to comply with safety standards and practices (Christian, Bradley, Wallace, and Burke 2009; Colley, Lincolne, and Neal 2013). In addition, research further supports a general, positive relationship between an individual's safety/risk perceptions and subsequent employee performance (McCaughey et al. 2014; Neal, Griffin, and Hart 2000). Organizations with a perceived positive employee safety climate—including safety training and safety knowledge—show evidence of enhanced employee safety behaviors, which aids in minimizing workplace hazards and reduces incidents of work-derived injury and illness (Burke et al. 2008; Neal, Griffin, and Hart 2000).

Moreover, employees who express high commitment to workplace safety also perceive high levels of environmental support for employee safety from supervisors, managers, and the organization (Carr, Schmidt, Ford, and DeShon 2003; McCaughey, Halbesleben et al. 2013). Employee safety climate has been found to be related to managerial attitudes, employee organizational commitment, retention rates, injury rates, and work performance (Carr, Schmidt, Ford, and DeShon 2003; Clarke 2006; Smith-Crowe, Burke, and Landis 2003).

From a holistic perspective, health psychologists argue that employee safety climate is a critical component of "healthy" work environments (Danna and Griffin 1999). Workplaces characterized by high injury risk, violence, high strain, and chronic stress have been linked to adverse health outcomes for the employees such as burnout, high injury rates, and depression (Clarke 2006; Danna and Griffin 1999), problems commonly found in health care organizations. Additionally, a workplace-derived injury or illness can shape employee climate perceptions and influence subsequent workplace performance/behavior (Colley, Lincolne, and Neal 2013; McCaughey et al. 2014).

Given the high injury/illness rates of health care workers in the United States and the negative effect a poor employee safety climate has on employee and organization outcomes, it would seem logical to focus attention on this issue and bring it to the forefront of organizational priorities in health care. Equally deserving focus is an integrative research agenda examining and integrating the factors of patient safety with facets of employee safety—thus providing organizations a synergistic opportunity to optimize safety outcomes for all.

Flin's (2007) review of the health care safety literature identified inconsistencies across safety climate definitions, the interchangeable use of the terms "safety climate" and "safety culture," the lack of specific theoretical work to delineate antecedents of employee and patient safety, and a lack of health care–specific studies examining patient safety and employee safety climate concurrently and their relationship with adverse safety events for both employees and patients. In identifying industry best safety practices and evaluating them with regard to health care studies, Flin proposes a Model of Safety Climate and Injury Outcomes (Figure 1). This model attempts to address the limitations previously noted, while accounting for the uniqueness of health care's employee/patient safety outcomes duality. It is important to note that Flin uses the term "safety climate" to encompass the dual ethos of employee safety climate and patient safety climate.

Flin's (2007) model suggests that the existing safety climate contributes to both motivation (e.g., expectations for outcomes of particular behavior) and unsafe behaviors (e.g., rule breaking and risk taking), resulting in errors that may lead to patient and/or worker injury. The frequency and degree of employee and patient injuries indicate the need for a specific health care model. This type of model would allow for the examination of the adverse event pathways to determine whether the processes contributing to errors and injury are the same for employees and patients.

FIGURE 1
Model of Safety Climate and Injury Outcomes (adapted from Flin 2007)

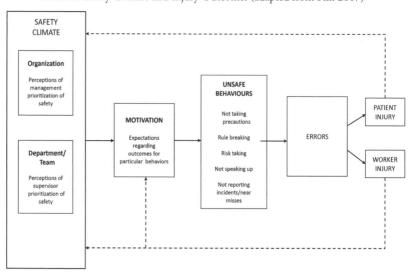

INTEGRATING PATIENT AND EMPLOYEE SAFETY CLIMATE

Flin's (2007) review of the safety climate literature is one of the first to propose similar antecedent pathways that lead to both patient adverse events (e.g., "never events," which are serious, but largely preventable, clinical events) (National Quality Forum 2011) and employee adverse events (e.g., back injury). The Model of Safety Climate and Injury Outcomes (Figure 1) takes information on safety climate from the extant literature and applies it to the health care sector, thus establishing an antecedent safety climate that is defined by employee perceptions of the prioritization of safety at two levels of management: the organizational level (senior management) and the department/unit level (supervisor). These beliefs may then serve as the primary antecedent for employee safety motivation and subsequent behaviors, which in turn may lead to errors that result in adverse safety events for patients and employees.

Similar to a cause-and-effect reaction, employee perceptions of safety serve as a motivational factor (the underlying expectations regarding the outcomes for specific safety behavior) that drives the employee to pursue and follow safe work practices (Figure 1). For example, an employee who perceives a low level of organizational support for safety may feel pressured to pursue a more expedient course of action and not follow a no-lift policy. This may result in the decision to perform a solo transfer/lift of a patient rather than use the provided equipment. The care provider who decides to perform a solo transfer may injure herself or himself or even drop the patient during the transfer. Employees in health care organizations are often faced with difficult choices; when pressed for time should one follow a more time-consuming safety protocol or engage in an action that may be more expeditious but puts the patient and care provider at increased risk for an adverse event or injury? Low commitment to safety procedures results in taking an unsafe action that may be the starting point for an adverse event (Flin 2007).

The simplicity of Flin's (2007) model coupled with its core facets of patient and employee safety climate provides a framework allowing health care organizations to influence individual care provider behavior. Integrating the model to examine both patient safety and the safety of care providers facilitates targeting safety improvement for both simultaneously.

Although Flin's (2007) model highlights the potential for integration, research examining safety climate has been slow to do so. There is, however, a movement arising in prominent institutions to recognize the synergistic relationship between the outcomes for employees and the patients for whom they provide care. The Joint Commission's monograph, *Improving Patient and Worker Safety* (2012), identifies synergies for addressing safety climate for patients and care providers. Specific to the health care industry, the Occupational Safety and Health Administration (OSHA) has identified organizational safety climate as the key foundation for linking patient and employee safety programs and outcomes (U.S. Department of Labor Occupational Safety and Health Administration, no date). Finally, the current president of the National Patient Safety Foundation, Tejal Gandhi (2015) has specifically linked the climate and environment of health care organizations to patient and care provider outcomes. These industry-leading institutions may yet provide the needed catalyst for a call to action regarding health care provider safety as *To Err Is Human* (1999) has done for patient safety.

This catalyst is critically needed given the staggering adverse event frequency at which health care industry employees are injured at work (U.S. Bureau of Labor Statistics 2013). With public reporting of adverse patient safety events, organizations are driven to acknowledge and address instances where patient safety is poor. Furthermore, they are now often financially penalized for adverse safety events by programs such as the Centers for Medicare and Medicaid's Hospital-Acquired Condition Reduction (HAC) program (Centers for Medicare and Medicaid Services, no date), a program that lowers hospitals' reimbursements for services as a result of poor performance in reducing HACs. These are but two examples of the drivers that motivate health care organizations to actively examine their patient safety performance metrics.

Occupational wellness statistics are not publicly reported by organizations, and public accountability is therefore absent. Were organizations required to publicly report on employee occupational wellness outcomes, it is probable they would demonstrate a more robust response to adverse employee safety events. Therein lies one of the most significant barriers to eliciting a greater response to employee occupational wellness and to integrate employee safety with patient safety—there is little impetus and motivation for organizations to take that step.

NEXT STEPS: INTEGRATING SAFETY OUTCOMES

With the growing commonality between the fields of patient and employee safety, a guiding framework is required to integrate and identify mechanisms that minimize adverse safety events for patients and care providers. While Flin's (2007) model is instrumental to understanding the individual pathways for employees and patients, it does not capture the multiplicity of workplace factors that have a role in whether an adverse safety event will happen. Such factors include staffing levels, process training, safety training, team cohesiveness, coworker support, and the environment for safety actions (such as stopping processes and error reporting). To address the complexity of the environment, a framework accounting for organizational influences on employee actions is critical to a research agenda linking patient and care provider safety.

One such framework was developed to capture workforce factors and to identify how organizational practices influence the quality of employee work life and the subsequent effect on employee on-the-job safety and health. Depicted in Figure 2, the framework developed by the National Institute for Occupational Safety and Health (NIOSH) facilitates the work of occupational safety and health researchers in examining factors contributing to employee illness and injury (Sauter et al. 2002).

In this framework, the pathways to employee adverse safety events (described in detail in the following paragraphs) are posited to be similar to patient adverse safety event pathways. The NIOSH framework offers a rich foundation from which to integrate patient safety and employee safety and has been found to be a valid foundation for occupational health and safety research (McCaughey, DelliFraine, McGhan, and Bruning 2013; McCaughey et al. 2015). A recent review of the antecedents of health care employee injury validated the framework's pathways for preventing adverse safety events in the health care environment (McCaughey et al. 2016).

The NIOSH framework proposes that occupational illness and injury occurs as a result of exposure to "psychological stressors" and "physical hazards." Psychological stressors include common work factors such as

FIGURE 2
NIOSH Organization of Work on Occupational Safety and Health Framework
(adapted from Sauter et al. 2002)

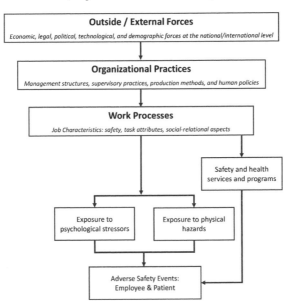

high demand/low control, role conflict, and fatigue. Physical hazards include ergonomics, exposure to pathogens, overexertion, and workplace violence. For example, a fatigued employee with uncertain job boundaries, who may believe he or she is not able to control the work environment, is likely to be at higher risk for unsafe work behaviors that result in patient and employee safety events. Further, employees exposed to contagious pathogens in the health care organization are at increased risk for a variety of hospital-acquired conditions related to the physical environment. Physical and psychological hazards exist in organizations that potentially foster adverse patient safety events in the same manner or pathway they do for employees.

Instances of adverse safety events happening are strongly influenced by two factors. For the first antecedent factor, the NIOSH framework identifies "organization of work" as external forces, organizational practices, and work processes that influence job design (Sauter et al. 2002). The outside or external level is the economic, legal, and regulatory forces influencing how health care functions at the organizational level. The organizational level is the structures and processes that lead and direct the organization. The work process level is the local job demands and conditions within a specific workplace. These factors are all aligned with the structures and processes driving improvements in patient safety climate.

When considering the external factors, much of the impetus for attention in patient safety has been driven by regulatory effects (i.e., CMS's value-based payment program and payment modifiers). As previously noted, these regulations act as a force that drives organizational policies and attention toward avoiding penalties for poor performance on specific patient safety outcomes (Colmers 2007). From the organizational level, factors encompass management and/or supervisory practices and overarching leadership within the organization. Management/supervisory practices include restructuring, downsizing, quality and process improvement initiatives, flexible work arrangements, and enacting high-performance work systems (Hofmann and Morgeson 1999). Leadership within an organization plays a critical role in driving employee commitment to following required safety processes (Hofmann, Morgeson, and Gerras 2003).

Across industries, the emergence of management safety actions/leadership as a dominant dimension of employee safety climate perceptions is well established (Flin, Mearns, O'Connor, and Bryden 2000; McCaughey, Halbesleben et al. 2013). Flin and colleagues (2000) examined the various safety climate scales used across industry sectors and found perceptions of management behavior and attitudes toward safety to be the most commonly assessed factor in safety climate studies. A similar review of safety climate scales used specifically in health care also found management to be the most commonly assessed safety climate factor, as well as being a significant positive factor in many of the studies' outcomes (Flin et al. 2006).

Previous research has found that employees with positive perceptions of leadership's safety commitment had more positive employee safety climate perceptions and lower reported injury rates (McCaughey, Halbesleben et al. 2013). The distinction between senior management and department/unit management is an important feature in studies of safety in health care given the structure of hospitals, which emphasizes care-providing units as the main model of care delivery (Singer, Gaba et al. 2009). Reviews of the patient safety literature also offer substantive evidence of the department/unit climate being a key factor in positive patient outcomes (Manser 2009; Sammer et al. 2010). Sammer and colleagues (2010) argue that a climate of optimal patient safety begins with strong leadership. Given its central role in safety climate perceptions, the importance of leadership directing organizational focus on safety structures and processes cannot be overstated (Hofmann and Mark 2006).

In addition to leadership, work designs and management practices are viewed as key antecedents for managing, preventing, or ameliorating workplace hazards that potentially lead to adverse safety events (i.e., psychological stress and physical hazards). Patient safety is optimized in local work environments that support and value teamwork, have open and honest communication (investigating safety issues), support a blame-free environment emphasizing that disclosure of errors and learning from adverse safety events is a norm, and use of evidence-based information to drive best practices in all facets of care provision (Sammer et al. 2010).

It is important to note that, for local work environments, the various levels are nested within one another so that a breakdown in patient safety at one level requires intervention at that level. For example, senior leadership translates the environment for the next level of leadership, and those mid-level managers translate the actions of senior leadership to the frontline employees—which in turn shapes their behavior.

Another antecedent to adverse safety event occurrence within the NIOSH framework is safety and health services and programs such as workplace safety programs, wellness initiatives, occupational training, teamwork efficiency training, conflict resolution training, leadership, and work–life balance initiatives. As shown in Figure 2, the organizational and work contexts exhibit specific job characteristics, which then expose employees to psychological stress and physical hazards that can result in adverse safety events for patients and employees (i.e., injury and/or illness). These hazards are potentially ameliorated by safety and health services and programs, which can function as a moderating influence that acts as a resource allowing employees to deal with psychological stress and physical hazards more effectively.

Many similar training and services programs aiding in optimizing patient safety can be found in the patient safety literature. Weaver and colleagues' (2013) systematic review of mechanisms that effectively promote patient safety found interventions such as team training on safety processes, use of communication tools, and interdisciplinary rounding (i.e., the planning and evaluation of patient care from various health care disciplines) are effective in promoting a climate in which care providers follow safety protocols. The efficacy of using simulation training to improve team performance in care provision has also been demonstrated (Nishisaki, Keren, and Nadkarni 2007). Process improvements such as automation, complexity reduction, and optimizing information processing are also recommended to improve patient safety outcomes (Nolan 2000). To address patient safety, these types of process improvements can be designed to prevent and detect errors—or even mitigate the errors if they are not detected before they occur (Nolan 2000).

In summary, the NIOSH model provides a framework to evaluate adverse safety event antecedents on multiple levels, assess the various ways job designs and managerial practices affect patient and employee safety climate, and identify mechanisms to reduce or prevent an adverse safety event from occurring (McPhaul and Lipscomb 2004; Sauter et al. 2002).

CONCLUSION

The purpose of this integration of the patient safety and employee safety climate literatures was threefold:

- To identify the industry impetus for the growing attention to patient safety climate while simultaneously examining the comparative inattention to employee safety climate
- To apply Flin's (2007) model as a framework to support the integration of the antecedents and facets of patient safety climate with employee safety climate in order to argue for a single model of employee behavior pathways that result in potential adverse safety events at the patient and employee levels
- To apply the NIOSH (Sauter et al. 2002) framework for examining an integrated safety climate for best safety practices by which health care organizations can extract valued direction in developing optimal safety environments that result in reduced adverse safety events and better outcomes for both patients and employees

This review of the existing literature provides initial support for the NIOSH model (Sauter et al. 2002) as a framework for integrating the patient and employee safety climate literature and thus capturing various mechanisms by which positive safety outcomes may be achieved (Landsbergis 2003; McCaughey et al. 2016). The NIOSH framework has the potential to be an effective mechanism for categorizing health care adverse safety event antecedents. It also adds to the existing patient safety climate and employee safety climate literature in two ways. First, the framework helps to categorize adverse event antecedents, thereby assisting organizations and researchers to identify the varying facets that contribute to care provider and patient adverse safety events. Second, until recently, relatively few studies have applied an integrative framework to assess adverse safety events for care providers and their patients. This has been one barrier for the comprehensive development of an adverse safety event prevention strategy.

The NIOSH Organization of Work on Occupational Safety and Health framework (Sauter et al. 2002) provides a foundation to test and develop theory within the health care management research domain (Landsbergis 2003). Further, the NIOSH framework affords various pathways to test the relationships between employees and patients and the antecedents to adverse safety events—and thus has the potential to contribute to evolving prevention strategies.

Reducing the excessive rates of adverse events experienced by care providers and patients is a critical need for health care organizations. Organizing safety climate studies around an evidence-based, conceptual framework offers managers and other leaders the opportunity to identify adverse safety event antecedents that are relevant to their organization and link safety programs to strategies to prevent adverse events. These links can present significant challenges for health care management when designing and structuring work processes, determining staff and support needs based on unit-specific work demands, and training organizational leaders to promote a positive, supportive workplace environment that prioritizes safety for all.

One of the goals of integrating research on patient and employee safety climate is the emergence of innovative interventions designed to improve the organizational environment and reduce adverse safety events for care providers and their patients. One way this goal may be accomplished is examining the dyadic relationship between care providers and patients and how that relationship impacts the safety climate.

In the end, this integration of synchronous safety antecedents is the next step in achieving health care's goal of preventing patient adverse events occurring while at the same time making the health care industry a safer place to work.

ACKNOWLEDGMENTS

The authors gratefully acknowledge the invaluable editorial suggestions and directions from Dr. Tim Vogus; this is a better chapter as a result.

REFERENCES

Aiken, L. H., W. Sermeus, K. Van Den Heede, D. M. Sloane, R. Busse, M. McKee, L. Bruyneel et al. 2012. "Patient Safety, Satisfaction, and Quality of Hospital Care: Cross Sectional Surveys of Nurses and Patients in 12 Countries in Europe and the United States." *British Medical Journal* 344: e1717. doi:10.1136/bmj.e1717.

Burke, M. J., S. Chan-Serafin, R. Salvador, S. Smith, and S. A. Sarpy. 2008. "The Role of National Culture and Organizational Climate in Safety Training Effectiveness." *European Journal of Work and Organizational Psychology* 17, no. 1: 133–52. doi:10.1080/13594320701307503.

Carr, J. Z., A. M. Schmidt, J. K. Ford, and R. P. DeShon. 2003. "Climate Perceptions Matter: A Meta-Analytic Path Analysis Relating Molar Climate, Cognitive and Affective States, and Individual Level Work Outcomes." *Journal of Applied Psychology* 88, no. 4: 605–19. doi:10.1037/0021-9010.88.4.605.

Centers for Medicare and Medicaid Services. No date. "Hospital-Acquired Condition Reduction Program (HACRP)." http://go.cms.gov/2a9GbAI.

Christian, M. S., J. C. Bradley, J. C. Wallace, and M. J. Burke. 2009. "Workplace Safety: A Meta-Analysis of the Roles of Person and Situation Factors." *Journal of Applied Psychology* 94, no. 5: 1103–27. doi:10.1037/a0016172.

Clarke, S. 2006. "The Relationship Between Safety Climate and Safety Performance: A Meta-Analytic Review." *Journal of Occupational Health Psychology* 11, no. 4: 315–27. doi:10.1037/1076-8998.11.4.315.

Colley, S. K., J. Lincolne, and A. Neal. 2013. "An Examination of the Relationship Amongst Profiles of Perceived Organizational Values, Safety Climate and Safety Outcomes." *Safety Science* 51, no. 1: 69–76. doi:10.1016/j.ssci.2012.06.001.

Collins J. W., A. Nelson, and V. Sublet. 2006. "Safe Lifting and Movement of Nursing Home Residents." DHHS (NIOSH) Publication No. 2006-117. Cincinnati, OH: National Institute for Occupational Safety and Health.

Colmers, J. M. 2007. "Public Reporting and Transparency." Presentation to the Commonwealth Fund/Alliance for Health Reform 2007 Bipartisan Congressional Health Policy Conference. http://bit.ly/2a9GYl7.

Danna, K., and R. W. Griffin. 1999. "Health and Well-Being in the Workplace: A Review and Synthesis of the Literature." *Journal of Management* 25, no. 3: 357–84. doi:10.1177/014920639902500305.

Flin, R. 2007. "Measuring Safety Culture in Healthcare: A Case for Accurate Diagnosis." *Safety Science* 45, no. 6: 653–67. doi:10.1016/j.ssci.2007.04.003.

Flin, R., C. Burns, K. Mearns, S. Yule, and E. M. Robertson. 2006. "Measuring Safety Climate in Health Care." *Quality and Safety in Health Care* 15, no. 2: 109–15. doi:10.1136/qshc.2005.014761.

Flin, R., K. Mearns, P. O'Connor, and R. Bryden. 2000. "Measuring Safety Climate: Identifying the Common Features." *Safety Science* 34, nos. 1–3: 177–92. doi:10.1016/s0925-7535(00)00012-6.

Gandhi, T. 2015. "The Changing Landscape of Patient Safety." Presentation at the MHA Patient Safety and Quality Symposium, Detroit, MI. http://bit.ly/2a9Hu2o.

Gomaa, A. E., L. C. Tapp, S. E. Luckhaupt, K. Vanoli, R. F. Sarmiento, W. M. Raudabaugh, S. Nowlin, and S. M. Sprigg. 2015. "Occupational Traumatic Injuries Among Workers in Health Care Facilities—United States, 2012–2014." *Centers for Disease Control and Prevention: Morbidity and Mortality Weekly Report* (Rep. 2015), 64: 405–10.

Health and Safety Commission Advisory Committee on the Safety of Nuclear Installations. 1993. *Organizing for Safety: Third Report of the ACSNI Study Group on Human Factors.* Sudbury, UK: HSE Books.

Hoff, T., L. Jameson, E. Hannan, and E. Flink. 2004. "A Review of the Literature Examining Linkages Between Organizational Factors, Medical Errors, and Patient Safety." *Medical Care Research and Review* 61, no. 1: 3–37. doi:10.1177/1077558703257171.

Hofmann, D. A., and B. Mark. 2006. "An Investigation of the Relationship Between Safety Climate and Medication Errors as Well as Other Nurse and Patient Outcomes." *Personnel Psychology* 59, no. 4: 847–69. doi:10.1111/j.1744-6570.2006.00056.x.

Hofmann, D. A., and F. P. Morgeson. 1999. "Safety-Related Behavior as a Social Exchange: The Role of Perceived Organizational Support and Leader–Member Exchange." *Journal of Applied Psychology* 84, no. 2: 286–96. doi:10.1037/0021-9010.84.2.286.

Hofmann, D. A., F. P. Morgeson, and S. J. Gerras. 2003. "Climate as a Moderator of the Relationship Between Leader–Member Exchange and Content-Specific Citizenship: Safety Climate as an Exemplar." *Journal of Applied Psychology* 88, no. 1: 170–78. doi:10.1037/0021-9010.88.1.170.

Institute of Medicine. 1999. *To Err Is Human: Building a Safer Health System.* Washington, DC: National Academies Press.

Joint Commission. 2012 (Nov.). *Improving Patient and Worker Safety: Opportunities for Synergy, Collaboration and Innovation.* Oakbrook Terrace, IL: The Joint Commission. http://www.jointcommission.org.

Joint Commission Resources (Joint Commission International). 2010. "Failure Mode and Effects Analysis in Health Care: Proactive Risk Reduction." http://bit.ly/2a9I3cB.

Landsbergis, P. A. 2003. "The Changing Organization of Work and the Safety and Health of Working People: A Commentary." *Journal of Occupational and Environmental Medicine* 45, no. 1: 61–72. doi:10.1097/00043764-200301000-00014.

Leigh, J. P. 2011. "Economic Burden of Occupational Injury and Illness in the United States." *Milbank Quarterly* 89, no. 4: 728–72. doi:10.1111/j.1468-0009.2011.00648.x.

Leigh, J. P., and J. P. Marcin. 2012. "Workers' Compensation Benefits and Shifting Costs for Occupational Injury and Illness." *Journal of Occupational and Environmental Medicine* 54, no. 4: 445–50. doi:10.1097/jom.0b013e3182451e54.

Liberty Mutual Research Institute for Safety. 2016. "2016 Liberty Mutual Workplace Safety Index." http://bit.ly/2c67DBS.

Manser, T. 2009. "Teamwork and Patient Safety in Dynamic Domains of Healthcare: A Review of the Literature." *Acta Anaesthesiologica Scandinavica* 53, no. 2: 143–51. doi:10.1111/j.1399-6576.2008.01717.x.

McCaughey, D., J. L. DelliFraine, G. E. McGhan, and N. S. Bruning. 2013. "The Negative Effects of Workplace Injury and Illness on Workplace Safety Climate Perceptions and Health Care Worker Outcomes." *Safety Science* 51, no. 1: 138–47. doi:10.1016/j.ssci.2012.06.004.

McCaughey, D., J. Halbesleben, G. Savage, T. Simons, and G. E. McGhan. 2013. "Safety Leadership: Extending Workplace Safety Climate Best Practices Across Health Care Workforces." *Advances in Health Care Management* 14: 189–217. doi:10.1108/s1474-8231(2013)00000140013.

McCaughey, D., A. Kimmel, T. Lukas, E. Walsh, G. Savage, and J. Halbesleben. 2016. "Antecedents to Workplace Injury in the Health Care Industry." *Health Care Management Review* 41, no. 1: 42–55. doi:10.1097/hmr.0000000000000043.

McCaughey, D., G. E. McGhan, E. Walsh, C. Rathert, and R. Belue. 2014. "The Relationship of Positive Work Environments and Workplace Injury." *Health Care Management Review* 39, no. 1: 75–88. doi:10.1097/hmr.0b013e3182860919.

McCaughey, D., N. Turner, J. Kim, J. L. DelliFraine, and G. E. McGhan. 2015. "Examining Workplace Hazard Perceptions and Employee Outcomes in the Long-Term Care Industry." *Safety Science* 78: 190–97. doi:10.1016/j.ssci.2015.04.013.

McPhaul, K. M., and J. A. Lipscomb. 2004. "Workplace Violence in Health Care: Recognized But Not Regulated." *Online Journal of Issues in Nursing* 9, no. 3: 7.

National Quality Forum. "2011 Serious Reportable Events in Healthcare—2011 Update: A Consensus Report." Washington, DC: National Quality Forum.

Neal, A., M. A. Griffin, and P. M. Hart. 2000. "The Impact of Organizational Climate on Safety Climate and Individual Behavior." *Safety Science* 34, nos. 1–3: 99–109. doi:10.1016/s0925-7535(00)00008-4.

Nishisaki, A., R. Keren, and V. Nadkarni. 2007. "Does Simulation Improve Patient Safety? Self-Efficacy, Competence, Operational Performance, and Patient Safety." *Anesthesiology Clinics* 25, no. 2: 225–36. doi:10.1016/j.anclin.2007.03.009.

Nolan, T. W. 2000. "System Changes to Improve Patient Safety." *British Medical Journal* 320: 771–73. doi:10.1136/bmj.320.7237.771.

Parker, C. P., B. B. Baltes, S. A. Young, J. W. Huff, R. A. Altmann, H. A. Lacost, and J. E. Roberts. 2003. "Relationships Between Psychological Climate Perceptions and Work Outcomes: A Meta-Analytic Review." *Journal of Organizational Behavior* 24, no. 4: 389–416. doi:10.1002/job.198.

Reiman, T., and C. Rollenhagen. 2014. "Does the Concept of Safety Culture Help or Hinder Systems Thinking in Safety?" *Accident Analysis and Prevention* 68: 5–15. doi:10.1016/j.aap.2013.10.033.

Sammer, C. E., K. Lykens, K. P. Singh, D. A. Mains, and N. A. Lackan. 2010. "What Is Patient Safety Culture? A Review of the Literature." *Journal of Nursing Scholarship* 42, no. 2: 156–65. doi:10.1111/j.1547-5069.2009.01330.x.

Sauter, S. L., W. S. Brightwell, M. J. Colligan, J. J. Hurrell Jr., T. M. Katz, D. E. LeGrande, N. Lessin et al. 2002. *The Changing Organization of Work and the Safety and Health of Working People.* U.S. Department of Health and Human Services, Centers for Disease Control and Prevention, National Institute for Occupational Safety and Health. Washington, DC: U.S. Department of Health and Human Services. http://bit.ly/2amAYc4.

Singer, S., S. Lin, A. Falwell, D. Gaba, and L. Baker. 2009. "Relationship of Safety Climate and Safety Performance in Hospitals." *Health Services Research* 44, no. 2p1: 399–421. doi:10.1111/j.1475-6773.2008.00918.x.

Singer, S. J., D. M. Gaba, A. Falwell, S. Lin, J. Hayes, and L. Baker. 2009. "Patient Safety Climate in 92 US Hospitals." *Medical Care* 47, no. 1: 23–31. doi:10.1097/mlr.0b013e31817e189d.

Smith-Crowe, K., J. J. Burke, and R. S. Landis. 2003. "Organizational Climate as a Moderator of Safety Knowledge-Safety Performance Relationships." *Journal of Organizational Behavior* 24, no. 7: 861–76. doi:10.1002/job.217.

U.S. Bureau of Labor Statistics. 2013. "Nonfatal Occupational Injuries and Illnesses Requiring Days Away From Work, 2012." http://www.bls.gov/iif.

U.S. Department of Labor Occupational Safety and Health Administration. No date. "Organizational Safety Culture—Linking Patient and Worker Safety." http://bit.ly/2amArGV.

U.S. Department of Labor Occupational Safety and Health Administration. 2011. "Statement from Secretary of Labor Hilda L. Solis on Reported Decline in Workplace Injuries and Illnesses." http://bit.ly/2amAbaX. Waehrer, G., J. Leigh, and T. Miller. 2005. "Costs of Occupational Injury and Illness Within the Health Services Sector." *International Journal of Health Services* 35, no. 2: 343–59. doi:10.2190/rnq3-0c13-u09m-tenp.

Weaver, S. J., L. H. Lubomksi, R. F. Wilson, E. R. Pfoh, K. A. Martinez, and S. M. Dy. 2013. "Promoting a Culture of Safety as a Patient Safety Strategy." *Annals of Internal Medicine* 158, no. 5: 369–74. doi:10.7326/0003-4819-158-5-201303051-00002.

About the Contributors

Ariel C. Avgar is an associate professor at the ILR School at Cornell University. His research focuses on two primary areas within employment relations. First, he explores the role that employment relations factors play in the health care industry. As such, he examines the effects of a variety of workplace innovations, including new technology, delivery of care models, and work practices, on patients, front-line employees, and organizational performance. Second, he studies conflict and its management in organizations with a focus on the strategic choices made by firms. His research has been published in a number of journals, including *Industrial and Labor Relations Review, Industrial Relations, British Journal of Industrial Relations, Ohio State Journal on Dispute Resolution, International Journal of Conflict Management, International Journal of Human Resource Management, Negotiation and Conflict Management Review, Advances in Industrial and Labor Relations*, and *Health Services Research and Medical Care*. He received a Ph.D. in industrial relations from the ILR School at Cornell University, a B.A. in sociology, and an LL.B in law from Hebrew University. He served as law clerk for the president of the Israeli National Labor Court before being admitted into the Israeli Bar.

Stephen Bach is head of the School of Management and Business and professor of employment relations, King's College London. His research interests include comparative public service employment relations, international migration of health professionals, and work reorganization in the public sector. He has led several EU-funded research projects on the consequences of austerity and on the role of service users in shaping employment practices. His research has been published in the *British Journal of Industrial Relations, Human Relations, Public Administration and Work*, and *Employment and Society*. His most recent book (edited with Lorenzo Bordogna) is *Public Service Management and Employment Relations in Europe: Emerging from the* Crisis. His other books include *The Modernisation of the Public Services and Employee Relations: Targeted Change* (with Ian Kessler) and *Managing Human Resources* (edited with Martin Edwards).

Jaeyong Bae is an assistant professor of public health in School of Health Studies at Northern Illinois University. He received his Ph.D. in health services research and health policy at Emory University. His research agenda focuses on the adoption of and outcomes from use of health information technology. His secondary research interests include health economics, physician incentives, patient safety, and quality management in health care. He is particularly interested in a rigorous assessment of the impact of electronic health records on the use and quality of health services.

Edmund R. Becker is a professor in the Department of Health Policy and Management at Emory School of Public Health in Atlanta. His research focuses on measuring and evaluating health care costs, outcomes, and prevention. Current projects include benchmarking and profiling hospital and physician cardiovascular performance and evaluating the impact of worksite and managed care health promotion activities on employee health behaviors. Recently, Becker was awarded a two-year PCORI grant—"Patient-Centered Care: What Factors Drive Outcomes in the Hospital Setting?—for which he leads a multi-university national research team focused on understanding the causes and consequences of exceptional patient experience in hospital care and racial and ethnic differences in outcomes using hospital patient satisfaction data. Prior to coming to Emory University in 1993, he was senior research associate at Harvard School of Public Health and project director on the Resource-Based Relative Value Scale (RBRVS) project—a seven-year national study revising Medicare's physician payment system. Becker's undergraduate training is in mathematics and sociology from Westminster College. He received his master's degree in sociology from Ohio University in 1973 and his doctorate in medical sociology from Vanderbilt University in 1981.

Simon Bishop is an assistant professor of organizational behavior, Nottingham University Business School. His research is primarily focused on the organization and management of health care. He completed his Ph.D. at the University of Nottingham, looking at the change in employment and ethos of staff moving between the public and private sectors. He has conducted studies on new types of health care organizations (such as independent sector treatment centers) and on organizations focused on closing the gap between research and practice in health care. An important theme of his research is the relationships between organizations—for example, partnerships and commissioning arrangements—and how they affect organizational management, work, and employment.

Paul F. Clark is director of and professor in the School of Labor and Employment Relations at Pennsylvania State University. Over the past decade, his work has focused on the employment problems facing registered nurses, including the nursing shortage, nurses' attitudes toward unions, and union efforts to win greater voice for nurses in decisions affecting patient care. He has also studied the phenomenon of international nurse recruitment and migration. His most recent research examines workplace partnerships between nurses unions and hospital administrations, which are aimed at improving the quality of care by giving RNs a greater voice in the health care workplace. He is the author or editor of six books and more than 60 articles in scholarly and professional journals.

Paul M. Cohen is a senior business consultant for Kaiser Permanente's Labor Management Partnership. He works with health plan and union leaders to support partnership teams and programs. Cohen has 30 years' experience as a business and health care writer, editor, and consultant. Before joining Kaiser Permanente in 2004, he was a senior editor of the *McKinsey Quarterly* and, prior to that, edited Tom Peters' newsletter *On Achieving Excellence* and *Leader to Leader*, the award-winning journal of the Peter F. Drucker Foundation for Non-Profit Management. He co-edited the book *Leader to Leader* and co-authored *Working Wisdom: Timeless Skills and Vanguard Strategies for Learning Organizations*.

Benjamin R. Dunford is an associate professor at the Krannert School of Management, faculty scholar at the Regenstrief Center for Healthcare Engineering at Purdue University, and a visiting professor at the School of Management, Seoul National University in South Korea. Dunford is a recognized teacher at master's and executive levels on topics such as leadership, compensation, employee engagement, conflict management, international negotiations and employee relations. His research is focused at the intersection of the organizational sciences and health care. On those topics, he has published more than 25 peer-reviewed journal articles, conference proceedings, and book chapters. His research has been cited in *The Economist*, as well as numerous major U.S. newspapers, and has been awarded for excellence by a number of academic journals and associations, including the Academy of Management, Labor and Employee Relations Association, Society for Industrial and Organizational Psychology, the *Journal of Healthcare Management*, and the *Journal of Applied Behavioral Science*. Dunford has consulted in a variety of industries including, media, restaurant, aluminum, and telecommunications but most extensively in health care. He earned his Ph.D. from Cornell University in 2004 and holds master's and bachelor's degrees in psychology from Indiana University–Purdue University Indianapolis and Brigham Young University, respectively.

Adrienne E. Eaton is professor of labor studies and employment relations and associate dean for academic affairs at the School of Management and Labor Relations at Rutgers, the State University of New Jersey. Her research focuses on labor–management partnerships, union organizing, and the impact of unionization on particular occupational groups such as public sector supervisors and other managerial workers, graduate student employees, and, most recently, informal workers. She's the co-author along with Tom Kochan, Paul Adler, and Robert McKersie of the book, *Healing Together: The Kaiser Permanente Labor-Management Partnership*, co-editor (with Susan Schurman and Martha Chen) of the forthcoming volume *Informal Workers and Collective Action: A Global Perspective*, and author of numerous articles published in journals such as *Industrial and Labor Relations Review, Industrial Relations, Labor Studies Journal,* and *Advances in Industrial and Labor Relations.* Eaton currently serves as co-director of the Center for Work and Health at Rutgers. She is a past president of the Rutgers Council of AAUP chapters, AAUP–AFT (the faculty, graduate student employee, and postdoc union at Rutgers University) and past member of the New Jersey Public Employment Relations Commission.

Jody Hoffer Gittell is professor of management at Brandeis University's Heller School for Social Policy and Management, executive director of the Relational Coordination Research Collaborative, and chief scientific officer of Relational Coordination Analytics, Inc. Her research explores how front-line workers contribute to quality and efficiency outcomes in coordination with each other, their customers, and their leaders, and how organizational structures support—or fail to support—this coordination. She has developed a theory of relational coordination, proposing that highly interdependent work is most effectively coordinated through relationships of shared goals, shared knowledge, and mutual respect, supported by frequent, timely, accurate, and problem-solving communication. Gittell's research is published in a wide range of scientific journals, including *Management Science, Organization Science, Academy of Management Review, Journal of Applied Behavioral Science, Industrial and Labor Relations Review, Health Services Research, Medical Care,* and *Journal of Air Transport Management.* She has published five books, including 2016's *Transforming Relationships for High Performance: The Power of Relational Coordination,* which shows how relational, structural, and work process interventions enable organizations to achieve sustainable systemic change. She received her Ph.D. from the Massachusetts Institute of Technology's Sloan School of Management.

Rebecca Kolins Givan is an associate professor of labor studies and employment relations in the School of Management and Labor Relations at Rutgers, the State University of New Jersey. She has published widely on employment relations in health care, comparative welfare states, and labor studies in journals such as *Social Forces, ILR Review,* and *British Journal of Industrial Relations.* Her recent book, *The Challenge to Change: Reforming Health Care on the Front Line in the United States and the United Kingdom* was published in 2016.

Brian Hilligoss is an assistant professor in the Division of Health Services Management and Policy in The Ohio State University College of Public Health. His research explores the dynamics of both clinical and administrative work and investigates how processes of organizing, communicating, and coordinating influence the quality and safety of health care. He has studied patient hand-offs, accountable care organizations, quality improvement, and translational science. Hilligoss specializes in qualitative methods, including ethnographic and field-based observational approaches to understanding organizational phenomena. He received his Ph.D. from the University of Michigan School of Information.

Tal Katz-Navon is an associate professor of organizational behavior at the Arison School of Business of the Interdisciplinary Center, Herzliya, Israel. She received her Ph.D in organizational psychology from Columbia University. Katz-Navon studies cross-level models of organizational climates, employee motivation, learning processes, autonomy, and voice that aim to improve employee and organizational performances. Among other efforts, her research integrates organizational behavior and health services research and is focused on quality improvement and clinical outcomes in health care. This research has been published in top journals: *Academy of Management Journal, Journal of Applied Psychology, Management Science, Journal of Organizational Behavior, Medical Care,* and more.

Sarah Lax joined Kaiser Permanente in 2014 as an administrative fellow and is currently an assistant department administrator in Specialty Care. In her role, she manages day-to-day clinic operations and implements regional strategic initiatives. She holds a bachelor of science degree in kinesiology from the University of Illinois at Urbana-Champaign and a master's degree in health care administration from the University of Illinois at Chicago. She entered the health care field because of her passion for total health and equitable care. Among her philanthropic endeavors, she is a member of the board of directors for the YWCA of Greater Portland and Impact Northwest. In her spare time, she enjoys playing in local volleyball leagues and exploring the great Northwest.

Peter Lazes is the director of health care programs and a research associate of the Joseph S. Murphy Institute for Worker Education and Labor Studies at the City University of New York. His programs provide labor union and management leaders with customized education activities, research, and consulting services to help implement strategic worker participation programs. His current work involves assisting hospitals and other health care organizations develop methods to improve patient care and reduce costs through intensive front-line staff engagement. Lazes has written more than 30 articles and produced videos on topics such as organizational change, innovation, and new work systems, new roles for unions, and strategies for keeping American jobs. His international activities include consulting and education programs in Ireland, Poland, Norway, and the United Kingdom. Other activities include strategic planning for unions, organizational change and leadership development, breakthrough processes to create integrated delivery systems, methods to encourage employee-driven innovation, and creating health care learning collaboratives between health care delivery systems to accelerate the spread of best practices to improve patient care and control costs. Lazes received his Ph.D. in clinical and industrial psychology from Union Institute and University.

Ann Scheck McAlearney is professor of family medicine and vice chair for research in the Department of Family Medicine at the Ohio State University. She has over 25 years of health services research experience and has authored over 150 peer-reviewed publications, 8 monographs, and 40 book chapters. McAlearney is currently studying the development of accountable care organizations, and her general research interests include the areas of primary care quality improvement, information technology innovations in health care, and organizational development. She received her undergraduate and graduate degrees from Stanford University and Harvard's T. H. Chan School of Public Health.

Deirdre McCaughey is an associate professor in the Department of Health Services Administration at the University of Alabama at Birmingham. She is also program director for graduate programs in health care quality and safety. Her research involves examining organizational factors, such as leadership and organizational culture in health care institutions, that influence health care provider and workforce well-being and subsequently optimize organizational patient safety and quality outcomes. McCaughey's research is published in journals such as the *Journal of Healthcare Management, Journal of Occupational Health Psychology, Journal of Applied Psychology, Safety Science,* and *Health Care Management Review.*

Laura E. McClelland is an assistant professor in the Department of Health Administration at Virginia Commonwealth University. She has expertise in health administration, organizational behavior, management, and organization theory. Her research interests include workplace compassion, employee well-being, and patient experience. Her research has been published in leading health services and management journals including *Health Services Research* and *Human Resource Management Review* and cited by Kaiser Health News and CNN. She received her

Ph.D. in organization and management from Emory University and B.S. degrees in management and economics from Villanova University. Previously, she was a management consultant for PricewaterhouseCoopers and IBM.

Gwen McGhan is an assistant professor in the School of Nursing at the University of Alabama at Birmingham. The focus of her research is on understanding and improving outcomes for family caregivers and health care providers of older adults in various settings using a person-centered approach—specifically the role of resources in maintaining caregiver well-being. McGhan has published her research in several journals and presented at regional, national, and international conferences. As part of her nursing background, she has clinical and administrative experience in both inpatient and outpatient settings.

Jessica N. Mittler is an associate professor in the Department of Health Administration at Virginia Commonwealth University. She studies the pursuit of patient-centered care and the transformation it requires for individuals and organizations. Her research is published in high-impact journals such as *The Milbank Quarterly, Medical Care Research and Review, Health Services Research, and Health Affairs.* Mittler earned her Ph.D. in health policy and medical sociology from Harvard, her master's in health services administration and public policy from the University of Michigan, and her B.S. in urban studies from Cornell University.

Eitan Naveh is an associate professor at the Faculty of Industrial Engineering and Management, Technion–Israel Institute of Technology, where he received his D.Sc. in quality assurance and reliability. His focus is on two streams of organizational research: errors in organizations and linkage between innovation and quality. Applying an interdisciplinary approach that combines aspects of behavioral sciences and engineering, he has contributed to the understanding of errors, innovation, and quality by revealing the hidden tensions resulting from multiple-priority situations and exploring their consequences. He primarily studies research and development teams in high-tech companies and medical teams in medical centers. His research has been published in the *Academy of Management Journal, Journal of Applied Phycology, Journal of Management, Journal of Operations Management, Management Science,* and other leading academic journals.

Matthew B. Perrigino is a doctoral candidate in the Organizational Behavior and Human Resources program at Purdue University's Krannert School of Management. He is also a research fellow at Purdue's

Regenstrief Center for Healthcare Engineering. His research interests include health care management and issues concerning the work–family interface.

Benjamin R. Pratt is a doctoral student in the Organizational Behavior and Human Resource Management program in the Krannert School of Management at Purdue University. He is also a research fellow at Purdue's Regenstrief Center for Healthcare Engineering. He also holds a master of science degree in sociology from Purdue University, a master of social work degree from the University of Houston, and a bachelor of arts degree in anthropology from Brigham Young University. Before coming to Purdue, Benjamin was a LEAH social work fellow at Baylor College of Medicine and was assistant chief of social work services in the VA Salt Lake City Health Care System. He is interested in the ways in which changes in health care professions impact individual stakeholders, health care organizations, and society in general.

Jim Pruitt is vice president of labor partnership and relations for the Permanente Federation. The federation represents the national interests of the Permanente Medical Groups—the physician-owned organizations that serve Kaiser Foundation Health Plan members. He has worked for Kaiser Permanente since 1974 in labor relations roles. He graduated from the University of California and received his master of labor and industrial relations at Michigan State University. Pruitt was elected to the executive board of the Labor and Employment Relations Association (LERA) for the 2011–2014 term. He is the past co-chair of the health care industry council for LERA. He has written on labor relations, generational differences, labor history, and sports and culture.

Cheryl Rathert is an associate professor in the Department of Health Administration at Virginia Commonwealth University. Her research centers on health care work environments, worker well-being, and patient experiences. Her research is published in leading health care journals such as *Medical Care Research and Review, International Journal of Nursing Studies, Health Expectations,* and *Health Care Management Review.* She earned her Ph.D. in organizational behavior from the University of Nebraska–Lincoln, M.S. in industrial and organizational Psychology from the University of Nebraska–Omaha, and her B.A. in Psychology from University of Nebraska–Lincoln.

Joan Resnick, at the time of writing her chapter for this volume, was a senior organizational development consultant for Kaiser Permanente's Northwest (KPNW) region in Portland, Oregon, but has since returned to a leadership role in federal service. Resnick brought to Kaiser Permanente the concept of relational coordination as a basic competency of how medical offices function. At KPNW, her focus was to engage leadership, labor partners, physicians, and staff to create a positive, measurable impact on culture and performance through a relational coordination survey. She also had her own consulting firm, Real Life Training and Consulting Group, which provided training to federal, state, and local governments in natural resource management, land use planning, and leadership and management.

Paula H. Song is an associate professor in the Department of Health Policy and Management in the Gillings School of Global Public Health at the University of North Carolina at Chapel Hill. Her research interests and publications cover areas such as health care financial management, accountable care organizations. and business case evaluation. She teaches graduate-level courses in health care finance and accounting. Song received her Ph.D. in health services organization and policy, and master's degrees in health services administration and applied economics, all from the University of Michigan.

Eliana Temkin is a senior consultant in learning and organizational effectiveness at Kaiser Permanente's Northwest (KPNW) region. In her role, she provides a wide variety of organizational effectiveness consultation services for KPNW, including the design and delivery of leadership development programs and change management resources. In addition, Temkin conducts individual assessments, coaches leaders, and facilitates meetings and retreats for all levels of leadership teams throughout the KPNW region. Examples of this facilitation work include coaching teams in their development in conflict management and mediation, change management, work-style assessments, and interpersonal communication skill building. She is experienced in assessing training needs and designing curriculum to meet those needs in the areas of team performance, service improvement, and leadership development. She is certified to administer the Hogan Assessment tool and as a facilitator for Facilitative Leadership and the Lominger Leadership and Team Architect Assessment. Temkin is currently working on a certification in evidence-based coaching for organizational leadership from Fielding Graduate University. She has a master's degree in organizational leadership from Gonzaga University.

Timothy J. Vogus is an associate professor of management at the Vanderbilt Owen Graduate School of Management. His research focuses on the cognitive (mindful organizing), cultural, motivational, and emotional processes through which individuals, work groups, and organizations enact highly reliable (i.e., harm-free) performance. He is especially interested in the role specific work practices play in enabling mindful organizing, ensuring reliable performance, and ensuring positive employee as well as organizational outcomes at the point of care delivery. More recently, he has begun to explore the role of organizational compassion practices and interpersonal processes in shaping the caregiver and patient experience of care delivery. His research has been published or is forthcoming in top industrial relations (e.g., *ILR Review*) management (e.g., *Academy of Management Annals, Academy of Management Review*), and health services (e.g., *Health Affairs, Health Services Research, Medical Care*, and *Medical Care Research and Review*) journals. He received a Ph.D. in management and organizations from the Ross School of Business at the University of Michigan and a B.A. in political economy and Spanish from Michigan State University.

Justin Waring is a professor of organizational sociology at Nottingham University Business School. He studied sociology and social policy at the University of Liverpool, followed by health care policy and management at the University of Birmingham. He is currently acting as a Health Foundation Improvement Fellow—part of a national program to instigate change in health care. He completed his doctorate in sociology at the University of Nottingham on the topic of social construction and control of medical errors. He is an expert in the field of patient safety and quality, as well as health care leadership more broadly. He is involved with a number of high-profile research projects seeking to improve the delivery of health care.

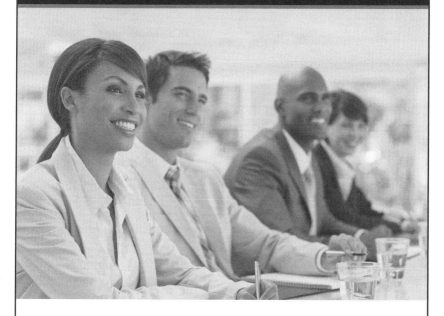
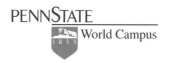

LERA Officers

President
Janice Bellace
University of Pennsylvania

President-Elect
Harry C. Katz
Cornell University

Past President
Bonnie Proutey Castrey
Dispute Resolution Services

Secretary-Treasurer
Craig Olson
University of Illinois at Urbana-Champaign

Editor-in-Chief
Ariel C. Avgar
Cornell University

National Chapter Advisory Council Chair
William Canak
Middle Tennessee State University

Legal Counsel
Steven B. Rynecki